DATE DUE

NOV 3 0 1994	
JAN 2 7 1996	
FEB - 1 1996	
JAN 2 9 1996	

GAYLORD   PRINTED IN U.S.A.

Toxicology of the Immune System:

A Human Approach

Toxicology of the Immune System:

A Human Approach

Robert Burrell, Ph.D.

Department of Microbiology,
West Virginia University,
Morgantown, West Virginia

Dennis K. Flaherty, Ph.D.

Environmental Health Laboratory
Monsanto Agricultural Group
St. Louis, Missouri

Leonard J. Sauers, Ph.D.

The Procter and Gamble Company
Cincinnati, Ohio

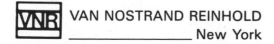 VAN NOSTRAND REINHOLD
_____ New York

Printed in the United States of America.

Van Nostrand Reinhold
115 Fifth Avenue
New York, New York 10003

Chapman and Hall
2-6 Boundary Row
London, SE1 8HN, England

Thomas Nelson Australia
102 Dodds Street
South Melbourne 3205
Victoria, Australia

Nelson Canada
1120 Birchmount Road
Scarborough, Ontario MIK 5G4, Canada

16 15 14 13 12 11 10 9 8 7 6 5 4 3 2 1

Library of Congress Cataloging-in-Publication Data
Burrell, Robert.
    Toxicology of the immune system : a human approach / Robert
Burrell, Leonard J. Sauers, Dennis K. Flaherty.
      p. cm.
    Includes bibliographical references and index.
    ISBN 0-442-00836-8
    1. Immunotoxicology. I. Sauers, Leonard J., 1958-
II. Flaherty, Dennis K., 1944-   . III. Title.
    [DNLM: 1. Immune System—drug effects. 2. Immune System—
immunology. 3. Immunologic Diseases—chemically induced.   QW 504
B969t]
RC582.17.B67 1992
616.97—dc20
DNLM/DLC
for Library of Congress   92-49664
                                                              CIP

Contents

	Preface	**xi**
1.	**Introduction**	**1**
	A. Scope	1
	B. Popular Perception	2
	C. Definitions	4
	D. Foundations of Immunotoxicology	5
2.	**Basic Immunology**	**9**
	A. Introduction	9
	B. Cellular Basis of the Immune Response	10
	1. B Lymphocytes	11
	2. T Lymphocytes	12
	3. Other Effector Lymphocytes	13
	4. Antigen-Presenting Cells	13
	C. Tissues and Organs of Immunologic Importance	14
	1. Thymus	15
	2. Spleen	16
	3. Lymphatics	17
	4. Lymph Nodes	18
	5. Lymphoid Nodules	18
	D. Immunoglobulin Gene Super Family	21
	1. Immunoglobulins	21
	2. Major Histocompatibility Molecules	26
	3. T-Cell Antigen Receptors	26
	4. CD4 and CD8 Molecules	26
	5. The CD3 Molecule	27
	E. Cellular Interactions of the Immune Response	27
	1. Cellular Interactions in Immune Response Induction	28
	2. Cellular Interactions in Effector Cell Recognition	31
	3. Immunoregulation	32
3.	**Basic Principles of Toxicology**	**33**
	A. Introduction	33
	B. Toxicology and the Role of the Toxicologist	34
	C. Expression of Toxic Effects	34
	1. Dose–Response Relationships	34
	2. Types of Response to a Xenobiotic Exposure	36
	C. Factors Affecting the Expression of Toxicity	39
	1. Dosing Regimen	39
	2. Characteristics of the Exposed Individual	40
	3. Characteristics of the Xenobiotic	43

v

    D. Risk Assessment Process   45
4. **Effector Mechanisms: Immunopharmacology**   **49**
    A. Introduction   49
    B. Cellular Activation   49
        1. Membrane Signaling   50
        2. Early Events   51
        3. Late Events   53
    C. Effects of the Nervous System on Immune Function   54
    D. Mediators of Immediate Hypersensitivity and Inflammation   57
        1. Preformed Mediators   57
        2. Synthesized Mediators   59
    E. Cytokines   62
        1. Cytokines That Mediate Innate Immunity   63
        2. Cytokines That Regulate Lymphocytes   67
        3. Cytokines That Activate Inflammatory Cells   69
        4. Cytokines Regulating Hematopoiesis   69
        5. Conclusions   71
5. **Effector Mechanisms: Expression of Immunity**   **79**
    A. Introduction   79
    B. Humoral Mechanisms   80
        1. Humoral Antibodies   80
        2. The Complement System   81
    C. Neutrophils and Phagocytic Mechanisms   87
        1. Chemotaxis   88
        2. Engulfment   88
        3. Metabolic Events   88
        4. Killing and Digestion Mechanisms   89
    D. Macrophages   90
    E. T-Cytotoxic and NK Cells   91
    F. Mast Cells and Basophils   93
    G. Eosinophils   94
    H. Platelets   96
    I. Endothelial Cells   96
    J. Integration   98
        1. Infectious Disease   98
        2. Tumors   100
6. **Mechanisms of Injury by the Immune System**   **104**
    A. Introduction   104
    B. Differentiation of Hypersensitivity from Toxicity   104
    C. IgE-Mediated Hypersensitivity   105
        1. Immediate Reactions   105
        2. Late-Phase Reactions   109
        3. Bronchial Asthma   110
    D. Cytotoxic Antibodies   113
    E. Immune Complex Disease   116
    F. Nonspecific Complement Activation   118
    G. Delayed-Type Reactions   120
        1. Mechanisms   121
        2. Assessment   123
        3. Other Forms of Delayed-in-Time Reactions   126
    H. Hyperplasia   127

I. Hypersensitivity-Like Reactions   127
J. Autoimmunity   128

7. Damage to the Immune System   **137**
A. Introduction   137
B. Primary Immunologic Deficiency Diseases   137
C. Vulnerable Points in the Immune System   140
   1. Stem Cells   141
   2. Macrophages/Monocytes   143
   3. B Lymphocytes   145
   4. T Lymphocytes   147
   5. NK Cells   149
   6. Neutrophils   150
D. Additional Considerations   152
E. Conclusions   154

8. Intentional Modulation of the Immune Response: Immunopotentiation and Immunosuppression   **158**
A. Introduction   158
B. Immunologic Enhancement   159
   1. Prototypes   159
   2. Mineral Compounds   160
   3. Bacterial Stimulants   160
   4. Muramyl Dipeptides   161
   5. Nontoxic Analogs of Bacterial Lipopolysaccharide   163
   6. Other Synthetic and Natural Peptides   163
   7. Liposomes   164
   8. Synthetic Polymers   165
   9. Miscellaneous Synthetic Immunostimulating Drugs   166
   10. Host Mediators   167
C. Immunosuppression   168
   1. Immunologic Tolerance   168
   2. Natural Means of Immunosuppression   169
   3. Therapeutic Immunosuppression   170
D. Conclusion   177

9. Assessment of Secondary Immunodeficiencies in Man and Animals   **181**
A. Introduction   181
B. Secondary Immunodeficiencies Associated with Other Diseases   181
C. Diagnosis of Secondary Immunodeficiency   183
   1. Laboratory Testing   183
   2. Antibody-Mediated Immune System   184
   3. Cell-Mediated Immunity   188
   4. Accessory Functions   194
D. Assessment of Immune Function in Animals   197
   1. Indirect Immunotoxic Effects   198
   2. Standard Toxicology Endpoints   199
   3. Flow Cytometry   200
   4. Antibody-Mediated Immunity   201
   5. Cell-Mediated Immunity   202

10. Relevance of Immunotoxicologic Findings to Human Immune Competence   **214**
A. Problems in Studying Immunotoxicology   214
B. Definition of How Immunotoxic Abnormalities Are Realized   215

C. Risk Factors: Allergy 219
D. Risk Factors: Pharmacological 220
E. Risk Factors: Environmental 222
F. Non-Antigen-Specific Immunologic Enhancement 224
G. Problems with Predicting and Interpreting Immunotoxicity 226
H. Problems in Extrapolating Experimental Animal Data
to Humans 228

11. Agents and Effects of Immunotoxicity **235**
A. Introduction 235
B. Clinical Effects of Immunotoxicology 236
1. Skin Manifestations 236
2. Manifestations of the Respiratory Tract 238
3. Ocular Manifestations 239
4. Gastrointestinal Manifestations 240
C. Selected Agents of Immunotoxicity 242
1. Polybrominated-Polychlorinated Biphenyls and Toxic Oils 243
2. Pesticides 247
3. Polycyclic Aromatic Hydrocarbons 249
4. Dioxins 250
5. Drugs 252
6. Anesthetics 256
7. Medical Devices 258
8. Cigarette Smoking 260
9. Substances of Abuse 262
10. Heavy Metals 265
11. Air Pollution 267
12. Mycotoxins 269
D. Selected Diseases with Immunotoxic Effects 269
1. Occupational Asthma 269
2. Anaphylaxis 272
3. Hypersensitivity Pneumonitis and Organic Dust
Toxic Syndrome 275
4. Multiple Chemical Sensitivity 276
5. Pneumoconiosis 279
6. Splenectomy 281

12. Regulatory Immunotoxicology **293**
A. Introduction 293
B. Food and Drug Administration 294
1. Immunotoxic Concerns within the FDA 294
2. FDA Drug Licensing 297
3. Immunotoxicity Testing 298
4. Risk Assessment 301
C. Environmental Protection Agency 301
1. EPA Approval for the Use of a Chemical
under FIFRA 302
2. EPA Approval of a Chemical under TSCA 302
3. Immunotoxicology Concerns of the EPA 302
4. Unreasonable Risk 305
5. Regulation of Compounds on the Basis of Immune
System Effects 305

D. Concerns about Current Immunotoxicity Testing   305
    1. Choice of Test Animal   306
    2. Validation of Ex Vivo Parameters   306
    3. Sensitivity of Ex Vivo Assays   306
    4. Predictive Nature of Rodent Ex Vivo Assays   306
E. Conclusions   307

Index   **311**

Preface

In the exponential pace of contemporary medical science, the topic of immuno-toxicology is a fairly late starter. The comparatively young science asks whether the negative impact of foreign substances, i.e., xenobiotics, can affect the host immune mechanisms in such a way as to lead to harmful changes in host responses and/or enhanced susceptibility to infectious disease and tumorigenesis. Toxicologists have been turning their attention toward the immune system for several years, and the immunologist has now begun to realize that subjects not previously of concern, i.e., pharmacology and toxicology, are exceedingly important in trying to understand how the normal immune system functions. Our intent is to provide a bridge between the two sciences with an introduction to the basic mechanisms by which environmental, occupational, and therapeutic agents may interfere with immunologic systems.

Pioneers in this field, most notably Vos, Sharma, Dean, and Luster, have helped focus the attention of the toxicology community on problems affecting the immune system, but similar efforts have not been made among the immunologists. One of the goals of this book is to approach the entire subject of immuno-toxicology from the viewpoint of the immunologist in order to bring greater attention of the subject to more from that field. In this task, we have been selective, not exhaustive, in our topic coverage and have attempted to present the coverage of each item in such a way that the reader gains an understanding of current concepts and knowledge in specific areas. We have tried to point out the best of studies, to identify gaps of missing information, and to suggest paths for future work.

Another goal has been to introduce microbiological principles of infection and host resistance to the field. There is abundant evidence that microbial processes or products may suppress or potentiate the immune system in such a way that subsequent exposure to a chemical substance produces an altered effect. The best example of the worst type of immunosuppression is indeed an infection, i.e., AIDS, and much has been learned from the study of AIDS that is applicable to how the immune system can be affected adversely. Finally, one of the best ways to assess the relevance of changes in immune parameters is to evaluate the effect of those changes on host resistance to infections.

Previous treatises in this field have centered on laboratory studies of experimental animals administered selected xenobiotics under controlled conditions and measured the effects on their various immune parameters. This text does not attempt to duplicate the coverage of this animal work already found in many standard reference works. Rather, our intent is to stress the effects of immuno-toxicity on the human immune system and on human well-being. That is not to say that animal work is ignored; rather, we have selected those studies that either point the way for further human studies or provide the most immediate relevance to the human situation. The biggest problem in assessing immunotoxicity is determining the relevance to human health. A large part of our attention in writing this book has been to address that question. Not only is an entire chapter devoted to the topic, we tried to make it a constant theme throughout the book.

After introductory chapters on principles of basic immunology, toxicology, and immunopharmacology, the text considers not only damage *to* the immune system but damage *by* the immune system because xenobiotics may bring about both forms of disturbance, and indeed some agents are capable of doing both. These chapters assess each kind of damage by type, citing the best-known human examples. The subject of controlled immunotoxicology, i.e., that achieved by purposely administered drugs for immunosuppression or immunopotentiation, is then covered inasmuch as the modes of action of these agents have been studied intensively and serve as good examples to point the way for future work on xenobiotics. The matter of how one assesses immune injury is given much attention, for not only is it important how to realize immune defects, it is equally important to try to achieve standard practices that will help prevent the disparity in results that characterizes so many studies in the field. A great amount of consideration is also given to the types of clinical populations in which these types of damage occur and the general organ systems that are affected. The coverage is next extended to consider classes of xenobiotics that either cause or are suspected of causing human immune injury. This chapter ends with a discussion of selected clinical conditions in which immune injury is either a proven factor or else has been putatively suggested as having a role in pathogenesis. Finally, an attempt has been made to discuss the matter of regulatory affairs in regard to assessing and defining immunotoxic reactions and risk assessment. With an increasingly litigious climate, chemical, pharmaceutical, and cosmetic manufacturers are concerned about risk assessment and safety in new products being developed.

The text is intended to be of benefit to toxicologists, immunologists, industrial hygienists, microbiologists, and those involved with chemical or biological regulatory affairs. In addition, clinical allergists and immunologists, pharmaceutical chemists, and many others working in the ethical drug, agricultural chemical, or cosmetic industries would benefit.

Thus, the text attempts to fulfill a need for some basic and critical information concerning a popular subject about which very little centralized material is available. We intend to present a unified source where immunotoxicologic information can be critically assessed in a uniform fashion. With an increasing environmental awareness, coupled with an inaccurate public perception of what environmental chemicals can and can not do, there is a need for a source of objective evaluation of just what risks may arise from such exposure.

Acknowledgments

The authors are indebted to numerous people who have aided in the preparation of this effort. Particularly helpful were those who reviewed drafts of various chapters and provided us with constructive critiques: Drs. William A. Beresford, James M. Sheil, William H. Houser, Mark J. Reasor, G. Frank Gerberick, Karen A. Kohrman, Thomas Fuhremann, Charles Healy, and Daryl Thake.

Special thanks are extended to Dr. Irvin S. Snyder for reviewing parts as well as for continued encouragement on the project.

The task would have been impossible without the thoroughly professional staff of Mrs. Marguerite Abel of the West Virginia University Health Sciences Library. We are certain that Allyson McKee, Sarah Burgess, Ada M. Bellay, Lena Lim, and Alex Lubman, all of whom provided invaluable services, are glad our project is completed.

We also wish to acknowledge the secretarial assistance ably provided by Mary A. Morris and Catherine A. Goldschmidt. Editorial assistance and encouragement from Carol Flaherty were particularly helpful. Bonny Starkey and Melvin C. Wilson provided all of the original illustrations except for those reproduced through the courtesy of Dr. Joseph A. Bellanti of Georgetown University School of Medicine and the W. B. Saunders Co.

Certain portions of this text have been expanded from tracts that were initially prepared in background support of a publication by the Office of Technology Assessment, United States Congress: *Identifying and Controlling Immunotoxic Substances* (Washington D.C., U.S. Government Printing Office, April 1991). We are especially indebted to the support and encouragement received from Dr. Roger C. Herdman, Director of the Health and Life Sciences Division, and Ms. Holly L. Gwin, Project Director.

Finally, the labors of our task were made considerably more pleasant by the delightful Assistant Editor in charge of our project, Ms. Judy Brief, who also happens to be the reason we chose Van Nostrand Reinhold to produce the book.

1
Introduction

A. SCOPE

The subject of immunotoxicology, like the offspring of any mixed union, is one not really claimed by either parent. Even with the explosive growth of immunology over the past two decades, which owes much of its understanding to almost every branch of medical and biological science, not one major textbook in immunology devotes space to the subject of immunotoxicology. The field of toxicology does somewhat better in acknowledging that the immune system, like any other organ or physiological system of the body, is subject to the deleterious effects of xenobiotics. However, until recently toxicologists have not been trained or even acquainted with basic immunology, and their approach has been traditionally and understandably a toxicologic one. The purpose of this text is to bring legitimacy to the marriage of these two reputable fields and, by providing a basic understanding of both sciences, to attempt to achieve a firm foundation for their new offspring.

The scope of modern immunology is quite wide, encompassing results obtained from many areas of medical science. Immunity originally meant freedom or protection from infectious or noxious substances. Although the term still includes such connotations, its modern meaning is much broader. The immune system can finely differentiate extremely small chemical differences in the prosthetic groups of antigens (epitopes), but it cannot predict potential harm somewhere in the future. For that reason the very same immune system response that will produce antibodies against a bacterial toxin will also form a similar response against something as innately unharmful as egg white or airborne pollen. Today the term immunity means an altered response to anything foreign, whether toxic, infectious, or not, and includes the induction of antigen-specific responses as well as non-antigen-specific inflammation.

Another misconception about immunity in reference to infectious disease (which is a relic from how early healers viewed the phenomenon of immunity) was the belief that immunity was absolute. It is now realized that immunity may result in degrees of protection as well as several other alterations of response to infectious agents. Immunity to diseases such as pertussis or typhoid fever is only realized by comparing incidence of mortality and clinical severity in immunized and unimmunized groups with equal exposure to the respective agents. Although one may have been immunized against these agents, clinical disease may still occur, but it takes a more benign course than in those with no immunity at all. Epidemiologic information may be the only evidence of the effectiveness of immunization when a lowered mortality in the immunized population may be realized. Infections may also take a different form in the immunized. The best

1

example is in the differences between primary and secondary tuberculosis. The pathology of the latter is quite different from the former, mostly because of the added presence of cell-mediated hypersensitivity to a protein constituent of the tubercle bacilli.

Altered immune reactivity to a substance may also take a harmful turn, as evidenced by the many forms of allergy and immune injury. In these cases, the response is quite the opposite of protection, and inflammatory disease is the result, but knowledge gained from the study of allergy has provided much insight into the nature of normal immune responses and inflammation biology. Nor is the immune system sophisticated enough to know when medical scientists are trying to do something clinically useful such as carrying out a blood transfusion or tissue homograft. The immune system may recognize antigens on these useful tissues as "foreign" also and mount an appropriate immune response resulting in either a serious side reaction or graft rejection. Much of the most fundamental insight into the nature of the immune response has been learned from the study of the transplantation rejection phenomenon. Turning that phenomenon around, immunologists have long been fascinated with the prospect of turning the immune response against harmful tumors. This has led to another area from which much knowledge of matters of modulation of the immune system has been acquired, immunopotentiation. Another clinical area from which much fundamental immunology has been learned, and one closer to the subject of this book, is that of immunodeficiency diseases, i.e., the absence or impairment of immunity. Through trying to find out what is wrong in patients with such diseases, much has been learned about how the *normal* immune response is supposed to work. This continues currently with the immunologic study of AIDS victims, which has been yielding much useful immunology information applicable to immunotoxicology.

B. POPULAR PERCEPTION

There is a great deal of current popular awareness of the major effects environmental influences can have on a variety of life processes. Such awareness comes from at least two major sources, the very same two sciences that have given birth to immunotoxicology. On the one hand, awareness of toxicology has arisen from public knowledge of the teratogenic effects of drugs like thalidomide or of infections such as toxoplasmosis or rubella. The possible carcinogenic effects of exposure to cigarette smoke, coal tar derivatives, radon, and other seemingly harmless agents such as artificial sweeteners or meat preservation nitrites have been in the public eye for so long that it is now difficult for us to evaluate critically the many carcinogenic claims made daily in our newspapers. In addition, there is growing public awareness of such controversial places or toxic exposures as Love Canal, Times Beach, agent orange, and multiple chemical sensitivities, where strong polarization exists with respect to understanding the factual bases of these incidents. Concern over the possibility of adverse effects of environmental agents has progressed beyond chemicals and extended to such ubiquitous items of modern life as video display terminals of computers, TV sets, and even electric blankets! Such media attention has been so constant and uncritical that the public is understandably frightened when it comes to facing modern technology.

Similarly, the public's awareness and understanding of the immune system have been captured by such newspaper accounts as those that detailed the life of

David, the "bubble boy," so-called because he lived his entire short life enclosed in a germ-free barrier because of an inherited immunologic deficiency disease (Williamson et al. 1977). But even more in the public eye since the early 1980s is the acquired immunodeficiency disease known as AIDS, resulting from an infective agent that alters the most fundamental immunologic functions (Follansbee et al. 1982). The question in many people's minds is that of determining if there are any environmental agents capable of inducing AIDS-type diseases in exposed individuals. Can exposure to environmental, food, medicinal, or cosmetic substances cause harm to the immune system, and if so, what might be the result? The media fan the flames of such fears by suggesting that there are phenomena like "chemical AIDS" lurking in our midst. Even the very concept of immunization has been challenged in recent years. The value of immunization against such childhood diseases as polio, whooping cough, diphtheria, and now measles and mumps has largely been unquestioned, but the public wonders about such problems as the association of the Guillain–Barré syndrome with the widespread influenza vaccination program of 1976–1977, or the dangers of giving living, attenuated vaccines to people who may have imperfections in their immune systems.

Conditions of hypersensitivity or hypersensitivity-like states are better known to the lay public. Everyone knows someone who has experienced hay fever, a poison ivy rash, or who has to avoid some food or medicine because of nuisance reactions caused by them. Rarer, but always newsworthy, are reports of fatalities from bee stings, a severe type of systemic allergic shock. Less well known in the popular idiom are other types of immune responses that damage the host and lead to diseases, e.g., rheumatic fever, glomerulonephritis, sympathetic ophthalmia. In each of these cases an otherwise normal immune response has resulted in self-inflicted damage to heart muscle, renal glomerular filters, or eye tissue, respectively. As news items about these curious events reach the public, there is even more understandable consternation about just how protective our immune system is. The line between hypersensitivity and immune toxicity is an extremely fine one. Both are the result of exposure to an environmental agent, both result in an undesirable alteration of immune function, and both lead to damage to the host, often by the same inflammatory systems. Since it is sometimes difficult to distinguish hypersensitivity from toxicity, both will necessarily receive our attention.

None of the above is to imply that the scientists interested in these topics are sufficiently informed and above fear and misinformation. On the contrary, immunologists and toxicologists have been traditionally trained in their own disciplines almost exclusively. Both have been exposed to genetics, biochemistry, and molecular and cellular biology, but curiously, until recently, neither has received much exposure to the other's subject. Scientists of either persuasion in the pharmaceutical, medical products, cosmetic, and environmental-chemical industries are continually being confronted by nontraditional problems that cross traditional disciplinary bounds. Matters of risk assessment, predicting toxicity and hypersensitivity, and limiting or eliminating exposure to such agents are questions that keep coming up and need the collective wisdom of both sciences to be properly evaluated. Physicians are largely in the dark when it comes to evaluating exposure to possible harmful environmental agents in relation to the patient's present condition. Unlike infections, where the time between exposure and clinical illness is short, exposure to an allergen or an immunotoxicant may have occurred so long ago or been so inapparent that the patient may be unaware of it. Even when a patient has an occupational history of working in the chemical industry, often the patient is found to have been exposed to dozens or more of different chemicals, and determining which one or combination was responsible for the present condition is nearly impossible.

C. DEFINITIONS

The most general definition of immunotoxicology considers any condition in which a substance inhibits, destroys, or exaggerates an immune component and also includes the study of any substance that interferes with the normal development of the immune system. The World Health Organization defines the subject as the specialty concerned with the adverse effects resulting from the interaction of the immune system with xenobiotics and includes the consequence of an activity of a substance or its metabolites on the immune system as well as the immunologic response to such a substance. The body may respond immunologically to a foreign substance in a variety of ways. If the substance is an antigen, i.e., capable of inciting one of various specific immune responses, that immune response may range from being measurable but of no biological effect to a killing or disposition of the foreign material by immune or inflammatory mechanisms invoked by the immune response, or it may lead to any number of processes characterized by an abnormal immune response (e.g., allergy or hypersensitivity) that inflicts harm on the possessor. Other substances, whether antigens or not, may lead to a toxic or damaging effect to the immune system. Situations or agents that may interfere with immunologic systems include environmental, occupational, or therapeutic agents, and one's reaction to these agents may or may not also include a genetic component. The significance of a genetic component to immune dysfunction is readily apparent when one considers the severe immunodeficiencies in a newborn suffering from impairment or absence of normal immune system components (Rosen, Cooper, and Wedgewood 1984), or the familial nature of asthma triggered by environmental inhalants (Marsh and Bias 1988). The former results from genetic or developmental anomalies prior to birth and may be manifest in several ways, the most serious of which is known as severe combined immunodeficiency disease, whereas the latter results from an environmental interaction in a genetically prone individual.

This text uses certain terms in very specific ways, which also require definition at this point. The word "specific" refers to specific immune responsiveness induced by antigens. Antigens are substances tha   ulate a specific immune response capable of recognizing and reacting with the antigen that induced that response; i.e., diphtheria toxin induces specific immune responses against diphtheria toxin, not to mumps virus, etc. These specific reactions involve recognition of the antigen either by soluble, humoral antibodies or by antigen-specific receptors on the membranes of certain classes of lymphocytes. The word "nonspecific" refers to those forms of immunity that recognize foreign material in a biochemical sense, do not require specific soluble or cellular recognition units, and do not require prior sensitization. It is important to recognize at the outset that both antigen-specific and nonspecific methods may elicit the same kinds of inflammatory or other undesirable consequences, but the initiation of these is by different recognition systems (see Fig. 1–1). Inasmuch as the major function of the immune system is to differentiate self from nonself, i.e., distinguish that

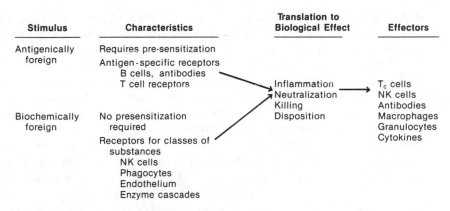

Stimulus	Characteristics	Translation to Biological Effect	Effectors

Antigenically foreign	Requires pre-sensitization
	Antigen-specific receptors
	    B cells, antibodies
	    T cell receptors
		Inflammation
		Neutralization
		Killing
		Disposition
			T_c cells
			NK cells
			Antibodies
			Macrophages
			Granulocytes
			Cytokines

Biochemically foreign	No presensitization required
	Receptors for classes of substances
	    NK cells
	    Phagocytes
	    Endothelium
	    Enzyme cascades		

FIGURE 1-1.   Diagrammatic scheme comparing the differences and similarities of antigen-specific and non-antigen specific means of activating the immune response. Once activated, both systems are translated into biological effects using the same inflammatory or effector systems.

which is foreign, the term "xenobiotic" (literally foreign to life) usually refers to agents that affect the immune system in any manner, positively or negatively. By convention, such substances referred to by this term are inanimate, but this text also deals with foreign animate objects such as microbial cell walls and toxins.

Our biggest specialized use of immunologic terms, *which may deviate from normal usage*, is in differentiating toxicity from hypersensitivity. Because of the nature of the subject matter of this text, the term toxicity refers to any alteration in the immune response and includes the terms "hypersensitivity" and "allergy," which refers to *any* type of immune injury (including autoimmunity), whether IgE-mediated or not. Hypersensitivity is more a case of enhanced tissue reactivity in a sensitized individual than an enhanced or heightened immune responses to antigens (although the latter may indeed also be present). Elevated responses in themselves are not necessarily harmful and on occasion are purposely sought.

Immunotoxicity also includes immunosuppression, which refers to any kind of decrease in immune function from foreign substances. To understand these sorts of abnormal decreases in immune function will require a familiarity with natural immunosuppression brought about by normal immunoregulatory systems. This subject receives attention as well. Those with immunologic expertise are advised to watch out for these specialized usages.

D. FOUNDATIONS OF IMMUNOTOXICOLOGY

Although there are innumerable reviews and texts dealing with allergy and other forms of immune injury, comparable coverage of immunotoxicity is lacking. Individual specialty papers of course may occur anywhere, but there are currently four major journals with "immunopharmacology" in their titles, one of which also includes the term "immunotoxicology." Aside from individual laboratory reports or case reports, only a few monographs or reviews and no texts on the subject are available.

Vos first called attention to the matter of immunotoxicology in 1977, when he compiled the first information available and concluded that current procedures for toxicity testing of chemicals underestimated the importance of the immune system. He called attention to the limited methods available at the time to assess potential risk of immunotoxicants and to the dearth of information concerning the mode of action of such agents. His article first suggested ways to deal with problems immunotoxicologists are still facing, e.g., a proper way of approaching immune functions systematically, how to extrapolate animal data to human situations, the difficulties of interpreting abnormal values, and warned against excluding the immune system from toxicologic evaluation.

Sharma and Zeeman (1980) reviewed a number of environmental chemicals but most importantly first pointed out a number of theoretical immunologic steps in which immunotoxicants might act. They also first pointed out the many possible sources of variability of results obtained in evaluation and outlined needs for future investigation. Somewhat later Sharma (1981) edited a two-volume collection of reviews of the immunotoxicologic literature that first presented basic immunologic and toxicologic considerations before taking up specific studies on an agent-by-agent basis. In so doing, he set up a classification of xenobiotics that largely still stands. Included in this review were the first mention of allergens in an immunotoxicity setting, attention to a source of immunotoxicity that is seldom mentioned today (ionizing radiation), and a discussion of methods available for immunotoxicity evaluation.

In 1983, an immunotoxicology workshop was jointly sponsored by the Toxicology and Pathology study sections of National Institutes of Health and by the National Institute of Environmental Health Sciences, and a collection of papers and abstracts presented at the 2–day meeting was published. Aside from some introductory overview presentations, the papers were mostly current reports of ongoing studies, and few critiques or syntheses were offered. Similarly, the Proceedings of the First International Symposium on Immunotoxicology, held at the University of Surrey, was published that same year (Gibson, Hubbard, and Parke 1983). This volume contains more reviews of selected but far-ranging topics and offers valuable syntheses and critiques in each. Many aspects of hypersensitivity were well covered, as were certain immunologic aspects of pathological responses to certain agents. Immune restoration (or immunomodulation as it is more often called now), which is the direct opposite of immunotoxicity, was now included as an additional means by which one can view the effects of outside agents on the immune response. Other important topics covered that do not receive much coverage in print today were those dealing with the use of immunologic data with implications in drug design, the relationship of immunosuppressive drugs and cancer, and the use of immunotoxicologic data in regulatory affairs. The Commission of European Communities held an international seminar on immunotoxicology in 1984, and the published proceedings contained similar papers by many of the same authors (Berlin et al. 1987). Their point of focus was on any type of adverse immunologic reaction resulting from contact with xenobiotics. These three references are the results of the first attempts to bring together scientists interested in this new specialty.

A somewhat different approach was offered by Li et al. (1983), whose volume is essentially a response from industry discussing the complications of trying to assess human risk to possible toxicants as well as developing standardization and validation procedures for toxicologic testing. Although this was not mainly an immunotoxicologic treatise, one subsection contained some reports devoted to the immune aspects of these concerns.

A series of papers edited by Mullen (1984) grew from a NATO Advanced Study Institute on Immunotoxicology. In the preface, Mullen examined the roots of immunotoxicology in detail and differentiated *IMMUNO*toxicologists from immuno*TOXICOLOGISTS* from the standpoints of training, orientation, and interests. He also made a strong case that pharmacokinetics and biotransformation should be given more attention. Even though that splendid suggestion was made in 1984, it has largely gone unheeded. Although the volume has not been as widely distributed as other collections, it contains a number of insightful papers.

Dean et al. (1985) edited a compendium of chapters dealing with a variety of immunotoxicologic subjects, mostly by different authors. It contains sections on basic immunologic responses, methods of assessment, immunotoxicity and immunopharmacology of therapeutics, and mechanisms of immunotoxicity of selected agents in man and animals. Some of the chapters are agent-oriented (e.g., polychlorinated biphenyls), whereas others are organ-system-oriented (e.g., immunotoxicology of the central nervous system). Most of the articles present unannotated reports of laboratory findings on animals. The most recent update on this subject by these authors appeared in 1990 (Dean et al. 1990). Most importantly, thanks to their efforts, at last immunotoxicology found its way into first-line textbooks in toxicology that have updated these topics in chapter form in various reference texts (Dean, Murray, and Ward 1986; Dean et al. 1989).

These same authors have also played an instrumental role in developing what has been called the tier approach to immunotoxicity evaluation of xenobiotics whereby the agent is subjected to a flexible and systematic battery of screening tests and, depending on results obtained, is then advanced to one of several tiers of increasing immunologic complexity. Such order out of chaos was important because of the plethora of hit-or-miss selection studies of the past, poor validation of methods, and lack of uniformity in test methods previously in use. The National Toxicology Program of the National Institute of Environmental Health Sciences initiated efforts to develop a validated, prioritized approach to immunotoxicity testing as early as 1979. A cooperative, intralaboratory project was sponsored wherein standardized methods were adopted and validated in such a tier approach. The results of this project and the current recommendations are given in their present form by Luster et al. (1988).

The most recent compendium to appear, and the only one until now with a human focus, is a multiauthored research text edited by Newcombe, Rose, and Bloom (1992). The aim of this volume is to approach the subject clinically. After a few brief background chapters, the rest deal in depth with a few specific agents (e.g., halothane, dioxins, organophosphorus) in a similar manner to the above volumes.

Finally, a rather unprecedented source of immunotoxicology information is available from an unexpected source. In 1983, a number of therapeutic and medical products industry scientists, faced with an increased realization of the prospect of immunotoxicity of their products and how to evaluate it, became concerned with the possibility of new regulatory procedures in a climate where no standard, validated evaluation program existed at the time. These scientists formed a loosely knit organization known as the Immunotoxicology Discussion Group. This unique association schedules timely meetings to disseminate news and discuss current results and problems in this field. The organization promotes forums that focus on immunotoxicology by stimulating interaction of scientists from a number of diverse fields. In so doing, it draws people from industry, academia, and government with mutual interests in these problems.

References

Anonymous. 1983. *NIH Immunotoxicology Workshop. Research Triangle Park, 1983.* Research Triangle Park: NIH/NIEHS.

Berlin, A., J. Dean, M. H. Draper, et al. 1987. *Immunotoxicology.* Drodrecht: Martinus Nijhoff.

Dean, J. H., J. B. Cornacoff, and M. I. Luster. 1990. Toxicity to the immune system: A review. *Immunopharm. Rev.* 1:377–408.

Dean, J. H., J. B. Cornacoff, G. J. Rosenthal, and M. I. Luster. 1989. Immune system: Evaluation of injury. In *Principles and Methods of Toxicology*, 2nd ed., ed. A. W. Hayes, pp. 741–60. New York: Raven Press.

Dean, J. H., M. I. Luster, A. E. Munson, and H. Amos. 1985. *Immunotoxicology and Immunopharmacology.* New York: Raven Press.

Dean, J. H., M. J. Murray, and E. C. Ward. 1986. Toxic Responses of the Immune System. In *Casarett and Doull's Toxicology. The Basic Science of Poisons*, 3rd ed., ed. C. D. Klaassen, M. O. Amdur, and J. Doull, pp. 245–85. New York: Macmillan.

Follansbee, S. E., D. F. Busch, C. B. Wofsy, et al. 1982. An outbreak of *Pneumocystis carinii* pneumonia in homosexual men. *Ann. Intern. Med.* 96:705–13.

Gibson, G. G., R. Hubbard, and D. V. Parke. 1983. *Immunotoxicology.* New York: Academic Press.

Li, A. P., T. L. Blank, D. K. Flaherty, et al. 1983. *Toxicity Testing. New Approaches and Applications in Human Risk Assessment.* New York: Raven Press.

Luster, M. I., A. E. Munson, P. T. Thomas, et al. 1988. Development of a testing battery to assess chemical-induced immunotoxicity: National Toxicology Program's guidelines for immunotoxicity evaluation in mice. *Fund. Appl. Toxicol.* 10:2–19.

Marsh, D. G., and W. B. Bias. 1988. The genetics of atopic allergy. In *Immunological Diseases*, 4th ed., ed. M. Samter, D. W. Talmage, M. M. Frank, et al., pp. 1027–46. Boston: Little, Brown.

Mullen, P. W. 1984. *Immunotoxicology. A Current Perspective of Principles and Practices.* Berlin: Springer-Verlag.

Newcombe, D. S., N. R. Rose, and J. C. Bloom. 1992. *Clinical Immunotoxicology.* New York: Raven Press.

Rosen, F. S., M. D. Cooper, and R. J. P. Wedgewood. 1984. The primary immunodeficiencies. *N. Engl. J. Med.* 311:235–42, 300–10.

Sharma, R. P. 1981. *Immunological Considerations in Toxicology.* Boca Raton: CRC Press.

Sharma, R. P., and M. G. Zeeman. 1980. Immunologic alterations by environmental chemicals: Relevance of studying mechanisms versus effects. *J. Immunopharm.* 2:285–307.

Vos, J. G. 1977. Immune suppression as related to toxicology. *CRC Crit. Rev. Toxicol.* 5:67–97.

Williamson, A. P., J. R. Montgomery, M. A. South, and R. Wilson. 1977. A special report: Four year study of a boy with combined immune deficiency maintained in strict reverse isolation from birth. *Pediatr. Res.* 11:63–64.

2

Basic Immunology

A. INTRODUCTION

Immunology is the study of altered host responses to stimulants or substances that are nonself. The science has classically concerned itself with recognizing nonself by antigen-specific or adaptive responses wherein the primary encounter with an antigen induces specific response characteristics that are magnified after the secondary encounter with that same antigen. Following secondary contact with an antigen, specific antibodies are often qualitatively different with respect to immunoglobulin class and binding capacity; they are produced faster, reach a higher maximum, and remain elevated for a longer period of time than is seen following only a single antigen encounter. This immunologic memory is called the anamnestic response and is one of the most fundamental characteristics of the immune response. Specific cell-mediated responses are similarly changed following secondary encounter with antigen. More antigen-specific and reactive lymphocytes are selected, resulting in greater lymphocyte functions on stimulation. Antigen-specific responsiveness involves antigen-presenting cells, the interaction of a number of types of lymphocytes, antigen processing and presentation within the context of special classes of cellular markers, regulation of effector cells and molecules, and somatic genetic generation of diversity.

Much of immunology is also concerned with innate or non-antigen-specific immunity in which similar inflammatory effectors are eventually activated. Innate immunity principally differs from antigen-specific immunity by the means of recognition of nonself. Innate immunity has evolved a limited repertoire of receptors that have been selected by evolutionary means to recognize certain foreign patterns. These receptors are not subject to somatic diversification (Janeway 1991). This is in sharp distinction to adaptive immunity in which there is a great somatic diversification of receptors capable of recognizing individual foreign molecules (antigens). Contemporary immunologists recognize that the innate, non-antigen-dependent mechanisms may also be changed by prior contact with a stimulant. Inflammatory cells become physiologically activated and primed by receptor activation to produce mediators, such that if in this period of heightened physiological responsiveness a secondary contact with a stimulant is made (not necessarily the same substance), an exaggerated inflammatory response is realized.

If immunology is defined as the body's reaction to foreign insult, then one must also consider substance-induced responses as the involvement of endothelial cells, activation of the complement and procoagulation cascades, vascular changes, cytokine generation, lysosomal enzyme release, the generation of toxic oxygen radicals, arachidonic acid metabolism, even the effect of cytokines on the

9

hypothalamus, among many others. It is such an interpretation of immunology that is followed in this text because all of these factors are important in responding to potentially noxious or infective agents and because xenobiotics can adversely influence any of these factors.

B. CELLULAR BASIS OF THE IMMUNE RESPONSE

For decades, the science of immunology was primarily concerned with the molecules of immunity, most notably antibodies and complement, for these substances were the most easily measurable evidences of immune function. Modern immunology recognizes the importance of these humoral substances as well as many soluble mediators or cytokines of cellular origin, but the focus is now on the sources of these substances, the cells themselves. Most of the cells of significance to immunologists arise from pluripotent stem cells, leading in turn to two main lineages, the myeloid and lymphoid cell lines. These stem cells not only need to replenish themselves but also must undergo various forms of differentiation leading to the various mature effector and regulator cells that characterize the immune response. Stem cells originate in the bone marrow of vertebrates, and how they differentiate depends on the microenvironment in which they develop and is greatly influenced by growth factors present. These growth factors affect specific cell types at certain points in their differentiation and maturation in a highly ordered sequence. Various colony-stimulating factors and certain interleukins are especially important in this regard. A graphic overview of this hemopoietic system is presented in Fig. 2-1, which shows the origins and relationships of the individual cell types important in immune responses.

The myeloid lineage gives rise to a wide diversity of cell types and includes such cells as granulocytes, mast cell types, platelets and their progenitors, and the various cells making up the monocyte–macrophage family. Mature cells of the lymphoid lineage include effector lymphocytes (B and T cytotoxic cells) as well as regulator lymphocytes (T helper and suppressor cells). Immunologically important cells of uncertain origin include NK cells, which resemble large granular lymphocytes without the distinguishing features of either T or B cells. In addition, contemporary immunologists regard such diverse cells as vascular endothelial cells and epithelial cells from a variety of organ sources as important in antigen presentation and as sources of immunologic cytokines.

Classically, hematological and lymphoid cells have been identified on the basis of morphology after standardized histological staining procedures. Today recognition goes far beyond morphological appearance and extends to functional significance of individual cell types. In some cases, merely the presence of a product serves to identify a cell. For example, demonstrating that cells secrete immunoglobulins identifies them as B lymphocytes or plasma cells. Often cell membrane markers or recognition units serve as a means of identification. The functions of these markers are often unknown, but they appear at different stages of a cell's development and are in themselves antigenic, which allows their identification with appropriate antisera. Fluorescent-labeled antisera specific for such markers make possible identification and even quantitation of specific cell types. There are at least 78 of these markers in humans, called CD (clusters of differentiation) antigens, and a standard nomenclature has been adopted to avoid confusion re-

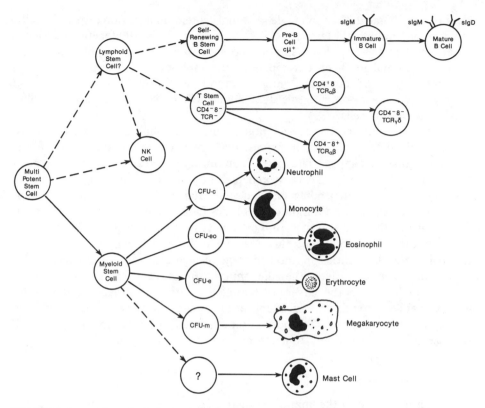

FIGURE 2-1.   A hypothetical overview of hemopoiesis showing proven (solid lines) and theoretical (broken lines) lineages of selected formed elements of immunologic importance. B-cell lymphopoiesis is better known and consists of several identifiable stages based on expression of various immunoglobulin structures, either in the cytoplasm (cIg) or on the cell surfaces (sIg). T- and NK-cell lineages are less well known, and a suspected lymphoid stem cell is hypothesized. At least three types of T cells can be demonstrated based on CD4/CD8 expression and type of TCR chains produced at the cell membrane surfaces. The CFUs are colony-forming units or proven progenitor clones of each of most of the myeloid elements.

sulting from a multiplicity of arbitrary designations (Erber 1990). Table 9-3 in Chapter 9 lists some of the more common CD antigens. At other times, a particular receptor for a cytokine, an immunoglobulin, or an activated complement component may serve to identify a cell type at a particular stage of its activity. By far the most common method of identifying classes of leukocytes, particularly lymphocytes, is through the phenotypic expression of a complex, polymorphic set of genes known as the major histocompatibility complex (MHC). Membrane antigens controlled by these genes not only have proven useful in typing individual tissues but are vital in functions related to the induction and expression of specific immune responsiveness as well.

1. B Lymphocytes

The humoral arm of the immune system is known as the B-lymphocyte, bursal-dependent, or bone-marrow-dependent system. In birds, the humoral mechanism is located in an outpocketing of gastrointestinal epithelium known as the Bursa of Fabricius. If this organ is removed soon after hatching, the chick will be deficient in development of lymph node germinal centers, maturation of plasma cells, and immunoglobulins. Mammals do not have such a centrally located analogous organ. Rather, the fetal liver, spleen, and adult bone marrow appear to be the sites of mammalian B-cell development. B lymphocytes that arise from these origins populate the secondary lymphoid organs, e.g., lymph nodes, spleen, and Peyer's patches, and, on antigenic stimulation, differentiate into immunoglobulin-producing plasma cells.

B cells are identified by the secretion of immunoglobulins on their cell membrane surfaces. Immature B cells express IgM precursor chains and/or IgD molecules, but following appropriate maturation through several steps and subsequent stimulation, there can be a class switch such that another immunoglobulin class may then be found, depending on its clonal origin. These differentiation steps are controlled by the elaboration of cytokines from the lymphoid microenvironment in which they arise. If mature B cells meet specific antigen for the immunoglobulin they are producing, this reactive cell type undergoes proliferative expansion and differentiation into end-stage plasma cells that do not reproduce. If they do not meet antigen, they die. Immunofluorescent staining of immunoglobulin molecules on the surface of lymphocytes by appropriate laboratory reagents enables recognition and quantitation of individual lymphocyte types in blood or lymphoid organs. The possession of specific immunoglobulins on B cell surfaces also facilitates their functioning as antigen-presenting cells.

2. T Lymphocytes

The other main arm of the immune system is referred to as the T-lymphocyte or thymus-dependent system. This component of the immune system is responsible for certain cell-mediated forms of immunity as well as many immunoregulatory functions. Since the development of T lymphocytes takes place in the thymus, thymectomy of neonatal animals renders them devoid of these types of immune function, and they succumb to secondary, intracellular infections.

T cells have been shown to play a critical role in the initiation, amplification, regulation, and expression of the immune response. One easy way in which human T cells were formerly identified was on the basis of a membrane receptor (CD2) that binds to sheep erythrocytes, forming easily seen rosettes comprised of both cell types. T cells may also be fluorescently stained with appropriate reagents specific for characteristic T-subtype markers.

T-cell precursors (lymphoblasts) migrate to the thymus from fetal liver, spleen, or adult bone marrow and mature in the required microenvironment found there. An intimate contact with thymic epithelial cells is necessary for maturation in addition to the T-cell colony-stimulating factors (growth and development hormones), thymosin, and thymopoietin. When the cells leave the thymus, most do not reenter but locate descendant clones in second-level lymphoid tissues such as the spleen and lymph nodes. Subsets of lymphocytes are directed and aided in this homing process by a class of cell membrane molecules known as addressins. When the cells are settled in the secondary level lymphoid tissues, thymic hormones act on them to assure continued maturation. Daughter cells circulate peripherally through these lymphoid tissues via both blood and lymphatic vessels. The life span of most T cells is short; if there is no contact with antigen, they die.

Several functional subtypes of T cells are known, e.g., helper cells, amplifier cells, suppressor cells, and cytotoxic (or effector) cells. Helper (T_h) and suppressor (T_s) cells are involved in the induction and regulation of both humoral and cellular responses and act in a competitive manner. The magnitude of a given response is in part determined by the relative balance of activities of these two cell types. T-helper and T-amplifier (T_a) cells share similar markings, and both have a positive influence on the immune response, but they differ in several respects with regard to kinetics of response to antigen, extent of thymic control, sensitivity to steroids, control by histocompatibility molecules, among others. T-helper cells act to initiate immune responsiveness to antigen, whereas T-amplifier cells enlarge or expand ongoing responses (Baker 1990). Cytotoxic cells (T_c) are responsible for various defensive or effector functions against antigen-specific targets. Some workers refer to special effector cells (T_{dth}) involved in delayed-type hypersensitivity. These are cytotoxic cells elaborating macrophage-activating lymphokines. Finally, there remains a theoretical cell population of T-memory cells, i.e., a small population of long-lived, resistant cells retaining the stamp of specific immune memory.

3. Other Effector Lymphocytes

Natural killer (NK) cells and lymphokine-activated killer (LAK) cells are distinctly different lymphocytes of uncertain lineage that seem to play a large part in defense against tumors and certain types of infections, particularly viral (Whiteside and Herberman 1989). The NK cells should be considered a mixed population of cell types. Although they lack typical T-cell CD markers, their nearly uniform larger size and greater density facilitate their laboratory isolation. Of the many functional types that go into any mixed NK-cell population, there seem to be at least two general functional types. Many NK cells exhibit membrane receptors for immunoglobulin heavy chains (Fc receptors). Hence, NK cells can bind to antibody-coated target cells. This close attachment serves as the means by which NK cells could kill targets, often those much larger than themselves, by direct contact.

This process, known as antibody-dependent cellular cytotoxicity (ADCC), is important with other classes of inflammatory cells but is not the major way NK cells kill tumor targets. The NK cells mainly recognize tumors through unknown means. The nature of the receptor is unknown, although it is dissimilar from any of the known immunoglobulin superfamily molecules. They seem to attack certain types of tumor cells involving a chemical means of recognizing unique molecules expressed by these tumors (Herberman, Reynolds, and Ortaldo 1986). The NK cells are not subject to antigen-specific induction or expansion, but are affected by a variety of environmental stimulants (some adversely). The LAK cells are mostly an artificial product of the laboratory bearing no distinctive CD marker in vivo. They are obtained by activating NK cells with the immunopotent cytokine interleukin 2 (IL-2). The possibility exists that LAK cells could be spontaneously produced in vivo during graft-versus-host reactions, a rejection process initiated when mature lymphocytes are transplanted to an immunologically incompetent recipient.

4. Antigen-Presenting Cells

Antigen presentation and processing are extremely important parts of the induction of the immune response. Those cells that first contact antigen and may further process the antigen are known as antigen-presenting cells (APC). Originally, these cells were thought to belong exclusively to the macrophage–monocyte lineage, but the range of recognized APC types has become much broader (see Table 2-1). In addition to tissue macrophages and peripheral blood monocytes, other APCs include astrocytes, Langerhans cells in the skin, which migrate to draining lymph nodes (where they become known as interdigitating cells), and follicular dendritic cells of lymph nodes and spleen. Other medullary interdigitating cells present self-antigen to T cells in the thymus, presumably where the body initially learns to distinguish self from nonself. Activated B cells are also able to present antigen to T cells, albeit by a different mechanism. Nonlymphoid cells from a variety of somatic areas are responsive to certain immunologic cytokines and produce the kind of MHC molecules necessary for antigen presentation, so presumably such cells should also be considered APC.

In addition to these antigen-specific functions, macrophages–monocytes are also important in defensive functions unrelated to antigen recognition. These cells are phagocytic and, in addition to processing and presenting antigens to T cells, kill and digest infectious or noxious substances. Moreover, these cells may become physiologically activated by lymphocyte products, thereby enhancing their effector functions. They also express surface receptors for such molecules as the Fc portion of certain immunoglobulins, which enable the cells to recognize and engulf antigen–antibody complexes more readily. Thus, they are important in both afferent and efferent immune pathways.

C. TISSUES AND ORGANS OF IMMUNOLOGIC IMPORTANCE

The supportive tissues in which lymphoid and myeloid elements mature and function are of prime importance in immunotoxicology, as it is often in these locations that xenobiotics exert their effects. Hemopoietic precursors are originally derived from embryonic mesenchyme, and the earliest precursor cells are found in yolk sac, later in the fetal liver and spleen, and finally in the bone marrow. Virtually all mammalian myeloid and lymphoid stem cells come from the widely dispersed bone marrow, primarily in the sternum, clavicle, ribs, and pelvis. Lymphoid stem cells from the adult bone marrow seed other organs and become committed at two levels. At one level, lymphocytes become committed toward

TABLE 2-1.   Antigen Presenting Cells

APC	Location	Phago-cytosis	Fc/C3 Receptors	MHC Class II	Present to
Monocyte–Macrophage lineage	Blood, tissues	+	+	Inducible	T + B
Follicular dendritic cells	Lymphoid tissue	–	+	–	B
Interdigitating dendritic cells	Lymphoid tissue	–	–	Constitutive	T
Marginal zone macrophages	Spleen, lymph nodes	+	+	Inducible	B
Langerhans cells	Skin	–	+	Constitutive	T
B/T lymphocytes	Various				
Endothelium Fibroblasts		–	±	Inducible	B/T

B- or T-cell lineages depending on in which organ they locate, e.g., the thymus, lamina propria, Peyer's patches, and antigen commitment occurs in secondary organs such as the lymph nodes or mature spleen.

1. Thymus

The thymus develops from the third and fourth branchial pouches of the embryonic pharynx, where it migrates caudally in most mammals and is infiltrated by precursors from bone marrow, yolk sac, and fetal liver. It contains no afferent lymphatic vessels or follicles. The thymus is partly divided by septa into sections called lobules, each of which consists of two regions, an epithelium infiltrated by lymphocyte precursors in its cortex and a medullary center with fewer lymphocytic elements (see Fig. 2–2). The medulla contains thymic corpuscles, which are concentric layers of swollen epithelial cells that may occasionally enclose a core

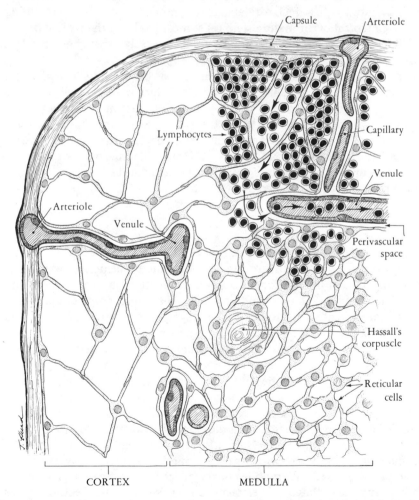

FIGURE 2–2.   A diagrammatic representation of the cellular organization of one lobule of the thymus. Lymphocytes are much more abundant in the outer cortex than in the inner medulla. (*From Bellanti, J. A. 1985. Immunology III. Philadelphia: W. B. Saunders. Reprinted with permission.*)

of keratin. The blood vessels are well insulated from the thymocytes, particularly in the cortices such that limited passage of cells and molecules is afforded.

Precursors arrive in the cortex, interact with epithelium, mature, then move into the medulla before departing in efferent blood or lymphatic vessels. Once they leave, most do not recirculate and only a very few ever return to the thymus. There is an enormous production of thymocytes in the cortex, but only about 1% survive. The selection for thymocyte death is a result of both positive and negative selection. Cells with receptors for "self" are negatively selected, and those not selected by antigen presentation die. In the thymus, a complete turnover occurs every 4–5 days. The T–cell generation time of 6.5–8.5 hr is very short compared to lymph node cells (three- to fivefold less). Those that live seed to either the spleen or lymph nodes. The thymus is more important at birth up to puberty, after which time it begins physiologically to decrease in size and structure (involution), but it can also prematurely involute with loss in function because of factors in the host environment. After puberty, further lymphocyte production and maturation take place in other organs. The main function of the thymus in adults is to safeguard damage to lymphoid tissue by maintaining and regulating maturation of mature stem cells, most likely by the release of maturational hormones. Macrophages may be found sparsely throughout the thymus, but interdigitating cells are found only in the medulla.

Thymectomy of experimental animals at or near birth results in well-recognized immunodeficiency disease characterized by a failure of the T-cell-mediated immune system to develop. After such thymectomy, immune competence may be restored in two ways, either by thymic transplant (which facilitates the regeneration of cells with recipient markers) or by lymphocyte infusion (characterized by proliferation of cells with donor markers). Human counterparts of experimental thymectomy are exemplified by spontaneous genetic or developmental failures of thymic growth, e.g., the DiGeorge syndrome.

2. Spleen

The spleen is a multifunctional organ that filters the blood of foreign particles, removes worn-out blood cells, converts hemoglobin to bilirubin, and is important in iron metabolism in addition to being a production source for lymphocytes. The interior consists of two kinds of pulp, the white pulp, containing numerous germinal centers or follicles where lymphocytes are produced, and an erythrocyte-laden background in the red pulp (see Fig. 2–3).

B cells mature inside these germinal centers, whereas T cells mature around the outside of the follicles or in periarteriolar sheaths. Many experimental procedures for evaluating xenobiotics utilize spleen-cell suspensions prepared by macerating excised organs, and such contain 25–35% B cells and 30–50% T cells. When lymphocytic precursors enter the spleen, T cells seem to associate with interdigitating cells, whereas B cells do so with follicular dendritic cells. The white pulp comprises nearly 20% of a "resting" spleen's weight but under immune challenge greatly increases, as do the number and size of germinal centers. The red pulp is packed with mobile phagocytic cells, and the linings of the sinuses contain many fixed phagocytic elements consistent with the clearance functions of this organ. Like the thymus, the spleen contains no afferent lymphatics.

It was once thought that surgical removal of the adult spleen was without consequence, but well-recognized risk factors are now known to jeopardize such

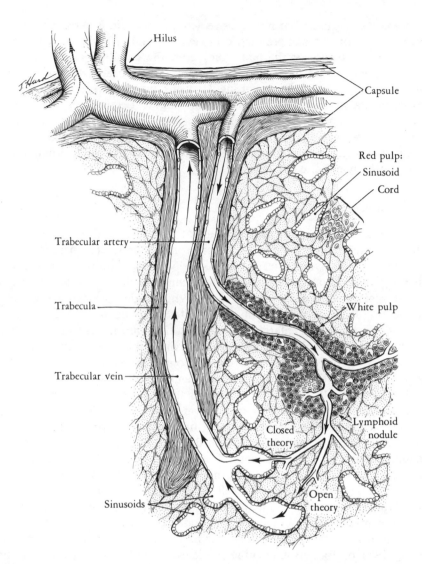

FIGURE 2–3.   Diagrammatic representation of the spleen showing the sinusoids, where clearance takes place, and the circulation in relation to the nodules of the white pulp, where lymphocytes mature.   (*From Bellanti, J. A. 1985. Immunology III. Philadelphia: W. B. Saunders. Reprinted with permission.*)

splenectomized individuals. These people are prone to suffer a greater incidence of certain types of life-threatening infections.

3. Lymphatics

The lymphatic system represents a second circulatory system of conducting vessels (lymphatic capillaries and lymphatics), loose aggregates of lymphoid tissues (nodules), and more highly organized and structured organs called lymph nodes. Through this system passes lymph, a collection of tissue fluids rich in globulins and lymphocytes. As this fluid passes through draining lymph nodes, the fluid becomes progressively enriched with more lymphocytes. Although there is nothing analogous to a muscular heart, movement of the fluid is enhanced by hemo-dynamic and perilymphatic pressure, osmotic tone, and ordinary body movement, i.e., the more exercise of the body, the better the capillary flow. The cellular contents empty back into the blood circulation via a thoracic duct, which in hu-mans is located where the internal jugular veins empty into the venous system. In experimental animals, cannulation of this duct is a convenient way to collect virtually pure suspensions of lymphocytes. After entry into the blood, these lymphocytes will eventually find their way into a lymph node, from which they may either stay in the circulating blood or else may reenter the recirculating pool of cells in the lymphatic circulation.

4. Lymph Nodes

Lymph nodes are highly organized organs of structural and lymphoid elements through which interact and pass two circulatory systems, i.e., there are both af-ferent and efferent lymphatics as well as blood vessels supplying and draining each node. Individual nodes consist of an inner medulla and an outer cortex containing germinal centers (see Fig. 2-4). When undergoing antigenic stimula-tion resulting from drainage of fluid from sites of inoculation and antigen cap-ture by APC, the nodes enlarge and may become painful. At this time, there is a great deal of DNA synthesis resulting from lymphoblastic activity taking place. The nodes consist of two main portions, an outer cortex and an inner medulla. The node is transected by reticular fibers extending from dividing struts (trabecu-lae). The stromal cells constituting this mechanical support may be an important source of lymphocyte growth or maturation-promoting substances. Within the cortex are a number of germinal centers of intense B-lymphocyte production. From these follicles extend medullary cords, also rich in B cells. In paracortical and subcortical areas there are looser, less organized collections of lymphocytes, which are T cells. If an excised lymph node is macerated and a suspension made of the lymphocytes, 10–20% are B cells, and 65–85% T cells.

The lymph nodes have two major functions. Just as the spleen serves to filter particulate matter from blood, lymph nodes perform a similar function on lymph. In this function, lymph nodes are particularly efficient, being capable of filtering 99% of foreign circulating particles. Lymph nodes are also a major source of antigen-committed lymphocytes, which enter the recirculating pool. As lymph node capillaries collect into postcapillary venules in the inner cortex, the vessels are lined by a specialized layer of cells termed the high endothelium (see Fig. 2-5). Lymphocytes are able to attach to and pass between endothelial cells or even directly through their cell membranes and enter free spaces within the node. They are then capable of interacting with interdigitating APC and/or en-tering the efferent lymphatic drainage, eventually to return to the circulation via the thoracic duct.

5. Lymphoid Nodules

Less-organized aggregates of lymphoid and other leukocytic elements occur as mucosal and submucosal collections in the respiratory, gastrointestinal, and geni-tourinary tracts as well as other specialized tissues such as the tonsils. Inasmuch as the development of these structures is very poor in germ-free animals, it is assumed that antigen stimulation is vital to their development. In these tissues,

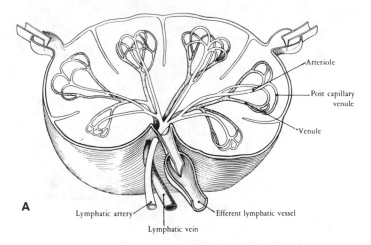

A

Arteriole

Post capillary venule

Venule

Lymphatic artery

Lymphatic vein

Efferent lymphatic vessel

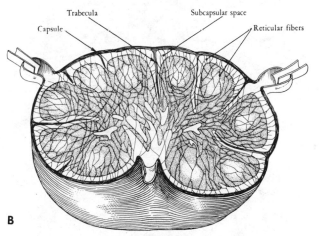

Trabecula

Subcapsular space

Capsule

Reticular fibers

B

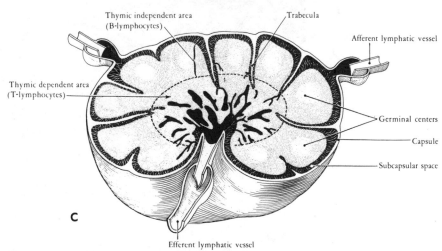

Thymic independent area (B-lymphocytes)

Trabecula

Afferent lymphatic vessel

Thymic dependent area (T-lymphocytes)

Germinal centers

Capsule

Subcapsular space

C

Efferent lymphatic vessel

FIGURE 2–4. Three schematic representations of a lymph node showing, from left to right, (A) the arrangement and association of densely packed germinal follicles as well as free lymphocytes and monocytes with reticulum fibers; (B) distribution of veins showing the arrangement of postcapillary venules in close approximation with germinal follicles; and (C) the arrangement of reticulum fibers showing the channels of the afferent lymphatics that allow lymphocyte traffic within the node. (*From Bellanti, J. A. 1985. Immunology III. Philadelphia: W. B. Saunders. Reprinted with permission.*)

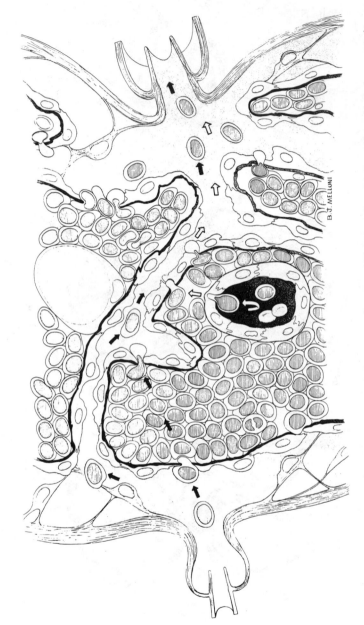

FIGURE 2–5. Schematic depiction of the circulation of lymphocytes within a lymph node. Lymphocytes are shown entering the node from the vascular bed by passage through the endothelium of the postcapillary venule and from the afferent lymphatic vessels. *(From Bellanti, J. A. 1985. Immunology III. Philadelphia: W. B. Saunders. Reprinted with permission.)*

Tlink output file : D:T1.PXT   Mon Aug 10 1992 05:17:07   Page 1

20

epithelium-related lymphoid concentrations are an important site of IgA synthesis. They originate in the connective tissue support of the epithelium, the lamina propria, but may spread into an underlying submucosal layer if one is present.

D. IMMUNOGLOBULIN GENE SUPERFAMILY

A fundamental way to understand the molecular characteristics and function not only of antibody (immunoglobulin) but of a variety of cell membrane molecules as well is to become acquainted with the structural similarities among them. They have several common characteristics: a highly conserved region of about 100 amino acids with a centrally placed disulfide cross-linkage that configures the chain into a stable fold; a carboxy-terminal portion of the chain that often extends through the plasma membrane into the cytoplasm; the attachment of a carbohydrate moiety; and often (but not always) the association of the basic chain with another similar or dissimilar chain. They probably arose by gene duplication and divergence from a single ancestral domain structure. These molecules function in three major ways: (1) recognizing an external stimulus (an antigen in the present context); (2) in some of these molecules, recognizing or signaling another cell; and (3) transducing signals internally into the cell bearing the molecule. In addition to the various classes of immunoglobulins, other members of this superfamily include CD3, CD4, and CD8 markers, both class I and class II MHC molecules, and the T-cell antigen receptor.

1. Immunoglobulins

Antibodies or immunoglobulins (Ig) are protein globulins found in the serum and various other external secretions that arise as a result of stimulation by antigen and are capable of reacting specifically with that antigen but not with dissimilar molecules. Immunoglobulins may be considered the effector molecules of humoral immunity, and although there are several classes, they all share certain similarities. All are glycoproteins in basic units of two pairs of peptide chains (see Fig. 2–6). Each of the larger chains has a molecular weight of approximately 50,000 (depending on Ig class) and is called the heavy (H) chain. These are joined by disulfide linkages at critical positions of cysteine residues. Each H chain is linked by similar disulfide bonds to a smaller light (L) chain of approximately 25,000 Da. Any particular immunoglobulin molecule therefore has one pair of identical H chains and a pair of identical L chains. The antibody-combining site is located at the amino-terminal end of the heavy and light chains, so that each immunoglobulin molecule has at least two antigen-reactive sites.

Digestion studies on IgG with enzymes have elucidated the functional components of antibodies. Papain cleaves antibodies into functional subunits, one of which, the Fab fragment, contains the light chain and the amino-terminal end of the heavy chain (Fig. 2–6). This Fab portion has been demonstrated to contain the antibody combining sites, and since the point of enzymatic digestion is beyond that which joins the heavy chains together, the result of such digestion is two univalent Fab fragments. The remaining parts of the heavy chains remain bound together into one unit by disulfide linkages, and this is termed the Fc fragment, that end of the immunoglobulin with other biological functions of that

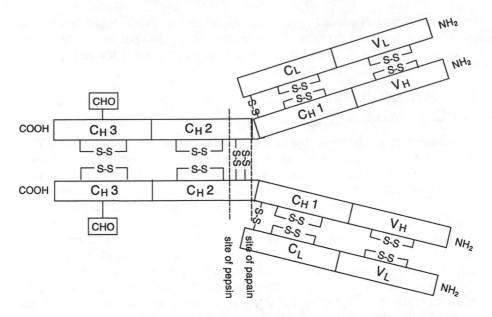

FIGURE 2–6.   A stylized drawing of an IgG₁ molecule showing the critical relationship of heavy and light chains, points of disulfide linkages, carbohydrate attachment, points of proteolytic enzyme attack, and organization of constant and variable domains.

particular class, e.g., binding of antibodies to cells, activation of the classical complement cascade, and passage through the placenta. When other proteolytic enzymes such as pepsin are used to digest IgG, the carboxy-terminal residues are digested away from the molecule below the interchain disulfide bridges, and the result is a molecule with functionally bivalent antigen-combining sites and nonfunctional Fc properties.

There are several different classes of humoral antibodies differing in chemical structure as well as in biological function. These are summarized in Table 2–2 and depicted in Fig. 2–7. Originally, these different classes were named according to their rate of migration in an electrophoretic field and ultracentrifugal sedimentation rates, but when knowledge of the structure and composition of the individual chains became available, a standard nomenclature was adopted. Each immunoglobulin class has a distinctive pair of heavy chains: γ chains for IgG, μ for IgM, α for IgA, δ for IgD, and ϵ for IgE. These chains differ chemically,

TABLE 2–2.   Summary of Major Immunoglobulin Features

Isotype	M. W.	Heavy Chain	Function Examples
IgG	150,000	γ (4 subclasses)	Mature, secondary responses Passes placenta
IgM	970,000	μ	Primary response antibody
IgA	160,000	α (2 subclasses)	—
sIgA	385,000	α	In all external secretions
IgD	184,000	δ	Important in ontogeny, cell differentiation
IgE	188,000	ϵ	Antihelminthic antibody; immediate-type hypersensitivity

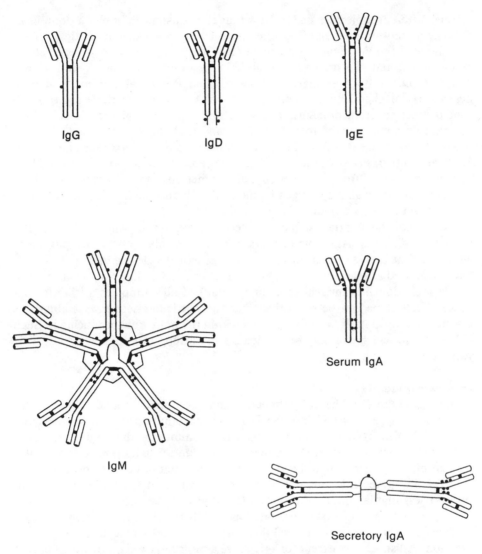

FIGURE 2-7.   Structural depictions of the major immunoglobulin classes showing light/heavy chain arrangements, position of J chains, attached carbohydrate groups (dark circles), and major interchain disulfide linkages. Only one IgG subclass, IgG₁, is depicted. Serum IgA may exist in polymeric forms in addition to the one shown here. The IgA molecule shown here is with a peptide extension important in linkage to a J chain. The IgE heavy chains are shown somewhat longer than other classes to reflect the added constant domains that ε chains are known to possess.

biologically, and serologically; i.e., when isolated chains from one species are injected into another species, antibodies specific for that particular type of chain are produced. Although there are five different kinds of heavy chains, there are only two kinds of light chains, κ and λ, and a pair of either may be found in each class. The light chains of a given molecule will be of the same type, but molecules with the other type may also be present in the same individual.

Much additional information concerning immunoglobulin structure has been obtained from amino acid sequencing studies. In the carboxy-terminal ends of light chains, a peptide of approximately 110 amino acids is rather constant among different molecules and is known as the constant:light chain domain or C_L. The amino-terminal end is extremely varied in sequence and for light chains is designated the V_L domain. Intrachain disulfide bridges enclose loops of 60–70 amino acids, and two of these in each light chain compose the V_C and V_L domains, respectively. A similar situation exists in the variable domain of each heavy class of chain, but the constant regions differ in that there are three to four distinct constant domains. The γ, α, and δ heavy chains each have three constant domains referred to as C_H1, C_H2, and C_H3 (Fig. 2-2). In both μ and ϵ heavy chains, there is a fourth constant domain at the carboxy terminus, C_H4. Fab fragments of heavy chains contain the variable domain and most of the first constant domain. Often particular biological functions can be located on individual domains; for example, antigen-bound IgM activates the classical complement pathway via the C_H3 domain of the μ chain.

Additional chain variation may be detected through the identification of allotypes and idiotypes. Allotypic markers, usually the substitution of a particular amino acid at a given point in a chain, are genetically determined and as such have been used as markers in population genetics studies. Individual variation in the variable domain (antigen-combining region) of all antibodies arising from a single B-cell clone can be so distinct that the particular sequence lending this distinction may in itself be antigenic even within the individual producing it. Such a distinction, which can only be defined by an antibody to it, is called idiotypic variation.

Immunoglobulin G

Immunoglobulin G is the most abundant immunoglobulin found in the serum, accounting for nearly 70–75% of the total. Normal adult serum levels range from 640 to 1,350 mg/100 ml. The IgG class of immunoglobulins is characteristic of the secondary (anamnestic) immune response and usually possesses a greater antigen-binding affinity than IgM. Human infants do not begin to produce their own IgG in appreciable amounts until about 7 weeks of age, although at birth they possess high amounts of maternal IgG that has been acquired transplacentally. The maternal IgG in the neonate has a half-life of approximately 45 days.

There are four subclasses of IgG that vary in structure, molecular weight, and function. All subclasses except for IgG_3 have a molecular weight of 146,000; that of IgG_3 is 170,000 because of its longer γ chain with more cysteine residues. Immunoglobulins G_1 and G_3 have Fc components that bind directly to Fc receptors on phagocytic cells and are also the only two IgG subclasses that can activate the classical complement pathway efficiently after antigen binding (IgG_2 does so less efficiently). Immunoglobulins G_2 and G_4 bind to the same receptors only after aggregation with large-molecular-weight antigens. The binding of antibody to the cell activates the cell and, in some cases, initiates phagocytosis.

Immunoglobulin M

Immunoglobulin M is composed of five basic units of heavy (μ chains) and light chains (κ or λ) covalently linked together by an additional peptide known as the J chain. The five-unit IgM molecule has a molecular weight of approximately 970,000 and makes up about 10% of the circulating immunoglobulin pool in normal ranges of 85–350 mg/100 ml of serum. The IgM antibodies are capable of activating the classical complement pathway and are produced early in the immune response. They can not pass the placenta, but they can be produced in utero following fetal contact with antigen. On a mole-per-mole basis, they can, of course, combine with more antigen, but their binding affinity is lower than that of IgG. They arise first in the course of immunization to many antigens and do not respond anamnestically (i.e., by an accelerated and higher elevation) as do IgG globulins. Some pathological antibodies such as most of the rheumatoid factors, cold agglutinins, heterophile antibodies, anti-DNA, many normal isoagglutinins of human blood groups, complete-type Rh antibody, leukoagglutinins, some thyroid antibodies, typhoid "O" antibodies, and the Wasserman antibody are typically all IgM.

Immunoglobulin A

Immunoglobulin A, consisting of α heavy chains, makes up about 15–20% of the normal pool of immunoglobulins and occurs in different forms depending on whether it is found in the serum or external secretions. The IgA found in circulating blood is either in basic monomeric units or in the form of dimers of basic units bound together by J-chains. The primary immunoglobulin found in body secretions such as saliva, tears, and colostrum is known as secretory IgA (sIgA), consisting of dimers to which a 70,000 secretory piece is attached. The IgA, like any immunoglobulin, is produced by plasma cells, but as it passes through the epithelial layer of the organ where it is produced, each IgA dimer picks up a secretory piece that has been synthesized by the epithelial cells. The secretory piece functions to inhibit enzymatic degradation of the antibody in the external milieu. There are two subclasses of IgA (IgA_1 and IgA_2), and about 90% is IgA_1 in the serum, whereas 60% of the IgA in secretions is IgA_2. The highest concentration of IgA_2 is found in tears and colostrum. These antibodies serve as the first line of specific defense against microorganisms that infect the respiratory and gastrointestinal tracts.

Immunoglobulin A does not fix complement by the classical pathway. It does not pass the placenta and so is not detectable at birth, although the free transport piece may be present. Human infants seem to be capable of synthesizing their own IgA beginning at 2 to 3 weeks of age.

Immunoglobulin D

Immunoglobulin D accounts for less than 1% of the total circulating immunoglobulin pool (3 mg/100 ml serum). Although its role in serum is uncertain, it seems to be an important part of B-cell differentiation prior to steps leading to class-specific clone development.

Immunoglobulin E

The IgE class of antibody has a chemical structure that is similar to IgG in that it consists of the basic two pairs of chains only. However, its molecular weight is slightly higher because its heavy chains (ϵ) are longer, possessing an extra constant domain. It also has a high carbohydrate content—12% compared to 2–3% for the IgG subtypes. Immunoglobulin E is normally present in all sera, but at extremely low concentrations (30–250 mg/ml mean in normal, nonatopic sera). The demonstration of both total and antigen-specific IgE requires the uses of secondary amplification methods (e.g., radioimmunoassays). The IgE has the ability to attach itself to mast cells and certain other leukocytes by means of binding between the unique domain on the Fc ϵ chains and specific receptors on cell membranes.

2. Major Histocompatibility Molecules

The MHC gene complex is a large family of genes located together on a single chromosome (chromosome 6 in humans, 17 in mice). These genes have been mapped in three classes, two of which concern us in this context: class I and class II. Their gene products are transmembrane glycoproteins that serve as useful markers for many types of cellular interactions. Since they are identified by immunologic techniques for organ transplantation, they are often also called major histocompatibility antigens (MHC). This gene family is extremely polymorphic, each class having 20–40 alleles. Figure 2–8 compares the structures of important immunoglobulin superfamily molecules with that of a stylized immunoglobulin.

The molecules of both classes consist of two chains, but only the heavy chain (the α) in the class I molecule is determined by genes in this complex. It is noncovalently linked to another, smaller chain of more constant structure, the β_2-microglobulin, which is encoded outside the MHC complex. The heavy chain consists of three domains, with α_1 and α_2 expressing allotypic variation. Class I genes determine markers in human HLA-A, HLA-B, and HLA-C regions and their K, D, and L counterparts in mice. Class I MHC molecules are more ubiquitous in location, being found on all nucleated cells as well as platelets and (in the mouse) erythrocytes.

Class II MHC molecules consist of pairs of noncovalently associated chains, α and β, each consisting of two external domains. Individual polymorphism is associated mostly with the β chain. Class II genes encode molecules from the I region of mice and the D region of humans. The similarity of these molecules with immunoglobulins refers not only to amino acid homology in the membrane-bound domains of each class but also to the way the variable portions of the MHC-encoded chains fold to form a cleft capable of noncovalently binding antigenic peptides. Class II molecules are found on lymphocytes and especially on some antigen-presenting cells (see Table 2–2).

3. T-Cell Antigen Receptors

Although MHC molecules bind antigen, the major antigen recognition units of T lymphocytes are distinctly different structures. These units are also composed of pairs of chains consisting of two globular domains each, with immunoglobulin homology being associated with the constant regions. These chains are covalently linked through disulfide bridges near the cell membrane. There are two sets of these T-cell receptors (TCR) differing in the type of chain composition, one set consisting of α and β chains, the other of γ and δ. The genes coding for these chains reside on different chromosomes from those of the MHC. Although the $\alpha{:}\beta$ receptors recognize antigen in a manner analogous to immunoglobulins, it is important to understand that they do so in the context of corecognition with MHC products. The function of the $\gamma{:}\delta$ receptor is unknown, but they have a different tissue distribution pattern, give rise to a smaller repertoire of receptor molecules, and seem to be more important against antigens of infectious origin or consequence (Born et al. 1991).

4. CD4 and CD8 Molecules

The characteristic molecule found on T-helper lymphocytes, CD4, is a single chain bearing three globular domains, two of which are variable. The molecule on the T-cytotoxic/suppressor lymphocytes, CD8, consists of a pair of smaller

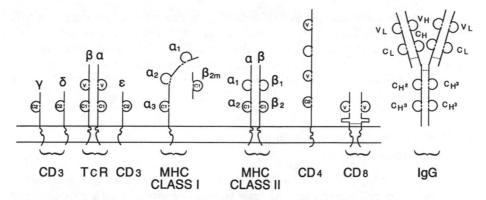

FIGURE 2-8.   Comparison of hypothetical structures of important members of the immunoglobulin superfamily molecules. Constant and variable domains are indicated by intrachain loops, most of which are closed by disulfide linkages. Most of these molecules are drawn showing carboxy-terminal chain extensions through the cell membrane into the cytosol. All amino-terminal portions of the chains are toward the top of the drawing.

chains with a single variable domain. It is believed that these units serve to stabilize the corecognition of antigen by T cells.

5. The CD3 Molecule

Both CD4$^+$ and CD8$^+$ T cells recognize antigen through their TCR in association with another complex present on both cell types, CD3. This complex consists of at least three different types of chains, γ, δ, and ϵ, noncovalently associated with each other but closely proximal to the TCR. It is believed that these molecules are involved in signal transduction on interaction of TCR with antigen.

E. CELLULAR INTERACTIONS OF THE IMMUNE RESPONSE

It is convenient to liken the immune response to that of a neurological reflex. In both there are afferent, central processing, and efferent limbs. In the afferent limb, antigen is taken up by APC, and this compares with the stimulus in a neurological response. Once taken up, the antigen is analyzed and processed in a variety of ways within the central limb and is presented to other types of cells for further action. In neither the nervous nor the immune system would this much activity be of consequence without a reflexive response. In immunologic terms, this response is how the immune system translates the immune recognition of antigen into some meaningful biological action or effector function (e.g., neutralization, killing, or disposition of a harmful agent) by means of its cooperating mediators and cells.

Cellular interaction occurs on at least two levels, and it is important to realize that xenobiotics can interfere with either type. One level has to do with the cellular interaction of antigen recognition, processing, and presentation to other cell types. Once suitable effector cells have been generated, there is an additional level of cellular interaction with immunologic and inflammatory cells to carry out the effector functions of the immune response. Much of this interaction is enhanced by cytokines, i.e., secreted molecules with biological activity. Many of these cytokines have multiple functions but in a given situation are more specific because of the specific microenvironment a particular cell type is in and the particular stage of differentiation or development that cell happens to be in at a given time. They function in a concerted, intricate network, and many owe their activity to the presence of additional stimuli. Cytokines are discussed in more detail in Chapter 4.

1. Cellular Interactions in Immune Response Induction

Antigen-presenting cells must first acquire contact with the antigen and take it up within their cell membranes. At least two major types of cells participate in antigen presentation, i.e., those of the macrophage–monocyte lineages and B lymphocytes. If the subsequent presentation is to be made to B cells (i.e., for T-cell-independent antigens), no further processing of the antigen is necessary; i.e., B cells recognize prosthetic groups on the intact antigenic molecule via specific immunoglobulins secreted by particular B-cell clones. However, if subsequent presentation is to be made to T cells, then the antigen must be processed or partially digested before parts of it are reexpressed on the cell membrane (Fig. 2–9). T cells recognize neoantigens processed by the APC from the native molecule.

For most antigens, presentation to T_h must occur in association with class II MHC molecules (Fig. 2–10). These molecules found on APCs, and lymphocytes are necessary for afferent induction of T-helper cells. Helper cells cannot recognize antigen on antigen-presenting cells in the absence of these molecules. When antigen reacts with immunoglobulin receptors on B cells, the complexes migrate to one pole of the cell, a process called capping, at which time the lymphocyte becomes activated. Antigen is internalized and processed in a manner similar to macrophages before it is reexpressed on the cell surface bound to MHC II molecules. In one sense B-cell antigen presentation is considered very efficient because the Ig receptors have a very high affinity for antigen and thus can function effectively in the presence of low antigen concentration (Myers 1991).

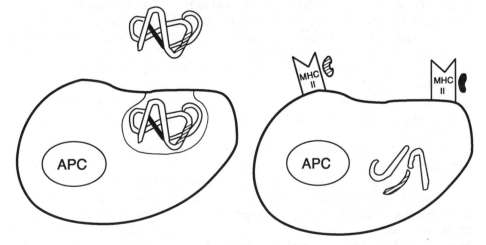

FIGURE 2–9.   Schematic drawing showing partial digestion of antigen by an antigen-presenting cell (APC) and certain peptide neoantigens being expressed on the cell membrane in context with class II MHC molecules.

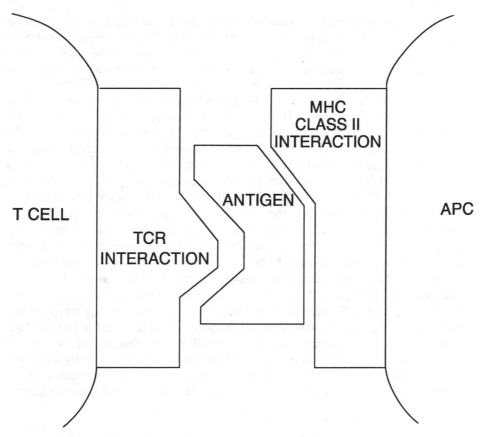

FIGURE 2-10.   Schematic detail of how an antigen is thought to be recognized simultaneously by a T-cell antigen receptor (TCR) from one cell and a class II MHC molecule from an antigen-presenting cell.

At this point, at least two kinds of signals are required: (1) those involving molecular recognition and (2) those involving cytokine stimulation. Antigen must be recognized as nonself by the T-cell antigen receptor (TCR) as well as the appropriate class II MHC molecule. This interaction is stabilized by either CD4 or CD8 and is in close contact with the CD3 complex, which serves to transmit the activation signal. The signals needed to activate T cells vary with the subset (CD4 or CD8) and the activation status (e.g., resting or activated) of the lymphocytes. In the activation process, qualitatively different signals are required for CD4 and CD8.

In addition, resting T cells require more signals than those already activated. TCR and MHC II stimulation alone will activate a certain amount of cell signaling by membrane perturbation but by itself is not enough. This activation must take place with a second signal provided by a cytokine produced by the APC, interleukin 1 (IL-1), which further activates a T-cell enzyme (protein kinase C) to stimulate the production of IL-2 and γ interferon (IFN-γ). In effect, the T cell receives processed antigen from the APC and then in essence "processes" the antigen again to interact with a B cell via the antigen and the class II MHC molecule. These cytokines amplify the above interactions in yet additional ways. For example, IFN-γ is a potent inducer of class II MHC molecules such that its release acts as a positive feedback signal. It also activates monocytes and synergizes with other mediators to promote B-cell differentiation into antibody-forming cells. Some of these cytokine influences are summarized in Fig. 2–11.

The influence of cytokines in these cellular interactions is very important to any type of immune cell interaction, and of these, IL-2 is one of the most important. In order for T cells to complete their development and become immunologically responsive, they require IL-2 from other, activated T cells. High-affinity IL-2 receptors do not appear unless the cells are first stimulated by antigen. The IL-2 receptor molecules consist of two chains, an α and a β, but the β chains are not present in the low-affinity receptors on resting cells. One of the responses to APC-generated IL-1 is for the T cells to produce the complete IL-2 receptor molecule. Thus, the T cell is subject to its own (autocrine) stimulation wherein stimulated T_h cells produce not only their own stimulating cytokine but the receptors for these cytokines as well. In addition, IL-2 activates NK cells and monocytes and promotes B-cell proliferation and differentiation. There are several other interleukins and cytokines involved in both afferent and efferent pathways of the immune response, and these are discussed in more detail in Chapter 4.

Because the expression of class II MHC molecules is so important to the induction of antigen-specific immune responses, the modulation of their expression, and the interference in these processes by xenobiotics, it is a most important area to consider in immunotoxicology. Some of the factors that are known to up-regulate the expression of these critical molecules are phagocytosis by APC and the production of certain key cytokines, e.g., IFN-γ and IL-4 (described in Chapter 4), which in itself is determined by cell associations in the microenvironment.

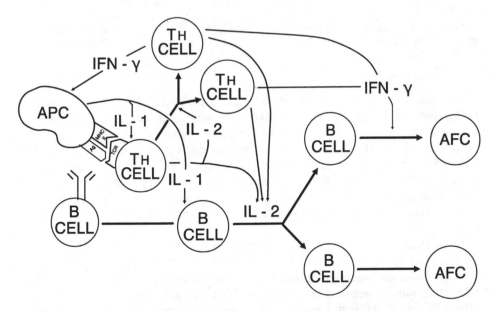

FIGURE 2–11.   Schematic representation of pathways of some of the key cytokines involved in immune response induction. In addition to the dual role of presenting antigen in a class II context to T_h cells and antigen to B cells, APC also produces IL-1, which activates B cells and stimulates T_h cells to produce IL-2. The IL-2 promotes B-cell proliferation as well as T_h-cell expansion. The IL-1-stimulated T_h cells also are caused to produce IFN-γ which acts as a positive feedback signal to stimulate APC to express more MHC molecules, and it also promotes B-cell differentiation into antibody-forming cells (AFC).

However, the effect of these molecules is selective: IFN-γ up-regulates expression of both MHC class I and II molecules while IL-4 increases expression of class II markers on antigen-presenting cells. Important factors that are known to down-regulate class II MHC molecule expression are certain types of tumor cells and the production of prostaglandin E_2. Since several xenobiotics have immuno-pharmacological consequences by affecting arachidonic acid metabolism, more attention will need to be paid to this mechanism of immunotoxicity.

2. Cellular Interactions in Effector Cell Recognition

As seen above, class II MHC molecules are important in afferent pathways, i.e., those leading to induction of immune responses. On the other hand, class I MHC molecules are important in the efferent pathways of the immune response, i.e., the carrying out of the effector mechanisms. Class I MHC molecules are found on all cell types and are important in such efferent responses as those needed to signal cytotoxic lymphocytes to recognize antigens. Such recognition usually implies that there is prior antigenic sensitization, that is, from the MHC class II antigen presentation pathway. Thus, any host with prior sensitization will lyse any self cell exhibiting foreign antigen in a class I MHC context by cytotoxic T cells with one important exception—cytotoxic lymphocytes will recognize foreign class I molecules as antigens directly without any requirement for pre-sensitization. The MHC class distinction may be seen in yet another way, in its interaction with cells with CD4 and CD8 molecules that must also be recognized in context with antigen in association with MHC. To oversimplify somewhat, CD4 on T_h cells interacts with MHC II of APC while CD8 on cytotoxic cells interacts with antigen in context of MHC I. These interactions are summarized in Fig. 2–12. The CD8 has also been a useful molecule for identifying T_s cells as well as T_c cells.

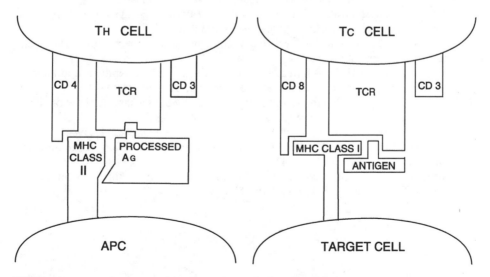

FIGURE 2–12. Summary schematic depicting differences in antigen presentation/recognition depending on MHC class context and whether immune response is being induced by afferent pathway or is being carried out by an efferent pathway.

Although T_c-cell activity is a major way specific immune recognition is translated into biological effector function, there are several other cellular interactions that are important in defensive/inflammatory functions. When certain antigen-presenting cells, particularly macrophages, make first antigen contact, the same process can be inflammatory. The liberation of inflammatory mediators into the microenvironment also plays a role in the subsequent type of immune responses seen.

3. Immunoregulation

The various types of antigen-specific immune responses are under several levels of control. Genes govern expression of antigen receptors, diversity of immunoglobulin production, amount of globulin production, as well as MHC molecules. Even more importantly, gene expression is often triggered by environmental influences. The ratio of T-regulator lymphocytes, the helper/suppressor cell ratio, is important in determining whether a response proceeds or is inhibited. A variety of hormones (e.g., steroids, neuropeptides) play an important role, as do the regulatory cytokines (interferons, interleukins, etc.). A number of external substances are also known to modify immune responses. If such modification is done in a positive way, the immune response is enhanced and several immune response adjuvants (e.g., alum, levamisole, transfer factor) are in use (Fudenberg and Whitten 1984). Agents that modify the immune response in a negative way are called immunosuppressants and, when purposefully administered, are vital in modern transplantation surgery (see Chapter 8 for more detail). Finally, external agents that affect the immune response in a negative way are considered immunotoxic and are the subject of this text.

References

Baker, P. J. 1990. Regulation of magnitude of antibody response to bacterial polysaccharide antigens by thymus-derived lymphocytes. *Infect. Immun.* 58:3465–68.

Bellanti, J. A. 1985. Immunology III. Philadelphia: W. B. Saunders.

Born, W. K., K. Harshan, R. L. Modlin, and R. L. O'Brien. 1991. The role of the γ:δ T lymphocytes in infection. *Curr. Opin. Immunol.* 3:455–59.

Erber, W. N. 1990. Human leukocyte differentiation antigens: Review of the CD nomenclature. *Pathology.* 22:61–89.

Fudenberg, H. H., and H. D. Whitten. 1984. Immunostimulation: Synthetic and biological modulators of immunity. *Annu. Rev. Pharmacol. Toxicol.* 24:147–74.

Herberman, R. B., C. W. Reynolds, and J. R. Ortaldo. 1986. Mechanism of Cytotoxicity by natural killer (NK) cells. *Annu. Rev. Immunol.* 4:651–80.

Janeway, C. A., Jr. 1991. To thine own self be true. *Curr. Opin. Biol.* 1:239–41.

Myers, C. D. 1991. Role of B cell antigen processing and presentation in the humoral immune response. *FASEB J.* 5:2547–53.

Whiteside, T. L., and R. B. Herberman. 1989. The role of natural killer cells in human diseases. *Clin. Immunol. Immunopathol.* 53:1–23.

3

Basic Principles of Toxicology

A. INTRODUCTION

Toxicology is often defined as the basic science of poisons and, in the present context, would concern poisons affecting the immune system. Since any substance is capable of producing injury under some condition, toxicology is really a basic science of dosage, which is the major characteristic distinguishing toxins from other substances. Inasmuch as this is an interdisciplinary text, a brief introduction to the principles of toxicology is included for those with primarily a nontoxicology background. In this chapter, only those principles of toxicology that are directly concerned with immunotoxicology are presented. For more detailed information on the general subject of toxicology, the reader is referred to more comprehensive textbooks in the area (Amdur, Doull, and Klaassen 1991; Hayes 1989; Loomis 1978).

B. TOXICOLOGY AND THE ROLE OF THE TOXICOLOGIST

Toxicologists have at their disposal many tools to assess the adverse effects that xenobiotics have on biological systems. These include information from direct observations of humans affected by the xenobiotic, effects in relevant experimental animal models of human exposure or human/animal in vitro culture systems, and retrospective/prospective epidemiologic studies. The toxicologist can also gain knowledge about the toxicity of a xenobiotic by evaluating structure/ activity relationships, pharmacokinetics following absorption, metabolic byproducts, and interrelationships with host factors and other environmental stimuli. From such data and consideration of the level of exposure, an assessment can be made about whether a xenobiotic will pose a health risk.

There are many subdisciplines of toxicology where research is directed at specific organ systems (i.e., hepatotoxicology, renal toxicology, neurotoxicology, immunotoxicology, reproductive toxicology, etc.) or specific classes of compounds (i.e., metals, pesticides, animal/plant toxins, etc.). In addition, toxicologists can specialize in many different areas, e.g., the treatment of poisonings (clinical toxicology), the medical/legal ramifications of xenobiotic exposure as a cause of death (forensic toxicology), effects of commercially available xenobiotics (industrial toxicology), or federal, state, and local governmental regulation of xenobiotics (regulatory toxicology).

C. EXPRESSION OF TOXIC EFFECTS

There are many characteristics of the xenobiotic or the affected individual interacting with genetic and environmental influences that ultimately determine the
precise nature of the resulting toxic response.

1. Dose–Response Relationships

When evaluating the lethality or toxicity of a specific xenobiotic, one observes
that not all members of a population respond to that xenobiotic to the same
degree. For example, as seen in Fig. 3–1, 170 mg/kg of the disinfectant hexachlorophene administered orally to rats causes death in only about 10% of the test
population that is exposed. However, as the dose is increased, a greater proportion of the population succumbs. This phenomenon, termed the dose–response
relationship, is a basic principle of toxicology and demonstrates that a relationship exists within a population between the dose of a xenobiotic and the response
of the individuals in that population to the xenobiotic. The dose–response relationship results from the inherent differences in responsiveness of individuals.
Given these individual differences in responsiveness, the dose–response relationship used to quantify the effects of a xenobiotic can be expressed in a statistical
way, i.e., by determining the dose that would kill 50% of individuals in a population. From the graph in Fig. 3–1, the LD_{50} of hexachlorophene in rats can be
determined to be approximately 220 mg/kg. It is used as a rough estimate of the
toxicity and as a useful means of comparing the toxicity of different xenobiotics.

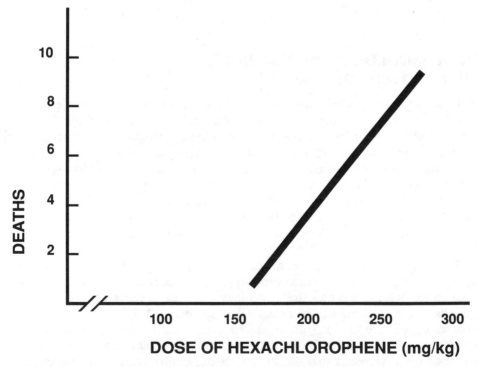

FIGURE 3-1.   Dose–response curve of the acute oral toxicity (as measured by lethality) of increasing doses of hexachlorophene. From this curve, an LD_{50} value of approximately 220 mg/kg
can be derived.   (*After Dashiell and Kennedy 1984.*)

At the present time, however, specific LD_{50} values are rarely determined on new xenobiotics. Alternative methods have been developed for approximating LD_{50} values with fewer animals, using computer modeling, or determining limit values (i.e., stating the LD_{50} in such terms as >5 g/kg or >10 g/kg). The switch to alternative methods has reduced the number of animals used in safety evaluations, and toxicologists have found them just as useful in risk assessment.

In the example above, the dose–response relationship was used to express lethality as a function of dose. The toxicologist can also use the dose–response relationship to evaluate a specific toxic or pharmacological effect of a xenobiotic as a function of dose. For example, metallothionein is a free radical scavenger (Bremner 1987) and has been shown to accumulate in the lungs of rats following exposure to paraquat. As seen in Fig. 3–2, rats exposed to 20 mg/kg of paraquat will accumulate approximately 2 µg of metallothionein per gram of wet lung. However, as the dose of paraquat increases to 30 µg/kg, the amount of metallothioneine in the lung increases to approximately 6 µg/g wet lung. Therefore, as the exposure to the xenobiotic increased, so did the degree of the effect observed, reemphasizing the presence of a relationship between dose and effect.

The LD_{50} and ED_{50} (effective dose$_{50}$) are important values to determine from the dose–response curve. The slope of this curve is also important. As can be seen in Fig. 3–3, compounds A and B have the same LD_{50}/ED_{50}, but the toxicity profiles of these materials are distinctly different. Based on their dose–response curves, the handling of these materials in an industrial or clinical setting would differ. Since the slope for compound B is steep, demonstrating that a major

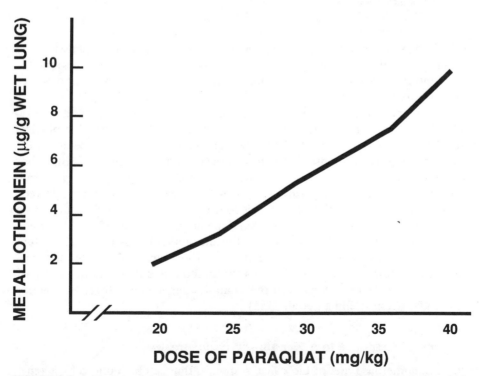

FIGURE 3–2.   Dose-dependent changes in the concentration of metallothionein in the lung 24 hr following exposure to various doses of paraquat. The level of metallothionein is expressed as micrograms per gram wet lung.   (*After Sato 1991.*)

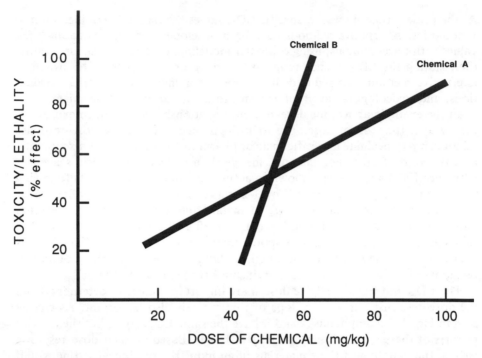

FIGURE 3-3.   Hypothetical curves illustrating the importance of the slope of a dose–response curve. Even though chemicals A and B have the same LD_{50}/ED_{50}, they differ significantly in the range of doses over which toxicity is observed and the severity of the toxic responses as a function of incremental increases in dose.

change in toxicity is seen with a small change in dose, one would strictly control exposure if it fell in this region of the curve. However, even though the slope for compound A is relatively flat, exposure would have to be controlled at doses of compound A that would not pose a concern with compound B.

Potency and efficacy are two characteristics of a xenobiotic that can be revealed by the dose–response curve. Potency refers to the degree of biological response as a function of the dose of a xenobiotic, whereas efficacy refers to the power or maximum response that can be induced. For example, chlorthalidone and methylchlothiazide are two diuretics used in the treatment of high blood pressure. Two hundred milligrams of chlorthalidone will induce the same diuretic response as 10 mg of methylchlothiazide. Therefore, methylchlothiazide is said to be 20 times more potent than chlorthalidone in inducing this effect. Although the dosages may be different, methylchlothiazide and chlorthalidone will induce approximately the same maximal effects. Therefore, their efficacy or "power" is the same. However, furosemide, another diuretic, is able to induce a higher maximum response as compared to the examples above. Therefore, furosemide is more efficacious (Gilman et al. 1985).

2. Types of Response to a Xenobiotic Exposure

There are numerous types of biological responses that can be induced by a xenobiotic. These responses can be therapeutic, adverse, or adaptive, immediate or delayed, localized or systemic, or allergic.

Therapeutic, Adaptive, or Adverse Responses

At appropriate doses, drugs provide a beneficial effect. However, in excessive doses, adverse effects can be observed. Using the furosemide example above, at therapeutic doses the drug is very effective at reducing blood pressure. However, at excessive doses, adverse effects such as metabolic alkalosis and hypotension can be observed. Sufficient exposure to an industrial chemical will generally cause a change in an individual that will lead to an adverse effect. Intuitively this is what one would expect, and the examples are numerous. Inhalation exposure to asbestos can cause mesothelioma, ingestion of toluene can cause ventricular fibrillation and shallow respiration, dermal exposure to chlordane can lead to hyperexcitability and convulsions, etc. However, not all exposures to xenobiotics lead to therapeutic or adverse changes. For example, following chronic low-level exposure to ethanol, DDT, or phenobarbital, the level of metabolizing enzymes in the liver is increased. This induction can manifest itself as a quantifiable change in liver size and weight. These changes are not necessarily adverse and represent an adaptive response in the exposed individual. They regress to normal when the agent is eliminated.

Similar observations are abundant in immunotoxicology, where, although various changes can be seen in immune parameters (e.g., a heightened IgG level or a depressed $CD4^+$ population), no adverse clinical effects necessarily accompany the changes. In allergy, the situation is a little different. The body, when exposed to foreign proteins such as pollen or insect venoms, will recognize these proteins as nonself and mount an immune response against them. Side effects of the allergic immune response can manifest themselves as sinusitis and nasal congestion, as observed in hay fever or mild allergy. Depending on the allergen, it can occasionally be much more severe, leading to anaphylaxis and death. One would surely consider these adverse effects. However, they could also be considered normal responses of a host defending itself from a foreign antigen.

Adaptation can lead to a decreased responsiveness to a chemical following repeated or chronic exposure. This decreased responsiveness has been given many terms including tolerance, tachyphylaxis, and desensitization. Although these terms are used loosely and interchangeably, they all refer to a diminishing response to repeated constant exposures to a xenobiotic. It can be explained by a variety of mechanisms, e.g., the induction of enzymes used to process or detoxify the xenobiotic (as in the example above with DDT, ethanol, or phenobarbital) or a decreased responsiveness of the target tissue. There are many adaptive mechanisms that can lead to decreased tissue responsiveness, e.g., an increase in the level of the targeted moiety, alteration in the receptor sites for the toxicant, increased repair of the damaged site of action, or alteration of absorption, distribution, and elimination of the toxicant (Hodgson and Guthrie 1980).

Adaptation to the pharmacological action of organic nitrates such as nitroglycerin is an example of decreased tissue responsiveness. Nitroglycerin relaxes vascular smooth muscle and is used in the treatment of angina. It functions by binding to nitrate receptors that are present in vascular smooth muscle cells. These nitrate receptors contain sulfhydryl groups, which reduce the nitrate to nitrite. The accumulation of nitrite in the smooth muscle cells is believed to cause the relaxation effect. Repeated administration of nitroglycerin leads to a hyporesponsiveness to the drug. The decreased responsiveness is believed to result from a nitrate-induced oxidation of sulfhydryl groups on the receptors leading to a decreased receptor affinity for the drug. This is of minimal importance in the treatment of angina, since the drug is administered intermittently and at low levels.

Another example of decreased tissue responsiveness is demonstrated by the example of chronic amphetamine exposure. Amphetamine is an indirect-acting sympathomimetic. This drug functions by displacing norepinephrine from storage in vesicles of the terminal axon swellings. When released, some of the displaced norepinephrine interacts with adrenoreceptors, inducing the biological response associated with the amphetamine exposure. Tolerance to repeated amphetamine exposure is observed when the pool of releasable norepinephrine is depleted. At that time, further administration of the drug has no effect, since the level of norepinephrine available for displacement has been reduced.

Another example of adaptation is seen in individuals who are occupationally exposed to large concentrations of carbon monoxide (i.e., tunnel workers, traffic officers in large metropolitan cities, etc.). The carbon monoxide exposure leads to a greater amount of carboxyhemoglobin in the blood and therefore to a decreased oxygen-carrying capacity. The body adapts to this decreased capacity by increasing the oxygen-carrying capacity of the blood through increased hemoglobin synthesis. Thus, these individuals will show an increased level of hemoglobin in the blood.

Immediate or Delayed
The biological response to a xenobiotic exposure is generally seen shortly after exposure. This is expected as the xenobiotic induces its effect when it reaches the target tissue. However, in some instances, the effect can be delayed. For example, exposure to the pesticide mipafox will lead to a neurotoxic-like response about 2 weeks after exposure has ended. The delayed response may be caused by an inhibition of metabolism in the nerve cell body present in the spinal tract. This inhibition leads to a decrease in the flow of nutrients to the long axons of the peripheral nerves, thus causing altered neuromuscular function in the upper and lower limbs. The toxic lesion induced by mipafox is immediate, but the expression of the response is delayed. Toxicologists are cautioned in using the term "delayed" in the immunologic sense, where very special mechanisms are implied with its use; these are discussed in greater detail in Chapter 6.

Localized or Systemic Effects
The biological response to a xenobiotic can be observed at the site of exposure, or the xenobiotic can be absorbed, travel via the bloodstream, and cause effects elsewhere in the body. For example, ingestion of high amounts of lead can lead to gastrointestinal irritation. This is a local effect observed at the site of exposure. However, ingestion of lead can also lead to toxicity to the central and peripheral nervous systems and changes in heme metabolism. These additional changes, termed systemic effects, result from absorption of lead from the gastrointestinal tract and its movement via the bloodstream to these other target tissues. Most materials induce both local and systemic effects. For example, inhalation of benzene can lead to inflammation in the lung (the site of exposure) and, following systemic absorption, toxicity to the kidney, liver, and hematopoietic and nervous systems.

Allergic
The immune response to many xenobiotics in certain people is often accompanied by inflammatory side reactions resulting from the combination of the allergen with the immune effectors in the body. In such instances, the body's immune

response is injurious and resembles a response to a toxin. "Poison ivy" is a common layman's term to describe one well-known type of allergic response. These types of allergic responses are one of the major focuses of this book and are addressed in Chapter 6.

C. FACTORS AFFECTING THE EXPRESSION OF TOXICITY

There are numerous factors in the nature of the xenobiotic or the responding individual that can affect the expression of a toxic response. These include dosing regimen, biological differences between exposed individuals, and the physical/structural form of the toxic substance.

1. Dosing Regimen

Before any xenobiotic can exert a toxic effect, it must reach a target tissue. The onset, duration, and intensity of a toxic effect result from the concentration of the xenobiotic at the target tissue and the speed at which the xenobiotic reaches that tissue. These effects are influenced by the route of exposure, dose level, and duration and frequency of exposure. Depending on route of exposure, significant differences can be observed in the absorption and metabolism of a xenobiotic. There are a variety of ways xenobiotics can enter the body, e.g., absorption through the gastrointestinal tract, skin, or lung following oral, dermal, or inhalation exposure. In addition, they can enter the body parenterally (other than the intestinal tract) through injection into a variety of compartments (i.e., intraperitoneal, intravenous, intramuscular, subcutaneous, intradermal, etc.). Generally, the descending order of effectiveness for route of exposure into the body is intravenous, inhalation, intraperitoneal, subcutaneous, intramuscular, intradermal, oral, and topical (Amdur, Doull, and Klaassen 1991). This order is dictated by the ease with which the xenobiotic is absorbed and enters the systemic circulation, which thus affects the speed it reaches and the concentration it attains at the target tissue. For example, a xenobiotic injected intravenously will generally induce greater toxicity than the same agent applied topically. Through intravenous exposure, higher blood and target tissue levels can be achieved much faster as compared to topical application with the subsequent need for absorption through the skin.

To illustrate this point further, the LD_{50} values for methylhydrazine are listed in Table 3–1 following exposure via a variety of routes. As can be seen, the route of exposure significantly influences the lethal response to the drug. In addition,

TABLE 3–1.   Effect of Route of Exposure on the LD_{50} Value for Methylhydrazine in the Rat

Route	LD_{50}
Oral	32 mg/kg
Dermal	183 mg/kg
Intraperitoneal	21 mg/kg
Subcutaneous	35 mg/kg
Intravenous	17 mg/kg

Source: Adapted from Sax and Lewis (1989).

the route of exposure can affect the metabolism of a xenobiotic. For example, xenobiotics absorbed orally pass through the liver before entering the systemic circulation. The liver can metabolize xenobiotics into either less or more toxic materials. Therefore, a xenobiotic administered orally could have a distinctly different toxicity profile from the same agent inhaled and entering the systemic circulation directly without initial metabolism. In practical settings, individuals are rarely exposed to a xenobiotic via one route of exposure. For example, in pesticide application to crops, both dermal and inhalation exposures can occur. In addition, when the crops are harvested, residues of the pesticides remain and are ultimately ingested by the population, resulting in oral exposure. In addition, pesticide residues can be found in the meat of animals grazing on treated fields.

The particular toxic effect that is observed is also based on the dose, duration, and frequency of exposure. Low-dose chronic exposure to a xenobiotic can have significantly different effects than high-dose, acute exposure. For example, an acute, high-level oral exposure to mercury leads to gastrointestinal toxicity, whereas chronic, low-level exposure leads to neurotoxicity. In addition, xenobiotic-induced cancer is an effect that generally requires a long latency time. A dose of a xenobiotic can be administered as a single bolus or as many smaller doses divided over time. This frequency of exposure can have an impact on the observed effect. A dose of xenobiotic delivered as a bolus will generally induce a greater toxicity than the fractionated dose. This is because higher blood and target tissue levels of the xenobiotic are achieved with the higher dosage level. In addition, the profile of toxicity may also differ.

2. Characteristics of the Exposed Individual

The toxic response that is observed following exposure to a xenobiotic can be different among members of a population. The varied responses arise from the inherent differences that exist among individuals. These include differences in species/strain, age, sex, health/nutrition status, and genetic make-up. Several examples have already been given of the importance of absorption and metabolism in regard to toxic effects. Differences in these properties are a major reason why different species/strains and individuals within a population respond differently to the toxic effect of xenobiotics.

The metabolism of a xenobiotic generally leads to detoxification and elimination. However, it is also possible for a xenobiotic that is biologically innocuous to be metabolized into a compound with a toxic potential, e.g., vinyl chloride or carbon tetrachloride. Moreover, the presence or absence of specific enzyme systems can have a profound influence on the toxicity of a chemical. These enzymes are proteins and are inherited based on Mendelian genetics. Therefore, the genetic make-up of a species/strain or individual determines the metabolizing enzyme profile and thus can affect the potential toxicity of a xenobiotic. Pharmacogenetics is the growing discipline that studies the relationship between genetic factors and the nature of responses to drugs. Metabolic enzyme systems are a predominant genetic factor. For example, the mouse can hydrolyze 6–propylthiopurine into mercaptopurine. Since mercaptopurine is a carcinogen, mice administered 6–propylthiopurine will develop cancer. On the other hand, humans hydrolyze 6–propylthiopurine at two positions leading to metabolites that are noncarcinogenic. Therefore, administration of 6–propylthiopurine to humans will not lead to a carcinogenic response (Hodgson and Guthrie 1980). Other examples where differences in the metabolizing enzyme profile have led to observed species-to-species variation in response to xenobiotic exposure are given by Jakoby (1980).

In the example above, the difference in metabolism was species specific. Differences can also be observed between individual members of the same species. For example, it has been shown that not all individuals respond to the antituberculosis drug isoniazid in the same way. The difference in response is based on the individual's N-acetyltransferase activity. N-acetyltransferase is a metabolizing enzyme and as a protein is inherited based on Mendelian genetics. Those with increased activity will exhibit resistance to the drug, whereas those with decreased activity will exhibit neuropathy from drug accumulation. Other examples of xenobiotics where individual-to-individual variation in toxicity is influenced by genetic factors include succinylcholine, nitrites, warfarin, quinones, and ethanol (Loomis 1978).

Several other interspecies differences exist that can affect the response to a xenobiotic. These can include differences in biliary excretion, plasma protein binding, capacity for DNA repair, or differences in the absorption rates and properties across the respiratory tract, gastrointestinal tract, and skin. Microflora in the gut can metabolize xenobiotics into inert or active materials. Therefore, the microflora profile of a species can influence the effects of ingested xenobiotics.

Based on the above, it is clear that no one animal species is adequate to characterize fully the toxicity of a xenobiotic and therefore completely correlate with humans. Therefore, the toxicologist generally uses the animal species that is the most sensitive in the parameter being studied or for which a sufficiently large data base is present. For example, rabbits are used for eye irritation studies because of their large, nonpigmented eyes and their tendency to be more sensitive to mild and moderate irritants than humans. Rats and mice are generally used to assess oral toxicity, since a large data base is available on these species and comparisons between xenobiotics can be made. Guinea pigs are used for allergy-based testing because of their unique sensitivity to contact and airborne allergens and their generation of allergic antibody.

In order to maintain the highest degree of consistency in toxicological evaluations, toxicologists will use inbred strains of animals as opposed to outbred strains. Inbred strains are generated by sequential inbreeding of a particular strain, leading to animals that are genetically identical. If an effect is seen in such a strain, it will be consistent and not related to some genetic default in the animal. In this way, the only variable in the experiment is the exposure to the xenobiotic. Outbred strains are formed by breeding of individuals in a population that are not closely related genetically. This leads to a genetic variability in 30–40% of the loci. Outbred strains are occasionally used in studies where a diverse population is needed. Some will argue that in toxicity testing, outbred strains are more appropriate since one increases the chance of having an animal in the test that will respond the same way as man. This is a difficult argument, since most of these studies are investigative, and the responses most pertinent to man are unknown. Therefore, inbred strains are generally used for most toxicity studies to assure consistency in the study. One exception is the use of outbred strains of guinea pigs for allergy testing.

The age of an individual can greatly affect the toxic response to a xenobiotic. As an individual gets older, metabolism is slowed and can influence toxicity as described above (Mann 1965). In addition, the degree of exposure can be altered by age. Younger animals generally have a higher respiration rate than older individuals. The significance of age on toxic responses can be demonstrated in Table 3-2, where the LD_{50} values for a variety of materials are compared between newborn and adult animals. Significant differences can be observed and should be kept in mind when evaluating any xenobiotic where there will be exposure to both young and old.

Also of major importance is the effect of xenobiotics on the developing embryo and fetus. Certain characteristics make the developing conceptus particularly susceptible to toxic insult. These include increased cellular proliferation, limited ability to detoxify xenobiotics, small numbers of cells, and a high percentage of undifferentiated cells. The placenta has a limited capacity to act as a barrier to the flow of xenobiotics to the conceptus. Therefore, since the developing conceptus shares its blood supply with its mother, xenobiotic exposure to the mother generally leads to exposure to the conceptus. In addition, some xenobiotics can concentrate in the milk and be delivered to the offspring through nursing. There is a subdiscipline of toxicology, termed developmental/reproductive toxicology, that is concerned with evaluating the effects of xenobiotics on the developing conceptus and determining the mechanism of teratogenic responses.

Generally, both males and females respond in the same way to a xenobiotic exposure. However, there are several differences between the sexes that can profoundly influence the observed effects. These include the levels of body fat and muscle mass, which can affect the distribution and excretion of xenobiotics. In addition, there are references in the literature documenting sex differences in the rate of drug metabolism, which can influence metabolic detoxifying/activating systems (Noordhoek and Rumke 1969). Also, anatomic differences in the reproductive system can allow for unique target tissues between male and female. In addition, the sex hormones themselves can be the target following a xenobiotic exposure. The impact of these differences is not well understood and is under investigation. Figure 3-4 illustrates how males and females can respond differently to xenobiotic exposure. In response to oxamniquine (a drug used against schistosomiasis), the acute oral LD_{50} in males is calculated to be 447 mg/kg. However, in females, the acute oral LD_{50} is calculated to be 57 mg/kg, about an order of magnitude less. Another example where gender can influence toxicity

TABLE 3-2.   A Comparison of LD_{50} Values for a Variety of Drugs in Newborn and Adult Rats

Drug	Strain	Age	LD_{50} (mg/kg)	Route
Chloramphenicol	Sprague–Dawley	1 day	602	Subcutaneous
		Adult	5447	
Clindamycin	Sprague–Dawley	1 day	245	Subcutaneous
		Adult	2618	
Isoproterenol	Charles River	1 day	610	Oral
		42 days	4282	
Digitoxin	Charles River	7 days	0.1	Oral
		Adult	56	
Phenobarbital	Wistar	1 day	121	Oral
		Adult	318	

Source: Adapted from Goldenthal (1971).

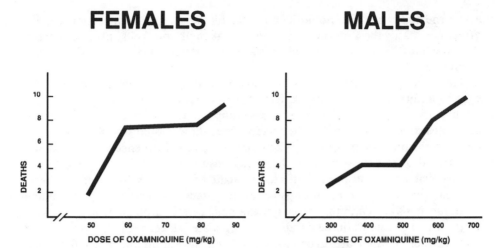

FEMALES   **MALES**

FIGURE 3-4.   Dose–response curves of the acute oral toxicity (as measured by lethality) of increasing doses of oxamiquine in male and female rats. The curves illustrate the difference in sensitivity of males and females to the toxicity of the drug.   (*After Gregory et al. 1983.*)

involves pregnancy. Beliles (1972) showed that intravenous exposures to either colchicine, chlorpromazine, or iron dextrin were more toxic to pregnant than nonpregnant mice, whereas oral exposure to aspirin was less toxic in the same comparison. The reason for the different toxicity profiles is currently unknown but may be hormonally based or related to altered compartmentalization of the xenobiotic.

The health/nutritional status of an animal can influence tremendously the effect that a xenobiotic will induce. Animals that are exhibiting decreased hepatic or renal function from poor health will have decreased abilities to metabolize or eliminate xenobiotics. Xenobiotics that require extensive detoxification via metabolism or are eliminated predominately via the kidney will demonstrate higher toxicities in these individuals. In addition, proteins and certain essential nutrients are necessary for proper function of detoxifying enzymes. Therefore, alteration of the health or nutritional status of the individual could allow for an exaggeration of the toxic response.

3. Characteristics of the Xenobiotic

As stated previously, in order for a xenobiotic to induce its toxic effect, it must reach a target tissue. There are several physical/chemical properties of a xenobiotic that can influence its ability to reach this tissue. These properties include molecular weight, degree of ionization, lipophilicity, viscosity, and concentration. These properties come into play in the absorption, distribution, metabolism, and excretion of a xenobiotic and will influence its potential biological burden and ability to induce a toxic effect. These characteristics influence how easily the xenobiotic can cross biological membranes, which are made up of lipid bilayers interspersed with protein. Generally, xenobiotics that are nonionized, of smaller molecular weight, and lipophilic can cross biological membranes more easily than those that are large, ionized, and hydrophilic. Since these parameters affect the ability of the xenobiotic to cross a biological membrane, they will also affect how easily the xenobiotic is excreted, taken up into cells, absorbed across the skin, lung, or gastrointestinal tract, or sequestered into various tissue compartments.

There are also characteristics of the structure of the xenobiotic that will influence its ability to induce a toxic effect. This is a newer area of toxicology and is the basis for the structure–activity relationships that are drawn between xenobiotics. Research has shown that the specific three-dimensional structure of a xenobiotic or the presence of specific functional groups can influence the toxicity that is observed. A recent overview of these relationships in regard to carcinogenicity, mutagenicity, skin and eye irritation, and acute oral toxicity has been published (Enslein 1989). These relationships have been used most extensively in the area of mutagenesis and carcinogenesis. For example, certain mutagenic responses can be traced to a xenobiotic being able to intercalate between DNA bases. Therefore, xenobiotics that are structurally flat (i.e., have minimal molecular thickness) and have a specific rectangular area are capable of inducing a mutagenic or carcinogenic response (Arcos and Argus 1974).

If there is exposure to multiple xenobiotics at one time, then it is possible for there to be some interaction between them. This interaction can lead to toxic effects that are either additive, synergistic, competitive, or potentiating. If the response is additive, then it would be equal to the sum of effects that would be observed following individual exposures. For example, liver toxicity can be quantified by measuring the level of serum liver enzymes. Assume 10 mg/kg of chemical A causes a serum liver enzyme level of 50 IU/liter, and 25 mg/kg of chemical B causes a serum liver enzyme level of 100 IU/liter. If the two chemicals were given together at the cited doses, then the serum liver enzyme level of the combined dose would be expected to be 150 IU/liter if the two chemicals acted in an additive manner. If the response is synergistic, then one observes an effect that is greater than the two individual responses. In synergistic responses, both compounds act to enhance the effect of each other. Using our example above, the serum liver enzyme level of the combined exposure to chemicals A and B could be 200 IU/liter or some value demonstrating an enhanced effect. A competitive response leads to an effect that is less than the individual responses. Using the example above, the serum liver enzyme level could be 35 IU/liter or some value that demonstrates a diminished response. In the case of a potentiating response, only one of the administered xenobiotics exerts a biological response. The other functions only to enhance that effect. Using the example above, one could administer chemical A and chemical D. Chemical D is innocuous and induces no toxicity. If chemical D potentiated the effect of chemical A, then the serum liver enzyme level of the combined exposure would be greater than 50 IU/liter.

From an immunologic standpoint, the concept of "priming" is relevant to this discussion. Priming refers to the first exposure that an individual receives to an antigen. This exposure leads to the primary antibody response. During this response, immunocompetent cells are stimulated, and memory cells are formed. Because of this priming, the host is able to mount a significantly increased response following the second exposure to the antigen. The secondary response is quicker in onset and results in a greater level of circulating antibody. Priming is the basis for deliberate immunization. Another type of priming is seen where one inflammatory mediator, e.g., γ-interferon, given prior to a second exposure to a different mediator, e.g., platelet-activating factor, greatly enhances the total inflammatory effect.

There are many reasons for the above interactive responses. One example is related to receptor interactions. For example, stimulation of β receptors will lead to an increase in cardiac activity, whereas stimulation of cholinergic receptors leads to the opposite effect. β-receptor agonists and antagonists given together would be expected to compete with each other, demonstrating a competitive response, whereas a β-receptor agonist and cholinergic receptor antagonist would be expected to enhance their effects. Interactive responses can also be based on alterations in distribution and metabolism. Repeated administration of phenobarbital will enhance the metabolic enzyme systems of the liver. Thus, it can be expected to decrease the effect of a concomitantly given chemical that requires these enzyme systems for detoxification or increase the effects of a chemical that requires these enzyme systems for activation. In addition, certain xenobiotics can affect absorption. For example, lead is absorbed poorly from the gastrointestinal tract; however, the chelator EDTA can bind to the lead, thereby increasing its solubility and subsequent absorption. Therefore, when given together, EDTA can increase the toxicity of lead.

The above concepts are exploited in the treatment of many poisonings. For example, ethanol is given as the treatment for methanol ingestion. Methanol is metabolized to formic acid, its toxic byproduct, by alcohol dehydrogenase. Ethanol acts to compete with the methanol for metabolism by the alcohol dehydrogenase and thus decreases the formation of the toxic metabolites. Charcoal gavage is used in the treatment of many oral poisonings and functions to bind the toxin, rendering it harmless and unavailable for absorption. Another example is naloxone, a narcotic receptor antagonist, which is used to reverse the effects of narcotic overdose by displacing the narcotic from its receptor.

D. RISK ASSESSMENT PROCESS

One of the responsibilities of the toxicologist is that of determining if a xenobiotic will represent a health risk to the exposed population. Risk is a relative term and is defined as the probability that some adverse effect will occur following a given exposure to a xenobiotic (Hodgson, Mailman, and Chambers 1988). To evaluate the risk associated with exposure to a xenobiotic, the toxicologist must (1) determine the toxicity of the xenobiotic and (2) quantify the level of exposure. To determine the toxicity of a xenobiotic, many in vivo and in vitro tests are available. These tests can evaluate target organ toxicity, teratogenicity, carcinogenicity, mutagenicity, irritation, sensitization, etc., and can be conducted using a variety of routes of exposure and lengths of exposure. Each of the tests is conducted to determine the types of toxicity that a particular xenobiotic can cause under particular exposure conditions. Specific animal models or validated in vitro tests are chosen based on their ability to accurately assess these effects. On completing these required tests, the toxicologist has available a complete assessment of the toxicity of the xenobiotic under the relevant routes of exposure and duration of exposure.

In addition to assessing the toxicity of a xenobiotic, the toxicologist must also quantify the level of exposure. For example, in quantifying the level of dermal exposure, surface area exposed, rate of absorption across the skin, duration of exposure, etc. are necessary factors in determining the systemic load. For inhalation exposure, the respiratory rate, tidal volume, particle size, absorption across the lung, vapor pressure of the xenobiotic, etc. are necessary parameters that must be measured to quantitate host exposure. For oral exposure, absorption across the gastrointestinal tract, level and daily water intake if the xenobiotic is a contaminant in drinking water, dose of the drug, etc. are necessary. When all factors are determined, the toxicologist can quantify exposure by a specific route or the total systemic exposure.

Once the toxicologist has assessed the toxicity of a xenobiotic and quantified the level of human exposure, the evaluation of health risk can begin. For all effects except cancer, the toxicologist can use subchronic and chronic toxicity studies to determine the level of exposure to a xenobiotic that does not cause an adverse effect in the animal tested. This level is termed the no-effect level (NOEL). Using the NOEL and taking into account variation between individuals and species, the toxicologist can set a safe level for exposure to humans. Variation between individuals and species is taken into account through the use of uncertainty factors. For example, it is assumed that a factor of 10 below the NOEL is sufficient to take into account variations among members of a population, and a factor of 10 is sufficient to take into account differences between animals and humans. Therefore, if reliable subchronic or chronic toxicity data are available, an exposure level 100-fold below the NOEL is sufficient to protect the human health in regard to systemic toxicity effects other than cancer. The uncertainty factors are only used as guidelines. These factors can be altered based on the quality and extent of the data base.

The toxicologist can use acute toxicity studies and dermal and eye irritation studies to determine potential systemic effects of an acute exposure or irritant potential, respectively. These types of evaluations are important in the case of a drug overdose, accidental ingestion of an industrial chemical by a child, chemical spill leading to a localized area of high exposure, or the accidental splashing of a chemical into the eye or onto the skin.

The above concepts are useful in addressing all toxicities but cancer. In regard to the carcinogenic response, the most conservative position is that there is no NOEL. It is assumed that any level of a carcinogen can cause cancer, since one molecule can alter DNA, thus potentially transforming a normal cell into a tumor cell. Therefore, concerning cancer, the toxicologist must estimate the dose that would cause a negligible risk, a most difficult task to judge. However, a value that has been chosen by the general scientific community, and one that regulatory agencies have recognized, is a value of less than one new cancer death per million individuals exposed. To estimate this level of a carcinogen, the toxicologist conducts a chronic bioassay. In this study, an animal is exposed to the xenobiotic through the relevant route of exposure for its lifetime. Following exposure, the carcinogenic response is quantified using the dose–response relationship. The toxicologist then uses a variety of statistical methods to extend the line of the dose–response relationship to that dose in which only 0.0001% of the population would demonstrate a carcinogenic response. This is the dose that would cause less than one in one million new cancers and is termed the virtual safe dose (VSD). There are many ways of determining this value that differ in their degree of conservatism.

When calculating an exposure level based on uncertainty factors or the VSD, it is important to realize that there is always some level of exposure to a xenobiotic that can be considered an acceptable risk. Humans have developed many defensive mechanisms to protect themselves against the adverse effects of xenobiotics. These include detoxifying enzymes, natural barriers to absorption (i.e., skin, lining of the gastrointestinal tract and lung, etc.), various components of the immune system, DNA repair systems, etc. These mechanisms provide a substantial protection against xenobiotic exposure.

The public understandably has a very difficult time grasping these technical concepts. Although impractical, the popular idea of a safe level of exposure is one that equates risk to zero. Instances such as trace levels of heavy metals in drinking water or low-level pesticide residues on fruits can bring a substantial outcry even if regulatory agencies assure safety. There are many causes for this confusion. To name a few: improved analytical methodology has allowed for detection of minute levels of toxins; toxic spills/contamination draw heavy media attention; litigation is increasing; expert scientists at times disagree on the safe level of exposure, leading to a lack of confidence by the public; the population for the most part has a limited technical background, and scientists often do a poor job explaining and communicating such matters to the public.

The solution to this problem rests with the education of the public. Toxicologists from industry, academia, and the government need to place more effort in conveying their discipline to the general public. Only through this communication can the public reestablish confidence in the scientific community and be assured of the safety of their surroundings. With the advances in modern toxicology and our continued understanding of the functions of biological systems, it is essential that we use our knowledge to develop risk assessments that will protect human health without establishing any unnecessary restraints.

References

Amdur, M. O, J. Doull, C. D. Klaassen. 1991. *Toxicology—the Basic Science of Poisons*. New York: Macmillan.

Arcos, J. C., and M. F. Argus. 1974. *Chemical Induction of Cancer*. New York: Academic Press.

Beliles, R. P. 1972. Influence of pregnancy on the acute toxicity of various compounds in mice. *Toxicol. Applied Pharmacol*. 23:537–40.

Bremner, I. 1987. Nutritional and physiological significance of metallothionein. In: *Metallothionein II*, ed. J. Kagi and Y. Kojima, pp. 81–107. Basel: Birkhauser-Verlag.

Dashiell, O. L., and G. L. Kennedy. 1984. The effects of fasting on the acute oral toxicity of nine chemicals in the rat. *J. Appl. Toxicol*. 4:320–25.

Enslein, K. 1989. An overview of structure–activity relationships as an alternative to testing in animals for carcinogenicity, mutagenicity, dermal and eye irritation and acute oral toxicity. In *Benchmarks: Alternative Methods in Toxicology*, pp. 59–78. Princeton: Princeton Scientific.

Gilman, A. G., L. S. Goodman, T. W. Rall, and F. Murad. 1985. *Pharmacological Basis of Therapeutics*. New York: Macmillan.

Goldenthal, E. I. 1971. A compilation of LD_{50} values in newborn and adult animals. *Toxicol. Appl. Pharmacol*. 18:185–207.

Gregory, M., A. Monro, M. Quinton, and N. Woolhouse. 1983. The acute toxicity of oxamniquine in rats: A sex dependant hepatotoxicity. *Arch. Toxicol*. 54:247–55.

Hayes, A. W. 1989. *Principles and Methods of Toxicology*. New York: Raven Press.

Hodgson, E., and F. E. Guthrie. 1980. *Introduction to Biochemical Toxicology*. New York: Elsevier/North-Holland.

Hodgson, E., R. B. Mailman, and J. E. Chambers. 1988. *Dictionary of Toxicology*. New York: Van Nostrand Reinhold.

Jakoby, W. E. 1980. *Enzymatic Basis for Detoxication*. New York: Academic Press.

Loomis, T. A. 1978. *Essentials of Toxicology*. Philadelphia: Lea & Febiger.

Mann, D. E. 1965. Biological aging and its modification of drug activity. *J. Pharm. Sci.* 54:499–504.

Noordhoek, J., and C. L. Rumke. 1969. Sex differences in the rate of drug metabolism in mice. *Arch. Int. Pharmacodyn.* 182:401.

Sato, M. 1991. Dose-dependent increases in metallothionein synthesis in the lung and liver of paraquat-treated rats. *Toxicol. Appl. Pharmacol.* 107:98–105.

Sax, N. I., and R. J. Lewis. 1989. *Dangerous Properties of Industrial Materials*. New York: Van Nostrand Reinhold.

4

Effector Mechanisms: Immunopharmacology

A. INTRODUCTION

Effector mechanisms are concerned with the translation of immune recognition into some form of relevant biological activity that results in either neutralization or disposition of an infectious or noxious agent, initiation of secondary inflammatory effectors, or the possibility of host injury arising from these processes. Once a foreign substance has been recognized by either antigen-specific or nonspecific means, a cascade of events, often redundant, is initiated through the elaboration of a wide variety of humoral or cellular mediators. Subsequent biological responses are put into effect through the agency of these mediators.

Immunopharmacology is a subdiscipline of immunology that is closely related to immunotoxicology. It concerns the study of the pharmacological basis for the humoral mediators that are involved in translating immune recognition into an end-stage immunologic response. Specific areas of investigation include the cytokines involved in the mechanism of lymphocyte activation and the physiological effects of many immunologic effector mediators (i.e., interleukins, tumor necrosis factor, interferon), inflammation (prostaglandins, thromboxanes, leukotrienes, platelet-activating factor), hypersensitivity (histamine and serotonin), and many others (neuropeptides, thymic peptides).

B. CELLULAR ACTIVATION

Two fundamental activities of the cell determine much of its subsequent cellular activities and how it is affected by external signals for activation and proliferation. These activities may occur simultaneously or independently. Proliferation is dependent on the basic cellular mitotic cycle, which can be divided into five stages as shown in Fig. 4–1: the resting stage (G_0), the stage when DNA replication occurs (S), the growth stage (G_1), a premitotic stage where the cell is preparing to divide (G_2), and the mitotic or cell-division stage (M). Many external signals may only be processed when the cell is in a specific phase, and this contributes to the orderly control of both affector and effector events.

Proliferation also depends on activation sequences being transferred to the nucleus from signals arriving on the cell membrane. Activation is a broad term used in many ways to denote the physiological activities of a cell that has been stimulated by some external signal. Physiologists use it in reference to increased respiratory burst and glucose utilization for energy production. In the present context, activation refers to the molecular events on the cell membrane that lead to the basic effector functions of that cell. Cellular activation begins with the binding of a ligand to a cell surface receptor. This binding induces a series of

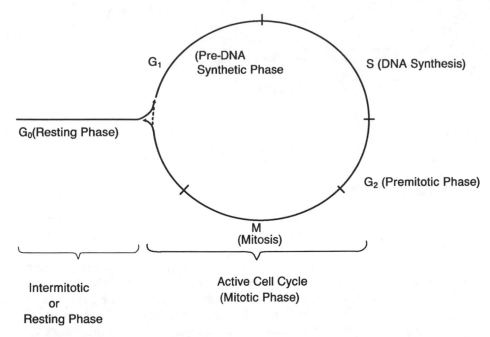

FIGURE 4-1.   Mitotic life cycle of a cell.

events that ultimately leads to a specific end-stage response that is determined by the cell that is stimulated. Examples of end-stage responses include contraction of a smooth muscle cell, secretion from an exocrine cell, degranulation of a mast cell, or, for lymphocytes, secretion of interleukins, expression of cell surface receptors, or the ability to lyse target cells.

Various second messengers propagate the activation signal. The specific second messenger that is formed depends on the receptor that is stimulated. For example, stimulation of β-adrenergic receptors leads to an increase of cAMP, and stimulation of cholinergic receptors leads to an increase in cGMP. Another second messenger system that has gained considerable attention is the one mediated by inositol trisphosphate and diacylglycerol (Berridge and Irvine 1984). Because this is the system that is responsible for the activation of a variety of immune cells, the primary emphasis of this section is placed here. Lymphocytes serve as an example, but a similar activation sequence is observed in mast cells, basophils, neutrophils, macrophages, and eosinophils following stimulation by a variety of agonists. The sequence of events involved in cellular activation is largely unknown. However, investigations have gained insight into several of the events, and a sequential order is becoming apparent. The cellular activation steps are presented as those associated with membrane signaling, early events that occur immediately following the propagation of the signal across the membrane, and late events. For more information, the reader is directed to reviews of the subject (Nel, Wooten, and Galbraith 1987; Hadden and Coffey 1990).

1. Membrane Signaling

Lymphocyte activation begins with the binding of either an antigen (as presented by the macrophage), a mitogen, or a cytokine to a specific surface receptor of the lymphocyte membrane that is associated with a MHC molecule (Lindahl-

Kiessling and Peterson 1969). The antigen-specific cell surface receptor of the T cell is a disulfide-linked heterodimer consisting of α and β chains of 49 and 43 kDa, respectively, that is noncovalently linked to the proteins of the T3-Ti (TCR-CD3) complex. The lymphocyte receptor for plant lectins such as phytohemagglutinin and concanavalin A has not been identified but is believed to be associated with the receptor that binds sheep erythrocytes. For mast cells, basophils, and B cells, activation is triggered by the crosslinking of membrane immunoglobulins, although there are other receptors as well. Membrane methyltransferases are activated that convert phosphatidylethanolamine (PE) to phosphatidylcholine (PC) by the addition of three methyl groups (Waxal 1983). The increased methylation causes a movement of phospholipids from the inner to outer membrane, leading to an increase in membrane fluidity. This process is believed to cause the opening of a calcium channel (Waxal 1983).

The increase in calcium causes an activation of phospholipase A (PLA) (Rittenhouse-Simmons and Deykin 1978). The PLA converts PC to arachidonic acid and lysolecithin (Dutta and Das 1979). The arachidonic acid is the basic substrate for the production of both prostaglandins by the cyclooxygenase pathway and leukotrienes by the lipoxygenase pathway (Flower and Blackwell 1976). These pathways and the biological significance of their products are outlined in more detail below.

Within the plasma membrane, phosphatidylinositol (PI), phosphatidylinositol 4-phosphate (PIP), and phosphatidylinositol 4,5-bisphosphate (PIP$_2$) are in equilibrium. When a ligand binds to the receptor, the equilibrium is shifted to the production of PIP$_2$. Concurrently, phospholipase C (PLC) is activated via the action of an intramembrane protein complex (G proteins). In this scheme, it is hypothesized that the antigen-receptor complex binds to the G proteins (α, β, and γ subunits) in association with guanine nucleotides. The subunits disassociate leaving an activated α subunit, which binds to PLC and activates it (reviewed by Nel, Wooten, and Galbraith 1987). This scheme is illustrated in Fig. 4-2. The activated PLC converts PIP$_2$ to diacylglycerol (DAG) and inositol trisphosphate (IP$_3$) (Michell and Allan 1975; Hui and Harmony 1980; Hasegawa-Sasaki and Sasaki 1981), which then act as the second messengers to propagate the signal through the cytosol.

2. Early Events

The DAG and IP$_3$ trigger parallel pathways that further activate the cell. The DAG activates protein kinase C (PKC), which is a cytosolic enzyme. To activate PKC, DAG, in conjunction with phosphatidylserine, forms a binding site in the membrane for PKC. The PKC translocates from the cytosol and binds to the membrane (Chen, Coggeshall, and Carrebier 1986). The PKC has two functional groups, one that is hydrophobic, which binds to the membrane, and one that is hydrophilic and faces the cytosol. The cytosolic portion contains the catalytically active unit. With this binding, the affinity of PKC for calcium, a necessary cofactor for enzyme activity, is reduced. This permits the activation of the enzyme with the low level of calcium that is available in the cytosol plus that which entered from the extracellular space following antigen/mitogen binding. The PKC functions to phosphorylate numerous protein substrates at seryl and threonyl residues. One of these proteins is involved in the membrane-bound Na^+/H^+ pump (Boron 1984). Phosphorylation leads to an increase in pump activity and

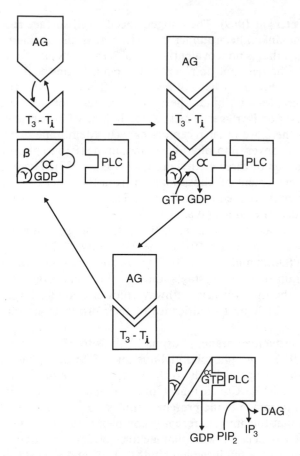

FIGURE 4–2.   Hypothetical scheme that attempts to explain the way signals are transferred across the membrane. Antigen (AG) binds to the T3–Ti receptor, and the complex then binds to the G proteins (α, β, and γ subunits) and guanine nucleotides. This process results in the dissociation of the α and β subunits. The α subunit, in conjunction with GTP, activates phospholipase C (PLC), which catalyzes the hydrolysis of phosphatidylinositol-4,5–bisphosphate (PIP_2) to diacylglyceral (DAG) and inositol trisphosphate (IP_3).   *(Based on Nel, Wooten, and Galbraith 1987.)*

a decrease in the cytosolic concentration of hydrogen ions. This leads to an increase in intracellular pH which is characteristic of activated cells. The PKC is also involved in the phosphorylation of several membrane receptors including the IL-2 receptor (Shackelford and Trowbridge 1984) and the T3–Ti (CD3–TCR) complex (Cantrell, Davies, and Crumpton 1985). It has also been shown to phosphorylate tyrosine protein kinase.

The other product formed by the action of PLC on PIP_2 is IP_3. The IP_3 functions to enhance the increase in concentration of intracellular calcium by binding to receptors on the endoplasmic reticulum and stimulating the release of stored calcium (Streb et al. 1983). A rise in intracellular calcium is an absolute prerequisite for cellular activation and functions to activate several calcium-dependent cytosolic enzymes, including acyltransferase, calcium ATPase, calcium-gated potassium channels, lipoxygenase, RNA-dependent DNA polymerases, calmodulin, and cGMP-dependent protein kinases.

The IP_3 is responsible for the initial rise in intracellular calcium that occurs approximately 20 sec after activation. However, it has not been demonstrated to be responsible for the sustained elevation in the level of intracellular calcium that lasts 2 to 4 hr following activation. The cause for the sustained peak is unknown but believed to be either an opening of a calcium channel in the plasma membrane, blockage of calcium uptake into intracellular stores, slowing of the pumps that extrude calcium out of the cell, or a combination of these.

In less than 2 min following antigen/mitogen binding, the permeability of monovalent cations increases (Quastel and Kaplan 1970), leading to membrane depolarization (Tsien, Pozzan, and Rink 1982). Meanwhile, lysolecithin activates guanylate cyclase, which converts GTP to cGMP, which activates cytoplasmic protein kinases that play roles in the increased de novo synthesis of PC, PI, and DNA (Whitefield et al. 1974). Other events observed in lymphocytes that occur within the first 30 min of activation include an increased uptake of potassium, glucose, amino acids, nucleosides, and phosphate along with an increased nonhistone protein binding to chromatin. There is also an increase in the activity of RNA polymerase I, histone kinase, histone acetylase, and phosphoribosylpyrophosphate synthetase. These early intracellular events are illustrated in Fig. 4-3.

3. Late Events

Within 2 hr, adenylate cyclase is activated, leading to the formation of cAMP (Smith et al. 1971), which also activates protein kinases that phosphorylate proteins involved in the synthesis and transcription of DNA (Juhl and Esmann 1979). The presence of cAMP in these late stages propagates the activation signal.

For many cells, cAMP is the second messenger that is formed during the initial stages of cellular activation. However, for lymphocytes, if cAMP is formed in these early stages, suppression of the activation signal is observed. There are several mechanisms by which cAMP can mediate this inhibitory effect. One possibility is the enhancing effect of cAMP on glucose metabolism through protein kinase C activation. As the blood level of glucose rises, intracellular levels of glucose-6–phosphate increase, and the latter inhibits further glucose uptake. This quickly depletes the energy supplies of the lymphocyte, and activation/mitosis is inhibited. Epinephrine, a hormone that greatly enhances cAMP production, is a very active lymphocyte inhibitor, whereas insulin, a hormone that promotes glucose entry into cells, increases the rate of mitosis. It is also possible that cAMP accumulation leads to a negative signal for IL-2 mRNA and IL-2 production. This would lead to a cessation of T-cell activation and the expression of end-stage responses. A similar effect is caused by PGE_1 and PGE_2. There is also evidence that cAMP can inhibit the phosphoinositide cycle and thus inhibit T-cell activity by preventing the formation of this vital second messenger.

Two signals are needed for activation of lymphocytes. The first involves antigen/mitogen binding, and the second is from IL-1 that is secreted by macrophage accessory cells. The IL-1, acting on lymphocytes that were primed from the antigen/mitogen signal, induces T cells to secrete IL-2 and express IL-2 receptors. The events that lead from the initial signal to the synthesis of IL-2, IL-2 receptors, or mitotic events are the least understood aspect of lymphocyte activation. However, it has been observed that changes do occur in the nucleus, which result in DNA, RNA, and protein synthesis.

During activation, only a few genes are utilized. The DNA synthesis begins approximately 24 hr after mitogen/antigen binding. An increase in the synthesis of ribosomal and transfer RNA is also observed, along with a tenfold increase

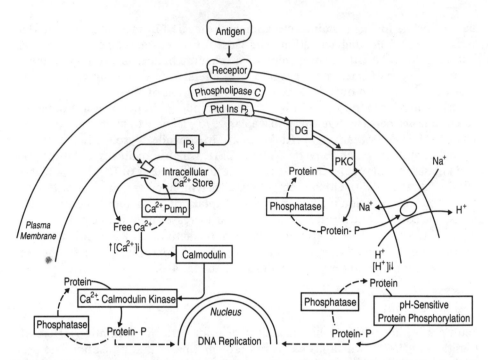

FIGURE 4-3.   A model of the early intracellular events that occur in lymphocytes following receptor-mediated activation. Inositol trisphosphate (IP₃) functions to cause a release of intracellular stores of calcium, and DAG functions to activate protein kinase C (PKC), which promotes phosphorylation of a variety of intracellular and nuclear proteins.   *(Based on Isakov et al. 1986.)*

in protein synthesis. As this is under way, the lymphocyte changes morphologically. The diameter of the cell doubles, the nucleolus appears, there are increased numbers of mitochondria and lysosomes, and there is decondensation of the heterochromatin.

C. EFFECTS OF THE NERVOUS SYSTEM ON IMMUNE FUNCTION

The immune system has traditionally been viewed as a distinct and independent organ system, partly because the peripheral leukocytes circulate independently, free from neurological fibers. However, the immune and nervous systems interact in a number of ways, which can be grouped into two lines of inquiry. One involves direct innervation of immunologic organs. Some of the early evidence that the immune and nervous systems had some interconnections included such interesting observations as unmyelinated nerve fibers found in the splenic white pulp associated with lymphocyte clusters; abnormalities in the number and function of lymphocytes can be found in animals with certain brain lesions; and the stimulation of postganglionic nerves supplying bone marrow augments production of lymphocytes (Besedovsky, del Rey, and Sorkin 1983a).

The other line of investigation has shown that immune function can be influenced by psychological and affective states, and, alternatively, the immune system can exert effects on behavior. These organic and psychological means of influencing immune events have in common the types of neurotransmitters and hormones released on stimulation that have effects on the immune system. It is important in these days of in vitro cytokine immunology to keep in mind that lymphoid and accessory cells also have receptors for corticosteroids, insulin, prolactin, growth hormone, estradiol, testosterone, vasointestinal peptide, substance P, somatostatin, dopamine, β-adrenergic agonists, acetylcholine, and endorphins (Besedovsky, del Rey, and Sorkin 1983b; Ader, Felten, and Cohen 1990; Khansari, Murgo, and Faith 1990) and that immune cells are under the influence of a wider variety of signals than even the myriad of immunologic cytokines known to affect them.

An example of an affective state having an influence over the immune system is stress, either physical or psychological (Stein 1989; Khansari, Murgo, and Faith 1990). Stress following the loss of a spouse, divorce, or even anxiety among medical students associated with impending examinations has been associated with alterations in immunologic parameters including decreased lymphoproliferative responses to mitogens, decreased NK-cell activity and interferon production, and an altered ratio of T-cell populations (Baker 1987). Similar effects have been found in laboratory animals that are stressed by multiple housing or restraint.

An example of the immune system regulating behavior is demonstrated by the MrL-Lpr/Lpr strain of mice, which demonstrates symptoms of an autoimmune disease (Grota, Ader, and Cohen 1987). When given the choice between water alone or water containing cyclophosphamide (an immunosuppressive drug used in the treatment of autoimmune diseases), these mice will voluntarily drink more of the cyclophosphamide-spiked water than control animals. Moreover, these animals will drink sufficient quantities to attenuate the autoimmune symptoms they are expressing. The investigators of these studies speculate that in these animals the brain may be acting on information received from a dysregulated immune system. Also, following immunization with sheep erythrocytes, mice exhibit a significant decrease in norepinephrine levels in the paraventricular nucleus of the hypothalamus. This decrease is very specific for this area of the brain and is localized in a key area that regulates autonomic and neuroendocrine outflow (Felten et al. 1987).

A description of physical interactions between the immune and neurological systems may be helpful in explaining these findings further. The immune system possesses extensive neural innervation, most of it indirectly (Bellinger et al. 1990; Reilly et al. 1976; Williams et al. 1981). Mediators released by the sympathetic, parasympathetic, and peptidergic systems innervate the primary (thymus and bone marrow) and secondary [lymph nodes, spleen, gut-associated lymphoid tissue (GALT)] lymphoid organs. Stimulating these receptors affects immunologic responses that are specific for the receptor stimulated.

Another example of the link between the immune and nervous systems involves hormone/cytokine and lymphoid cell/neural cell interactions. It has been shown that cells of the immune system produce neuroendocrine hormones and possess receptors for these hormones (Smith et al. 1983; Williams et al. 1976). Their interaction exerts profound effects on cells of the immune system. In addition, several cytokines have been shown to modulate the activity of neuroendocrine tissue. These actions are summarized in Table 4-1 (Weigert and Blalock 1987).

Briefly, IL-1, IL-2, and IL-6 have been shown to modulate the activity of the hypothalamus and pituitary, stimulating the secretion of corticotropin-releasing factor (CRF) and adrenocorticotropic hormone (ACTH) (Woloski et al. 1985;

TABLE 4-1.   Action and Sites of Action of the Hormones and Cytokines Involved in the Interaction Between the Immune System and the Nervous System

Cytokine/Hormone	Site of Action	Effect
IL-1	Hypothalamus	Stimulates secretion of CRF
IL-2	Pituitary	Stimulates ACTH release
IL-6	Hypothalamus	Stimulates secretion of CRF
	Pituitary	Stimulates ACTH release from pituitary cell line
Thymosin	Whole animal	Elevates levels of ACTH and glucocorticoids
β-Endorphin	Lymphocytes	Stimulates NK cells
	Monocytes/macrophages	Stimulates chemotaxis
Enkephalins	Lymphocytes	Stimulates T-cell rosette formation, T-cell activation at low doses
Glucocorticoid	Neutrophils	Stimulates neutrophil egress from bone marrow stores
	Monocytes/macrophages	Causes monocytopenia, inhibits IL-1 synthesis and secretion
	Lymphocytes	Causes lymphocytopenia, inhibits IL-1 secretion, inhibits nonspecific Ig production, suppresses NK-cell activity
Catecholamine	Lymphocytes	Depresses proliferative response to mitogens
Prolactin	Macrophages	Enhances activation
	Lymphocytes	Increases IL-2 production
Growth hormone	Macrophages	Enhances activation
	Lymphocytes	Enhances antibody synthesis
Ocytocin/vasopressin	Lymphocytes	Enhances T-cell proliferation
Substance P	Lymphocytes	Increases proliferation in culture
	Macrophages	Increases phagocytosis
	Mast cells	Increases histamine release
Somatostatin	Macrophages	Enhances activation
	Mast cells	Increases histamine release

Source: Adapted from Bateman et al. (1989) and Khansari, Murgo, and Faith (1990).

Naitoh et al. 1988). α-Interferon has been shown to induce steroid production by adrenal glands, induce melanin secretion by melanocytes, increase the beat frequency of cardiac cells in vitro, and induce opiate-like effects. The effects induced by interferon mimic those of the hormones that naturally mediate these responses (Blalock and Smith 1980).

Many examples exist to indicate that the cells of the immune system are sensitive to these neuroendocrine hormones. Glucocorticoids induce a general depression of immune function by inhibiting IL-1 synthesis, IL-1 and IL-2 secretion, and NK-cell activity, induce monocytopenia and lymphocytopenia, and stimulate neutrophil egress from bone marrow stores. β-Endorphins, enkephalins, growth hormone, and prolactin induce a general enhancement of immune function characterized by enhanced macrophage activity, T-cell activation and proliferation, and antibody synthesis (reviewed by Bateman et al. 1989). Catecholamines also depress immune function.

In addition, two sensory neuropeptides, substance P and somatostatin, which are both present in peripheral and central nervous systems, have been shown to modulate immunity and hypersensitivity (McGillis, Organist, and Payan 1987). Briefly, substance P can stimulate the proliferation of T lymphocytes in culture, stimulate IgA release from Peyer's patches lymphocytes, activate macrophages, and cause histamine and LTC_4 release from mast cells. Somatostatin inhibits the release of histamine from mast cells but stimulates macrophage activity. How these neuropeptides act in concert in modulating immunologic reactions is unknown. Vasoactive intestinal peptide (VIP) activates adenylate cyclase, leading to cAMP-dependent protein kinase C phosphorylation of a protein that possibly inhibits T-lymphocyte functions (O'Dorisio, Wood, and O'Dorisio 1985).

Based on the brief review of this area, one can understand how stress can lead to a depression in immunologic functions as described earlier. Stressful situations stimulate adrenocortical secretion, leading to increased serum glucocorticoid levels and activation of the sympathetic nervous system with subsequent release of catecholamines. Glucocorticoids and catecholamines have both been shown to depress immune function. The hypothalamus has been considered the efferent arm of the visceral brain and as such receives information from peripheral systems including cytokines produced by the immune system (e.g., thymosin fraction 5, thymopoietin, and IL-1) (Khansari, Murgo, and Faith 1990). After integrating the signals, the hypothalamus responds by adjusting sympathetic activity and endocrine secretion.

Investigation into the intimate ways the immunologic and neural systems interact has elicited some of the most profound questions in contemporary biology. One of the most intriguing molecular genetic questions in immunology is how the tremendous diversity in immunoglobulin variable domains is achieved through somatic recombination of genes. This phenomenon also has a counterpart in the brain through the demonstration of recombinational activating genes (RAG-1) in those areas of the brain containing the densest concentrations of neurons (Alt, Rathbun, and Yancopoulos 1991). It is possible that these genes might function by allowing neurons to generate a similar wide diversity in function and by participating in maintaining order in a very complicated system.

D. MEDIATORS OF IMMEDIATE HYPERSENSITIVITY AND INFLAMMATION

The mediators involved in immediate hypersensitivity and inflammation can be either preformed and released during effector cell degranulation or synthesized as a consequence of arachidonic acid metabolism by various cell types as a result of receptor–agonist interaction (as described above). Both types of mediators cause a variety of biological responses that, although in their strongest expression are typical of hypersensitivity and inflammation, are the essential molecules of the efferent immune system in general. The predominant mediators and their function and physical characteristics are summarized in Table 4–2 and discussed further below. For more information, the reader is directed to several review articles on the subject (Holgate, Robinson, and Church 1988; Schwartz and Austen 1984, 1988; Burrall, Payan, and Goetzl 1988).

1. Preformed Mediators

Mediators released from the granules of mast cells and basophils vary with the species but include histamine, serotonin, and eosinophil chemotactic factor of anaphylaxis (ECF-A). They are released from cytosolic granules into the extracel-

TABLE 4-2.   Mediators of Hypersensitivity and Inflammation

Mediator	Biological Activity Performed
Histamine (β-imidazoyl ethylamine)	Vasodilation, increased capillary permeability, bronchoconstriction
Serotonin (5-hydroxytryptamine)	Vasoconstriction, increased capillary permeability, bronchoconstriction
Eosinophil chemotactic factor of anaphylaxis (ala-gly-ser-glu) (val-gly-ser-glu)	Eosinophil chemotaxis, increased number of C4 and C3b receptors
PGE_2	Vasodilation, increased vasopermeability, bronchodilation, suppression of lymphocyte and PMN function
PGI_2 (prostacyclin)	Suppress platelet adherence and aggregation, vasodilation
$PGF_{2\alpha}$	Bronchoconstriction, vasodilation, increased vasopermeability
PGD_2	Bronchoconstriction, vasodilation, increased vasopermeability
Thromboxane (TxA_2)	Bronchoconstriction, stimulate platelet adherence and aggregation, vasoconstriction
Slow-releasing substance of anaphylaxis (LTC_4, LTD_4, and LTE_4)	Bronchoconstriction, increased vasopermeability, stimulate airway mucous secretion, decreased pulmonary compliance
Platelet-activating factor	Bronchoconstriction, increased vasopermeability, activation of neutrophils, vasoconstriction

Source: Modified from Holgate, Robinson, and Church (1988) and Burrall, Payan, and Goetzl (1988).

lular space following coupling by allgegen to membrane immunoglobulins. These mediators are discussed more extensively in Chapter 5.

Histamine (β-imidazoyl ethylamine) is one of the most extensively studied mediators present in the granules of the mast cells and basophils. It is synthesized from the amino acid histidine through the action of histidine decarboxylase (Schayer 1963) and is ionically bound to the carboxyl groups of heparin in the mast cell granule (Uvnas, Aborg, and Bergendoff 1970). Histamine is present in serum at approximately 0.2–0.4 ng/ml (Dyer et al. 1982) and approximately 3–8 pg is found in each human mast cell (Schulman, Kagey-Sobotka, and MacGlashen 1983; Fox, Dvorak, and Peters 1985).

Once released from the granule, histamine exerts its effect via H_1 and H_2 cell surface receptors. These receptors are found throughout the body, and their locations are summarized in Table 4–3. Of importance to hypersensitivity and inflammatory reactions is the stimulation of H_1 receptors on the smooth muscle cells

TABLE 4-3.   Distribution of Histamine Receptors

Organ	Receptor Type	Response
Bronchi	H_1 predominant H_2 small fraction	Bronchoconstriction
Arteries		
Large	H_1	Contraction
Small	H_1 and H_2	Relaxation
Heart	H_1 and H_2	Positive chronotropic and inotropic effects, increase coronary blood flow, prolongation of A–V conduction time
Mast cells	H_2	Feedback control of histamine release

Source: Modified From Reinhardt and Borchard (1982).

of the lung and the endothelial cells of blood vessels. This stimulation leads to contraction of bronchial smooth muscle and bronchospasm as seen with inhalation of an allergen and to an increase in vasopermeability and vasodilation. These vascular changes are the cause of the wheal-and-flare response and flushing of the skin that are seen in dermal reactions to allergens. Severe dilation of the arterioles can also lead to a drop in blood pressure, a signal of systemic anaphylaxis.

Other effects of histamine that are mediated by the stimulation of H_1 and H_2 receptors include increased secretion from salivary and mucous glands, enhanced expression of C3b receptors on eosinophils (Anwar and Kay 1978), and down-regulation of lymphokine production, lymphocyte proliferation, and interferon production (Melmon, Rocklin, and Rogenkranz 1981).

Another preformed mediator, serotonin (5–hydroxytryptamine), is synthesized by hydroxylation and decarboxylation of tryptophan (Clark, Weissbach, and Udenfriend 1955). It is not present in human mast cells but is present at up to 1 $\mu g/10^6$ cells in rat mast cells (Moran, Uunaxs, and Westerholm 1962). In addition to its release from mast cells and basophils during hypersensitivity reactions, it is also released from human platelets by platelet-activating factor (PAF) and thromboxane A_2 (TxA_2) (described below).

The role of serotonin is not fully understood in regard to human hypersensitivity and inflammatory reactions. It has been shown to be a potent vasoconstrictor in human skin and can cause an increase in postcapillary venular permeability and bronchoconstriction in rats. It increases phagocytic responsiveness to chemoattractants, increases fibroblast growth, and stimulates collagen formation (Schwartz and Austen 1988).

One major product of mast cell activation is eosinophil chemotactic factor A (ECF-A), which consists of two tetrapeptides, val-gly-ser-glu and ala-gly-ser-glu, each having a molecular weight of approximately 400 (Turnball, Evans, and Kay 1977; Goetzl and Austen 1975). In addition to chemotaxis, these peptides are also able to increase the number of C4 and C3b receptors on eosinophils and therefore increase their degree of phagocytosis (Anwar and Kay 1977, 1978). Eosinophils secrete a variety of mediators important in defense against infection as well as in both inflammatory and anti-inflammatory processes (see Chapters 5 and 6).

2. Synthesized Mediators

As a result of perturbation to the lipid membrane bilayer, two large families of lipid mediators, arachidonic acid metabolites and the family of platelet-activating factor molecules, are rapidly synthesized. These products in turn are quite biologically active and influence many of the effector immune responses. Moreover, many of them participate in regulatory functions of the immune response. When certain cells are stimulated, phospholipase A_2 converts membrane phospholipids to arachidonic acid. The arachidonic acid is then converted to the leukotrienes (LT) via the addition of hydroperoxyl groups by lipoxygenase. In addition, through the action of cyclooxygenase, arachidonic acid is converted to the prostaglandins (PG) and thromboxane (Tx). These metabolic pathways are summarized in Fig. 4–4. Although the biological functions of these mediators differ, the one thing they share in common is that they are rapidly generated and released.

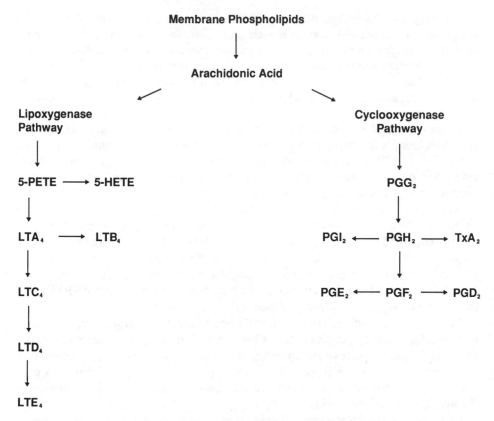

Membrane Phospholipids

Arachidonic Acid

Lipoxygenase Pathway

Cyclooxygenase Pathway

5-PETE $\longrightarrow$ 5-HETE

PGG$_2$

LTA$_4$ $\longrightarrow$ LTB$_4$

PGI$_2$ $\longleftarrow$ PGH$_2$ $\longrightarrow$ TxA$_2$

LTC$_4$

PGE$_2$ $\longleftarrow$ PGF$_2$ $\longrightarrow$ PGD$_2$

LTD$_4$

LTE$_4$

FIGURE 4–4.   Pathways for the metabolism of arachidonic acid into mediators of immediate hypersensitivity. The lipoxygenase pathway leads to the production of the leukotrienes. The cyclooxygenase pathway leads to the production of the prostaglandins and thromboxane.

Prostaglandins

The primary PGs that are formed are PGD$_2$, PGI$_2$ (prostacyclin), PGE$_2$, and PGF$_2\alpha$. The primary thromboxane formed is TxA$_2$. Prostaglandins exert a variety of biological responses, depending on the specific PG, that are either end-organ or cellular effects. Prostaglandin F$_{2\alpha}$ and PGD$_2$ cause contraction of smooth muscle and increase vasopermeability and vasodilation. Prostaglandin E$_2$ causes the same vascular effects but causes a relaxation of smooth muscle and suppression of lymphocyte (Rappaport and Dodge 1982) and PMN functions, whereas TxA$_2$ causes bronchoconstriction and vasoconstriction. Similar mutually antagonistic effects may also be seen at the cellular level. For example, PGI$_2$ suppresses platelet aggregation and adherence, but TxA$_2$ stimulates these functions, and both are believed to operate in a functionally opposing balance system.

Prostaglandin E$_2$ is often considered a major immunosuppressive molecule of humoral immunity. At physiological doses and when present at certain specific times of B-cell activation, PGE$_2$ (as well as a variety of lipoxygenase metabolites) directly suppresses B-cell function and later stages of proliferation (Behrens and Goodwin 1989); when it is present at other times in the B-cell growth cycle, the effect may be stimulatory. Some explanations for the nonuniformity in reported immunosuppressive effects may be that only certain subpopulations may be

PGE_2 sensitive or that suppressor activity may be inhibited, depending on the experimental setup and microenvironment conditions.

Prostaglandins can even modulate their own pathway after certain forms of cell stimulation. For example, exogenous PGE_2 can greatly enhance the ability of bacterial LPS-stimulated alveolar macrophages to produce $PGF_2\alpha$ but exerts no effect on the cells by itself (Tanamoto, Schade, and Rietschel 1989).

The activity of cyclooxygenase is classically inhibited by aspirin, indomethacin, and other nonsteroidal anti-inflammatory agents. In the broadest perspective, such clinically useful drugs would be considered immunotoxic.

Leukotrienes

The major leukotrienes that are formed are LTB_4, LTC_4, LTD_4, and LTE_4; LTC_4, LTD_4, and LTE_4 collectively make up what was once thought to be a single substance, slow-releasing substance of anaphylaxis (SRS-A). Leukotrienes are produced in different quantities by mast cells, neutrophils, eosinophils, and macrophages. The leukotriene family functions to constrict smooth muscle, increase vascular permeability, increase airway mucus secretion, decrease peripheral blood flow, and inhibit lymphocyte responses to mitogens. For example, LTC_4 is a more potent bronchoconstrictive agent than histamine, but human mast cells produce about 30 times more of the latter on a molar basis. It is also a potent stimulus for the secretion of mucus in the airways.

Leukotriene B_4 is the primary eicosanoid product of neutrophils, monocytes, and alveolar macrophages and is a potent chemotactic factor for these same cell types. It inhibits proliferation of $CD4^+$ T cells but enhances that of $CD8^+$ cells. Leukotriene is also a monocyte activator. With intradermal injection, it can promote neutrophil infiltration into local tissue sites. The mechanism is believed to be via a direct effect on endothelial cells, where the adherence capacity for the neutrophils is enhanced.

Platelet-Activating Factor

The other family of membrane phospholipids activated by a variety of signals is the platelet-activating factors (PAF). Like prostaglandins and leukotrienes, PAF (1–o-alkyl-2–acetyl-sn-glyceryl-3–phosphorylcholine) is formed by the action of phospholipase A_2 and acetyltransferase on membrane phospholipids. The PAF is found in a variety of cells including platelets, neutrophils, macrophages, and endothelial cells. It is generally agreed that the functions of PAF are mediated via cell surface receptors, because high-affinity binding sites have been found on platelets (Valone and Goetzl 1982) and neutrophils (O'Flaherty et al. 1986). In addition to being potent platelet-aggregating/activating agents, they are also mediators of vasoactive amine release, hypotension independent of that produced by released amines, increased vascular permeability, bronchial constriction, and cell necrosis (Braquet et al. 1987). The PAF also activates a wide range of inflammatory cells, is chemotactic for eosinophils and neutrophils, increases aggregation and degranulation of neutrophils, induces production of superoxide, and is many times more potent than histamine in altering endothelial permeability. Although PAF has a very short half-life, it has long-term effects because it is made continuously and because of its stimulation of other cytokines, e.g., IL-1, whose effect lasts much longer (Barthelson, Potter, and Valone 1990).

These two important families of lipid mediators may even interact. In certain instances, PAF contributes to eicosanoid release in vivo following bacterial lipopolysaccharide (LPS) exposure (Olson, Joyce, and Fleisher 1990), and it is likely that in addition to leukotriene regulation, these products enhance other important activities, e.g., calcium uptake, PKC activation, and enhanced release of superoxide anion. Other ways in which PAF can indirectly influence subsequent reactivity is by down-regulating β-adrenergic receptor densities in the airways (Agarwal and Townley 1987) and by increasing the intracellular accumulation of an IL-1 precursor (Barthelson, Potter, and Valone 1990).

E. CYTOKINES

The immune system is very complex and, to be effective, requires a coordinated interaction among a number of different cells. The tremendous advances in cellular immunology have been achieved through various in vitro studies of isolated lymphocyte or macrophage cell populations under very defined conditions. From these studies, it has been learned that all stages in development, growth, proliferation, and activation take place through the controlled intracellular elaboration of numerous cytokines. This coordinated interaction is achieved through several mediators that function to promote growth, differentiation, functional activation, and communication between cells.

Powerful techniques of molecular biology have facilitated the sequencing and even molecular cloning of many of these molecules as well as their individual receptors. The development of monoclonal antibodies specific for these pure entities provided an additional means to study their definitive actions. Much of the information comes from the study of murine systems, although many of these cytokines have been confirmed for humans as well. Although much of the following discussion refers to murine immunology, experience has taught that the murine system should continue to point the way for human studies. It is important to realize that much of the knowledge concerning cytokines has been obtained working with purified material on single cell types. Strictly speaking, results from such studies only show *potential* activity. An additional concern is that most of the information has been obtained through the study of in vitro systems, and comparatively little is known of how these cytokine functions are coordinated in vivo when they are subject to additional controls by endocrine hormones, neurotransmitters, cAMP regulation, and the like. Administering IL-2 to immunodeficient or cancer patients seemed like a good idea until actual in vivo administration showed how serious the toxic side reactions to other organ systems induced by this substance could be.

Cytokines are released during the effector phase of cellular stimulation, and although they are important in translating immune recognition (either antigen-specific or nonspecific), they are also important in regulating other functions of immune cells; i.e., cytokines produced by one cell type may affect the production of cytokines by other cell types. In fact, the elaboration of one cytokine may in turn affect the production of a highly integrated cascade of cytokine production, where those produced later in the cascade have various effects on those produced earlier. These effects could be either down-regulating or synergistic. Once bound or even transcribed, the cytokine often sends a signal regulating its own expression. In yet other instances, these cytokines essentially function as growth factors for other cells. Their production is brief and transient, and much work has been directed to the various types of stimulation that induce mRNA transcription. Indeed, it is at this level that immunotoxicologists should pay close attention.

In the following discussion, the cytokines have been grouped into families according to the principal function of each after the method of Abbas, Lichtman, and Pober (1991), although many cytokines function in other categories as well. Some of them enhance stimulation of other lymphocytes, thereby providing an amplification mechanism to antigen-specific immunity. In addition to their lymphocyte- and monocyte-stimulating roles, many of these protein hormones serve a regulatory role as the means for controlling the functions of many accessory cells. The major way cells of the immune system communicate is in fact through cytokines. These mediators include the interleukins (general discussion can be found in Mizel 1989, and Muraguchi et al. 1987), interferons, colony-stimulating factors, tumor necrosis factor, and several others.

1. Cytokines That Mediate Innate Immunity

These mediators are released by mononuclear phagocytes that have been stimulated by either infectious or inflammatory agents. These agents are extremely important in innate or constitutive protection against bacterial and viral agents but may also be elaborated as a result of antigen-specific, T-cell immune responses as well.

Interleukin 1

Interleukin 1 (IL-1) has been the most extensively studied interleukin because it was the first one discovered and because it induces such a wide variety of proinflammatory, immunoregulating, and nonimmunologic activities. For a detailed discussion of IL-1, the reader is directed to reviews by Dinarello (1989) or di Giovine and Duff (1990). There are two forms of IL-1, IL-1α and IL-1β (Auron et al. 1984; Lomedico et al. 1984). Although these forms are distinctly different polypeptides that are coded for by different genes, they stimulate the same receptors, share the same biological activities, and are crystallographically similar (Kilian et al. 1986). Interleukin 1β is the predominant polypeptide formed during most responses. The IL-1 receptor is an 80–kDa glycosylated peptide that spans the cell membrane (Paganelli, Stern, and Kilian 1987) with a molecular structure suggesting that it is in the immunoglobulin family (Simms et al. 1988).

Interleukin 1 is produced by a variety of cells including neutrophils, fibroblasts, epithelial cells, keratinocytes, astrocytes, endothelial cells, epidermal cells, smooth muscle cells, and microglial cells (Oppenheim, Kovacs, and Matsushima 1986). It induces a multitude of effects in a variety of immunologic and nonimmunologic cells. These effects are summarized in Table 4–4. Briefly, IL-1 functions as a comitogen in the activation and growth of T and B cells (Gery and Waksman 1972) and increases the binding of natural killer cells to target tumor cells (Herman et al. 1985). Through its interaction with endothelium, IL-1 promotes procoagulant production, thereby increasing adhesion for inflammatory cells.

Interleukin 1 regulates the production of lymphokines and expression of lymphocyte receptors. It can also stimulate the production of interferon (Van Damme et al. 1985), granulocyte–macrophage colony-stimulating factor (Bagby et al. 1986), IL-3, IL-6 (Van Damme et al. 1987), and platelet-activating factor.

The role of IL-1 in inflammatory reactions is mediated mainly by its ability to stimulate arachidonic acid metabolism in all target cells leading to the formation of leukotrienes, thromboxane, and prostaglandins. Since it is produced by a

TABLE 4-4.   Biological Activities of Interleukin 1

Cell	Biological Effects
Neutrophil	Neutrophil activation and induction of neutrophilia
Macrophage	Macrophage activation
T cell	Chemotaxis, increased IL-2 production, increased expression of IL-2 receptors
B cell	Chemotaxis, B-cell growth
NK cells	Chemotaxis augments natural killer cell activation
Tumor cells	Cytostatic and cytotoxic for certain cell lives
Fibroblasts	Increased collagen synthesis, increased proliferation and prostaglandin release, induces cachexia
Brain	Induces slow-wave sleep, pyrogenic
Liver	Increases production of certain acute-phase proteins
T cells/macrophages	Increases synthesis of hematopoietic CSFs
Bone	Bone resorption
Pancreas	Cytotoxicity

Source: Modified from Sauder (1989).

wide variety of infectious diseases, IL-1 is considered to be a major means of nonantigen-specific immunity.

In addition, when administered to animals, IL-1 induces a variety of systemic effects (summarized in Table 4-5). Briefly, IL-1 is the classic endogenous pyrogen, and it increases the production of acute-phase proteins in the liver (Bauman et al. 1984), decreases systemic arterial and central venous pressure (Okusawa et al. 1987), decreases appetite, and alters sleep patterns.

Interleukin 6
Interleukin 6 (IL-6) is produced by T cells, B cells, Kupffer cells, hepatocytes, pancreatic β cells, monocytes, endothelial cells, mesangial cells, keratinocytes, and stimulated fibroblasts (Vitetta et al. 1985; Lotz et al. 1989; Campbell et al.

TABLE 4-5.   Systemic Effects of Administered Interleukin 1

Central nervous system	Metabolic
Fever	Hypozincemia, hypoferremia
Brain PGE_2 synthesis	Decreased cytochrome P450 enzyme
Increased ACTH	Increased acute-phase proteins
Decreased REM sleep	Decreased albumin synthesis
Increased slow-wave sleep	Increased insulin production
Decreased appetite	Inhibition of lipoprotein lipase
	Increased sodium excretion
	Increased corticosteroid synthesis
Hematologic	Vascular wall
Neutrophilia	Hypotension
Nonspecific resistance	Increased leukocyte adherence
Increased GM-CSF	Increased PGE synthesis
Radioprotection	Decreased systemic vascular resistance
Bone marrow stimulation	Decreased central venous pressure
Tumor necrosis	Increased cardiac output
	Increased heart rate
	Decreased blood pH
	Lactic acidosis
	Chemoattractant

Source: Modified from Dinarello (1989).

1989; May et al. 1989; Zhang, Lin, et al. 1989). A detailed discussion of the biological effects of IL-6 is given by Heinrich, Castell, and Anders (1990), Wong and Clark (1988), and Wolvekamp and Marquet (1990).

Interleukin 6 plays a key role in inflammatory reactions, having been shown to increase the synthesis of the major acute-phase proteins from adult human hepatocytes. These include the C-reactive protein, serum amyloid A, hapto-globin, α_1-antitrypsin, α_2-macroglobulin, and fibrinogen (Castell et al. 1989). Interleukin 6 can also act as a pyrogen.

Interleukin 6 plays a key role in the terminal differentiation of B cells into Ig-secreting cells (Kishimoto 1987). This observation has been shown both in vivo and in vitro, where IL-6 augments murine antigen-specific antibody responses (Takatsuki et al. 1988). In addition, IL-6 stimulates T-cell proliferation by induc-ing the expression of the IL-2 receptor and enhances the generation of T-cyto-toxic cells (Billiau et al. 1989). It can also activate NK cells (Luger et al. 1989). Cells rarely respond to IL-6 alone but require a second signal, usually from IL-1, before responding (Billiau et al. 1989).

Interleukin 6 also plays a critical role in hematopoiesis by stimulating the dif-ferentiation of stem cells, inducing granulocyte–macrophage colony formation (Clark 1989), and stimulating erythropoiesis (Ulich, Del Castillo, and Guo 1989). Interleukin 6 was initially called interferon β_2 because of its antiviral activity. It has been shown to inhibit mengo virus and herpes simplex II virus (Zilberstein et al. 1986) and to induce specific interferon-activated genes such as 2′,5′-oligo-A-synthetase (Zilberstein, Ruggieri, and Revel 1985).

The production of IL-6 is stimulated by IL-1 (Zhang, Klein, and Gataille 1989), IL-2 (Kasid, Direchor, and Rosenberg 1989), TNF, interferons, bacterial products such as LPS, growth factors, and viral products (Sehgal et al. 1988; Navarro et al. 1989). The IL-6 receptor has a molecular weight of 80,000 and one highly conserved 90–amino-acid domain that indicates it is a member of the immunoglobulin superfamily (Yamasaki 1989).

Interleukin 8
Interleukin 8 (IL-8) refers to a large family of proteins ranging from 8 to 10 kDa. The prototype was originally isolated from LPS-stimulated human monocytes. It activates neutrophils, leading to enzyme release and a respiratory burst (Bag-giolini, Walz, and Kunkel 1989) and is chemotaxic for both neutrophils and lymphocytes (Larsen et al. 1989). Interleukin 8 is produced by activated mono-cytes and macrophages (Strieter et al. 1990) and is released from epithelial cells (Steiter, Kunkel, et al. 1989), fibroblasts (Streiter, Phan, et al. 1989), and synovial cells (Watson, Lewis, and Westwick 1988) following stimulation with IL-1 or tumor necrosis factor.

Tumor Necrosis Factor
Tumor necrosis factor (TNF) is produced predominantly by activated macro-phages but has also been shown to be produced by lymphocytes, keratinocytes, and endothelial cells. Although it was originally isolated from endotoxin-challenged mice and shown to induce a hemorrhagic necrosis in transplanted tu-mors (Carswell et al. 1975), its effects range well beyond that original definition. It is sometimes called cachectin because of its association with the wasting pro-cess characteristic of chronic diseases such as malignancies. By itself, it is ex-tremely inflammatory in that its release is one of the major cytokines triggered

by bacterial endotoxin (Burrell 1990), and it is one of the most important mediators of septic shock (DeForge et al. 1990). Yet, in smaller, controlled amounts it
is responsible for many immunomodulating activities. Tumor necrosis factor can
induce the production of hematopoietic colony-stimulating factors, IL-3 and IL-
6, along with activating T cells to increase the expression of IL-2 receptors and
major histocompatibility antigens (Zucali et al. 1987). Tumor necrosis factor also
exerts effects on hematopoietic stem cells in various ways, activates PMNs, and
stimulates endothelial cells to induce procoagulant activity. It shares many of the
same properties as IL-1 (Le and Vilcek 1987), i.e., many of the same properties
that were listed for IL-1 in Tables 4–4 and 4–5 are also true for TNF. Although
the biological effects of IL-1 and TNF are often indistinguishable, the two cytokines act synergistically in the immunologic response when given together.

Interferons
The interferons, first identified by their ability to protect cells against viral rein-
fections, are a heterogeneous family of proteins of two classes. Type I or viral
interferon consists of two species and is induced by infection. One variety, IFN-
α, is produced primarily by leukocytes, whereas the other, IFN-β, is produced by
fibroblasts. There is a great degree of heterogeneity among these molecules. Type
II or immune interferon consists of IFN-γ and is produced by lymphocytes on
separate genes in response to specific antigens or nonspecific mitogens. It is important to point out that this generalization is valid only for humans. The types
are not so neatly segregated in mice, where both IFN-α and IFN-β are mixed.
For a review of the structure and function of interferons, the reader is directed
to Zoon et al. (1987).

γ-Interferon has been isolated from T lymphocytes and natural killer cells and
exists in two forms, which differ in their degree of glycosylation. The cellular
origin of IFN-γ depends on the type of stimulus received. Although both CD4$^+$
and CD8$^+$ T cells produce IFN-γ in response to alloantigens or mitogens, soluble
antigens tend to stimulate mostly helper (CD4$^+$) cells. Its production is dependent
on the presence of IL-1 and IL-2; however, if IL-2 is the stimulus, NK cells are
the major IFN-γ producers.

In order to be functional, the interferons must first bind to membrane receptors, which differ in type, number, and specificity for each IFN. After internal-
ization, gene expression is effected through de novo RNA and polypeptide
synthesis to enable different functions. The most widely known function of IFN-
γ is that of a neoplastic cell growth inhibitor, although this is most likely done
in concert with other cytokines. Most other functions are stimulatory.

One of its major functions as a T-cell-derived product is to activate macrophages, which enhance oxidative metabolism, induce expression of high-affinity
Fc receptors for monomeric IgG, modulate tumoricidal activity, and potentiate
IL-1 production. The IFN-γ also induces IL-2 receptor activity on T cells, which
enhances their proliferation, producing even more IFN-γ in the process. All three
types of interferon enhance expression of class I MHC markers, and IFN-γ also
induces higher densities of these as well as type II MHC expression than the
others. The IFN-γ can also affect maturation of B-cell differentiation.

The biological effects exerted by the interferons are very similar but differ in
their dose–response curves and degree of cytostatic actions. These effects include
protection against viral infections, regulation of cell growth, modulation of cell
differentiation, and altered expression of different genes. Interferons are pro-

duced when the cell comes into contact with viral, bacterial, or fungal extracts, mitogens, polycarboxylates, or polynucleotides.

The molecular mechanisms involved in the antiviral effects of IFN were extensively reviewed by Clemens and McNurlan (1985). Inteferon can interfere with viral protein synthesis, regulation of cell growth, and cell differentiation. It stimulates the production of a protein kinase and 2,5–oligoadenylate synthetase. These enzymes function to degrade mRNA/rRNA and to inhibit translation, respectively. It is assumed that the antiviral activity is linked to this enzyme induction. The IFNs can also inhibit the progression of a cell through the cell cycle or prolong the length of time a specific stage continues. This inhibition is probably mediated by one or all of several events that have been shown to be caused by IFN, including inhibition of growth factor/receptor interactions, inhibition of DNA polymerase activity, inhibition of lipid synthesis, and tyrosinase activity. It is important to understand that many interferon effects are secondary and that they often act as cofactors with other cytokines.

2. Cytokines That Regulate Lymphocytes

These cytokines mainly regulate activation, growth, and differentiation of lymphocytes in response to antigen recognition. In fact, it is through these cytokines that T-helper cells function.

Interleukin 2

Interleukin 2 (IL-2) is a product of T cells that must interact with its specific receptor to be effective. The IL-2 receptor is a dimer consisting of two polypeptide chains—an α subunit of 55 kDa and a β subunit of 75 kDa (Dukovich et al. 1987). Resting cells have small numbers of these receptors with virtually no β chains. Once activated, the β chains are synthesized in a greater amount and form high-affinity dimers with the α chains. The affinity of either chain is very low in the unassociated state. When a cell is stimulated to secrete IL-2, it is bound to its IL-2 receptor, which stimulates growth and elaboration of more IL-2 in an autocrine manner.

Interleukin 2 is mitogenic for T cells once they have expressed the IL-2 receptor and stimulates the progression from G_1 to S phase in the cell division cycle. It is also mitogenic for a variety of lymphoid cells including NK cells, B cells, and lymphokine-activated killer (LAK) cells. The IL-2 increases the rate of synthesis of RNA for the cellular oncogene c-*myc* and the transferrin receptor, which is responsible for the transport of zinc into the cell (Depper et al. 1985; Blazsek and Mathe 1984). It also stimulates the secretion of TNF and IFN-γ from lymphoid cells (Miedema et al. 1985; Nedwin et al. 1985).

Because of its ability to augment LAK-cell activity, IL-2 has been suggested as a viable therapy in the treatment of cancer. Some of the more positive clinical trials showed that the injection of IL-2 into certain types of tumors or administration of IL-2–activated LAK cells to patients results in a complete or partial remission for varying times (Kohler et al. 1985; Pizza et al. 1984). However, systemic administration of IL-2 yielded minimal benefits (Lotze et al. 1985). Treatment with IL-2 resulted in serious side effects, which included pulmonary edema, fluid retention, dyspnea, and a decrease in peripheral blood leukocytes. Continued work on the proper route of administration and a greater understanding of the mechanisms behind the induced side effects are essential before widespread application of IL-2 as a therapeutic agent can proceed.

Interleukin 4

Interleukin 4 (IL-4) is synthesized and secreted by activated T cells. It has a specific receptor with a molecular weight of 140,000 (Paul and Ohara 1987). A detailed discussion of IL-4 is given by Paul and Ohara (1987). Interleukin 4 functions as an activating factor for resting B cells by enhancing the expression of membrane class II major histocompatibility complex molecules (Roehm, Liebson, and Zlotnick 1984; Peschel et al. 1989) and promotes the expression of IgG_1 and IgE by cells stimulated by bacterial LPS (Vitetta et al. 1985; Coffman et al. 1986). It can also increase the size of B cells and enhance MHC class II expression (Dennis et al. 1987). Interleukin 4 can also stimulate and maintain the state of activation in T cells by stimulating the progression of the cells from G_0 to G_1 and enhancing the production of IL-2 and IL-2 receptors (Mitchell, Davis, and Lipsky 1989). It can also increase the proliferative rate in mast cells costimulated with IL-3 (Mosmann et al. 1986). Conversely, IL-4 may possess some antiinflammatory activities, since it can suppress the synthesis of tumor necrosis factor, IL-1, and PGE_2 by macrophages (Hart et al. 1989).

Interleukin 9

Interleukin 9 (IL-9) is derived from T-helper cell clones that were isolated from the lymph nodes of antigen-primed mice (Uyttenhove, Simpson, and van Svick 1988). It is very specific in its actions. It has been shown to promote the long-term growth of only T-helper cells, independent of IL-2 and IL-4. It is inactive in maintaining growth of cytotoxic T-cell clones. Interleukin 9 has also been shown to enhance the response of bone-marrow-derived mast cells to IL-3.

Interleukin 10

Interleukin 10 (IL-10) is a B-cell-derived T-cell growth factor. It was isolated from subclones of the murine B cell lymphoma CH12.LX (Suda et al. 1990) and is believed to play a major role in the development of T cells in the thymus. It has been shown to induce the proliferation of specific subsets of mature T cells (CD4 and CD8) along with day-15 fetal thymocytes. Interleukin 10 does not induce this proliferation alone but only in the presence of IL-2 and IL-4 (MacNeil et al. 1990). Its relevance to biological systems has yet to be determined.

Transforming Growth Factor β

Transforming growth factor β belongs to a family of polypeptides that function to control (promote or inhibit) growth and survival of a variety of target cells depending on other factors present in the microenvironment. It is produced by a variety of cells in culture in an inactive form that is later converted by enzymatic means to the active form. Its main in vitro effect on lymphocytes is to inhibit T-cell proliferation in response to antigen or mitogen, and it also down-regulates the effects of inflammatory cytokines on macrophages, neutrophils, and endothelial cells. This is a major cytokine produced by what are generally regarded as suppressor cells.

3. Cytokines That Activate Inflammatory Cells

From the standpoint of translating immune recognition into meaningful biological action, these cytokines may be the most important. They are derived from activated T cells and are mainly responsible for regulating the effects of accessory cells, particularly those involved in cell-mediated immunity.

Interleukin 5

Interleukin 5 (IL-5) functions in the growth and activation of B cells (Kishimoto 1987). It is secreted by T cells and activated by B cells (Gordon et al. 1984). Interleukin 5 functions to induce the proliferation, maturation, and secretion of IgM, IgG, and IgA from B cells (Nakajima et al. 1985), to synergize with IL-2 to induce cytotoxic T cells and the expression of the IL-2 receptor (Takatsu 1987), and to promote maturation of eosinophils (Sanderson et al. 1988).

Lymphotoxin

Lymphotoxin belongs to the same family of molecules as TNF (see Paul and Ruddle 1988 for a review). It competes for similar receptor sites and exhibits similar activities. Often lymphotoxin is referred to as TNF-β to distinguish it from the latter, TNF-α. Lymphotoxin is synthesized only by activated T CD4$^+$ cells, whereas TNF can be produced by a variety of cells, especially activated macrophages. It is produced locally in cytotoxic reactions, mediating cell lysis, and formerly was believed to be the main agent for accomplishing this effect, but the majority of cell lysis is now thought to be promoted by direct cell contact and subsequent pore formation. Since lymphotoxin kills B cells presenting antigen as well as the cells that produce it, it might have some local immunoregulatory role. It also regulates activation of neutrophils and their interaction with endothelial cells. Neutrophil adhesion to endothelial cells and subsequent diapedesis through capillary walls is a primary inflammation event. All of lymphotoxin's functions are largely enhanced by IFN-γ.

MIF

At one time the major method of assessing in vitro correlates of cell-mediated immunity was by assessing the inhibition of migration of macrophages in the presence of antigen-stimulated lymphocytes. This technique is still useful for immunotoxicologic assessment. Briefly, short lengths of capillary tubes filled with lymphocyte–macrophage suspensions were placed in dishes of nutrient medium and incubated overnight. Normally, macrophages would migrate from the end of the tubing into the medium, and the area of the migrated cells from the tip was compared against similar tubes incubated in the presence of antigen. If lymphocytes specific for the test antigen were present, a lymphokine would be released that would inhibit the macrophage migration and result in a greatly reduced area of migration from the capillary tips. In spite of it being among the first cytokines discovered, its molecular characterization and in vivo significance remain unknown. It may participate in aiding retention of macrophages in local inflammatory microenvironments.

4. Cytokines That Regulate Hematopoiesis

These cytokines are primarily involved in stimulating progenitor stem cells to develop and expand and are produced from a variety of cell sources. Here, perhaps more than anywhere else, the cytokines must act in a carefully concerted sequence of steps. A given cytokine may be inhibitory at one stage of a cell's development yet stimulatory at another stage. They interact in an intricate network of other cytokines, and indeed, the presence of a given cytokine at a particular time in relation to the presence of other signals will influence the production or the effect of another cytokine. Thus, the immediate microenvironment becomes immensely important in regulating the development of these important cells and should be a very important target for immunotoxicologic interest.

Interleukin 3
Interleukin 3 (IL-3) is a T-cell product involved in the growth and differentiation of hematopoietic progenitor cell types including granulocytes, macrophages, megakaryocytes, mast cells, red blood cells, T cells, and B cells (Ihle and Weinstein 1986). It can act directly on progenitor cells in vitro and is capable of inducing differentiation into erythroid and multiple myeloid lineages (Suda et al. 1986). It can also induce the expression of the Thy-1 marker on cultured murine bone marrow cells (Schrader, Battye, and Scollay 1982). An overview of the biological properties and biochemistry of IL-3 has been given by Moore (1988). The IL-3 receptor is a 65-kDa protein (Park et al. 1986), although other higher-molecular-weight surface proteins have been detected that also have an affinity for IL-3 (Isfort et al. 1988).

Interleukin 7
Interleukin 7 (IL-7) is a bone marrow stromal cell product that functions as a regulatory cytokine in lymphocyte growth and differentiation. It acts as a growth-promoting factor for B progenitor cells (Goodwin et al. 1989) and is also mitogenic for T cells via its ability to induce IL-2 production and the expression of IL-2 receptors (Morrissey et al. 1989). Interleukin 7 also enhances the development of cytotoxic T-cell and lymphokine-activated killer-cell activity (Alderson, Sassenfeld, and Widmer 1990).

Colony-Stimulating Factors
The term colony-stimulating factor (CSF) refers to the method by which these cytokines are demonstrated, i.e., by stimulating the formation of cell colonies in bone marrow cultures. At lower concentrations, these cytokines may modify functions of mature cells, depending on target, concentration, and other microenvironment conditions (Pimental 1990). They can stimulate phagocytosis, prostaglandin synthesis, protease secretion, and expression of cytolytic activity. Specific CSF molecules affect specific stem cell lineages to develop into a particular, mature cell type that concomitantly excludes that stem cell from developing into other types. Many other lymphokines, e.g., IL-3, have essentially CSF functions. Figure 2–1 in Chapter 2 illustrates a general overview of hematopoiesis, indicating at what points specific CSF cytokines most likely act. They are named according to the final, differentiated cell type stimulated. Granulocyte-macrophage CSF (GM-CSF), as the name indicates, acts on stem cells at an earlier stage of commitment, but at an even earlier stage in humans than in mice. Activated macrophages recruit T cells (via IL-1) and activate endothelial cells and fibroblasts, all of which produce GM-CSF. It mimics some of the actions of IFN-γ. Monocyte–macrophage CSF (M-CSF) acts on progenitors already committed to become macrophages, whereas granulocyte CSF (G-CSF) acts on progenitors already committed to form neutrophils. This latter CSF circulates in the periph-

eral circulation, unlike the others, and thus serves as a signal between distant inflammatory events and the bone marrow. Often the presence of certain foreign substances, e.g., bacterial LPS, will cause an immediate leukopenia (from sequestration of neutrophils in capillaries), which is then followed by a leukocytosis caused by a release of new cells from the bone marrow.

5. Conclusions

Even this oversimplified outline of the many mediators involved in immune function and regulation must seem tremendously complex. Such findings have prompted many immunologists to question the significance of all of the apparent trivia and wonder if there is any meaning to all of it (Mosmann 1991). On the one hand, anything so complex would seem more susceptible to malfunction by a xenobiotic interfering with just one of the numerous key components, which in fact is exactly what the HIV agent does. The counterargument is that the extreme versatility and sophistication of the many interconnecting components provide insurance against virulent mutants of infectious agents. Since these agents evolve rapidly in their short generation times, clones with slightly different antigen expressions or virulence factors can arise quickly. Were the immune system relatively simple, ample opportunity would be afforded for such mutants to evade the defenses. The task of the modern immunotoxicologist is to sift through all of these details in search of the most relevant applications to impaired responses.

References

Abbas, A. K., A. H. Lichtman, and J. S. Pober. 1991. *Cellular and Molecular Immunology*, pp. 228–43. Philadelphia: W.B. Saunders.

Ader, R., D. Felten, and N. Cohen. 1990. Interactions between the brain and immune system. *Annu. Rev. Pharmacol. Toxicol.* 30:561–602.

Agarwal, D. K., and R. G. Townley. 1987. Effect of platelet-activating factor on beta-adrenoreceptors in human lung. *Biochem. Biophys. Res. Commun.* 143:1–6.

Alderson, M. R., H. M. Sassenfeld, and M. B. Widmer. 1990. Interleukin 7 enhances the cytolytic T lymphocyte generation and induces lymphokine activated killer cells from human peripheral blood. *J. Exp. Med.* 172:577–87.

Alt, F. W., G. Rathbun, and G. D. Yancopoulos. 1991. DNA recombination in the brain? *Curr. Opin. Biol.* 1:3–5.

Anwar, A. R., and A. B. Kay. 1977. The ECF-A tetrapeptide and histamine selectively enhance eosinophil complement receptors. *Nature* 269:522–24.

Anwar, A. R., and A. B. Kay. 1978. Enhancement of human eosinophil complement receptors by pharmacologic mediators. *J. Immunol.* 121:1245–50.

Auron, P. E., A. C. Webb, L. J. Rosenwasser, et al. 1984. Nucleotide sequence of human monocyte IL-1 precursor cDNA. *Proc. Natl. Acad. Sci. U.S.A.* 81:7907–11.

Bagby, G. C., C. A. Dinarello, P. Wallace, et al. 1986. Interleukin 1 stimulates granulocyte macrophage colony stimulating activity release from vascular endothelial cells. *J. Clin. Invest.* 78:1316–23.

Baggiolini, M., A. Walz, and S. L. Kunkel. 1989. Neutrophil activating peptide-1/interleukin 8, a novel cytokine that activates neutrophils. *J. Clin. Invest.* 84:1045–49.

Baker, G. H. B. 1987. Psychological factors and immunity. *J. Psychosom. Res.* 31:1–10.

Barthelson, R. A., T. Potter, and F. H. Valone. 1990. Synergistic increases in IL-1 synthesis by the human monocytic cell line Thp-1 treated with PAF and endotoxin. *Cell. Immunol.* 125:142–50.

Bateman, A., A. Singh, T. Krawl, and S. Solomon. 1989. The immune–hypothalamus-pituitary–adrenal axis. *Endocrinol. Rev.* 10:92–109.

Baumann, H., G. P. Jahreis, D. N. Sauder, and A. Koj. 1984. Human keratinocytes and monocytes release factors that regulate the synthesis of major acute phase plasma proteins in hepatic cells from man, rat, and mouse. *J. Biol. Chem.* 259:7331–42.

Behrens, T. W., and J. S. Goodwin. 1989. Control of humoral immune responses by arachidonic acid metabolites. *Agents Actions* 26:15–21.

Bellinger, D. L., D. Lorton, T. D. Roman, et al. 1990. Neuropeptide innervation of lymphoid organs. *Ann. N.Y. Acad. Sci.* 594:17–33.

Berridge, M. J., and R. F. Irvine. 1984. Inositol triphosphate, a novel second messenger in cellular signal transduction. *Nature* 312:315–21.

Besedovsky, H. O., A. E. del Rey, and E. Sorkin. 1983a. What do the immune system and the brain know about each other? *Immunol. Today* 4:342–46.

Besedovsky, H. O., A. E. del Rey, and E. Sorkin. 1983b. Neurocrine immunoregulation. In *Immunoregulation*, ed. W. Fabris, E. Garaci, J. Hadden, and N. A. Mitchison, pp. 315–39. London: Plenum Press.

Billiau, A., J. Van Damme, J. Ceuppens, and M. Baroja. 1989. Interleukin 6, an ubiquitous cytokine with paracrine as well as endocrine functions. In *Lymphokine Receptor Interactions*, ed. D. Fradelizi and J. Bertoglio, pp. 133–42. London: John Libby Eurotext.

Blalock, J., and E. Smith. 1980. Human leukocyte interferon—structure and biological relatedness to adrenocorticotropic hormone and endorphins. *Proc. Natl. Acad. Sci. U.S.A.* 77:5972–78.

Blazsek, I., and G. Mathe. 1984. Zinc and immunity. *Biomed. Pharmacother.* 38:187–93.

Boron, W. F. 1984. Cell activation, the basic connection. *Nature* 312:312.

Braquet, P., L. Touqui, T. Y. Shen, and B. B. Vargaftig. 1987. Perspective in platelet-activating factor research. *Pharmacol. Rev.* 39:98–145.

Burrall, B. A., D. G. Payan, and E. J. Goetzl. 1988. Arachidonic acid-derived mediators of hypersensitivity and inflammation. In *Allergy—Principles and Practice*, ed. E. Middleton, Jr., C. E. Reed, and E. E. Ellis, pp. 164–78. St. Louis: C. V. Mosby.

Burrell, R. 1990. Immunomodulation by bacterial endotoxin. *CRC Crit. Rev. Microbiol.* 17:189–208.

Campbell, J., A. Cutri, A. Wilson, and L. Harrison. 1989. Evidence for IL-6 production by and effects on the pancreatic beta cell. *J. Immunol.* 143:1188–91.

Cantrell, D. A., A. A. Davies, and M. J. Crumpton. 1985. Activator of protein kinase C down regulation and phosphorylation of the T3/T cell antigen receptor complex of human T lymphocytes. *Proc. Natl. Acad. Sci. U.S.A* 82:8158–62.

Carswell, E., L. Old, S. Kassel, et al. 1975. An endotoxin induced serum factor that causes necrosis in tumors. *Proc. Natl. Acad. Sci. U.S.A.* 72:3666–70.

Castell, J. V., M. J. Gomez-Lechm, M. Davis, et al. 1989. Interleukin 6 is the major regulator of acute phase protein synthesis in adult human hepatocytes. *FEBS Lett.* 242:237–39.

Chen, Z. Z., K. M. Coggeshall, and J. C. Carrebier. 1986. Translocation of protein kinase C during immunoglobulin mediated transmembrane signaling in lymphocytes. *J. Immunol.* 136:2300–04.

Clark, C. T., H. Weissbach, and S. Udenfriend. 1955. 5-HT decarboxylase—preparation and properties. *J. Biol. Chem.* 210:139–48.

Clark, S. C. 1989. Interleukin 6—multiple activities in regulation of the hematopoietic and immune systems. *Ann. N.Y. Acad. Sci.* 557:438–43.

Clemens, M., and M. McNurlan. 1985. Regulation of cell proliferation and differentiation by interferons. *Biochem. J.* 226:345–60.

Coffman, R. L., J. Ohara, M. W. Bond, et al. 1986. B-cell stimulatory factor-1 enhances the IgE response of lipopolysaccharide-activated B cells. *J. Immunol.* 136:4538–41.

DeForge, L. E., D. T. Nguyen, S. L. Kunkel, and D. G. Remick. 1990. Regulation of the pathophysiology of tumor necrosis factor. *J. Lab. Clin. Med.* 116:429–38.

Dennis, G. J., J. Mizuguchi, V. McMillan, et al. 1987. Comparison of the calcium requirement for the induction and maintenance of B cell class II molecule expression and B cell proliferation. *J. Immunol.* 138:4307–12.

Depper, J. M., W. J. Leonard, C. Drogula, et al. 1985. Interleukin 2 augments transcription of the interleukin 2 receptor gene. *Proc. Natl. Acad. Sci. U.S.A.* 82:4230–34.

di Giovine, F. S., and G. W. Duff. 1990. Interleukin-1: The first interleukin. *Immunol. Today* 11:13–20.

Dinarello, C. A. 1989. Interleukin-1 and its biologically related cytokines. *Adv. Immunol.* 44:153–205.

Dukovich, M., Y. Wano, L. T. B. Thuy, et al. 1987. A second human interleukin-2 binding protein that may be a component of high affinity interleukin-2 receptors. *Nature* 327:518–22.

Dutta, J., and A. Das. 1979. Phospholipase A hydrolysis and separation of the products in a single plate. *J. Chromotogr.* 173:379–87.

Dyer, J., K. Warren, S. Merlin, and D. D. Metcalf. 1982. Measurement of plasma histidine—description of an improved method and normal values. *J. Allergy Clin. Immunol.* 70:82–87.

Felten, D. L., S. Y. Felten, D. Bellinger, et al. 1987. Noradrenergic synpathetic neural interaction with the immune system: Structure and function. *Immunol. Rev.* 100:225–60.

Flower, R. J., and G. J. Blackwell. 1976. Importance of phospholipase A in prostaglandin biosynthesis. *Biochem. Pharmacol.* 25:285–91.

Fox, C. C., A. M. Dvorak, and S. P. Peters, 1985. Isolation and characterization of human intestinal mucosal mast cells. *J. Immunol.* 135:483–491.

Gery, I., and B. H. Waksman. 1972. Potentiation of the T lymphocyte response to mitogens. *J. Exp. Med.* 136:143–55.

Goetzl, E. J., and K. F. Austen. 1975. Purification and synthesis of eosinophilotactic tetrapeptides of human lung tissue. Identification as eosinophil chemotactic factor of anaphylaxis. *Proc. Natl. Acad. Sci. U.S.A.* 72:4123–27.

Goodwin, R. G., S. Lupton, A. Schmierer, et al. 1989. Human interleukin 7: Molecular cloning and growth factor activity on human and murine B-lineage cells. *Proc. Natl. Acad. Sci. U.S.A.* 86:302–6.

Gordon, J., S. C. Ley, M. D. Melamed, et al. 1984. Immortalized B lymphocytes produce B-cell growth factor. *Nature* 310:145–47.

Grota, L., R. Ader, and N. Cohen. 1987. Taste aversion learning in autoimmune MrI-Ipr/Ipr and MrI +/+ mice. *Brain Behav. Immunol.* 1:238–50.

Hadden, J. W., and R. G. Coffey. 1990. Early biochemical events of lymphocyte transformation. In *Immunopharmacology Reviews*, Vol. 1, ed. J. W. Hadden and A. Szentivanyi, pp. 273–376. New York: Plenum Press.

Hart, P. H., G. F. Vitti, D. R. Burgess, et al. 1989. Potential anti-inflammatory effects of interleukin 4: Suppression of human monocyte tumor necrosis factor, interleukin 1, and prostaglandin E$_2$. *Proc. Natl. Acad. Sci. U.S.A.* 86:3803–7.

Hasegawa-Sasaki, H., and T. Sasaki. 1981. Phytomitogen-induced stimulation of de novo synthesis of phosphatidylinositol, phosphatidic acid and diacylglycerol in rat and human lymphocytes. *Biochem. Biophys. Acta.* 666:252–58.

Heinrich, P. C., J. V. Castell, and T. Anders. 1990. Interleukin 6 and the acute phase response. *Biochem J.* 265:621–36.

Herman, J., C. A. Dinarello, M. C. Kew, and A. R. Rabson. 1985. Role of IL-1 in tumor-NK cell interactions: Correction of defective NK cell activity in cancer patients by treating target cells with IL-1. *J. Immunol.* 135:2882–92.

Holgate, S. T., C. Robinson, and M. K. Church. 1988. Mediators of immediate hypersensitivity. In *Allergy—Principles and Practice*, ed. E. Middleton, Jr., C. E. Reed, and E. E. Ellis, pp. 135–63. St. Louis: C. V. Mosby.

Hui, D. Y., and J. A. Harmony. 1980. Phosphytidylinositol turnover in mitogen activated lymphocytes. *Biochem. J.* 192:91–98.

Isakov, N., W. Scholz, W., and A. Altman. 1986. Signal transduction and intracellular events in T-lymphocyte activation. *Immunol. Today* 7:271–277.

Juhl, H., and V. Esmann. 1979. Purification and properties of cAMP dependent and independent histone kinases from human leukocytes. *Mol. Cell. Biochem.* 26:3–18.

Kasid, A., E. Director, and S. Rosenberg. 1989. Induction of endogenous cytokine mRNA in circulating peripheral blood mononuclear cells by IL-2 administered to cancer patients. *J. Immunol.* 143:736–39.

Khansari, D. N., A. J. Murgo, and R. E. Faith. 1990. Effect of stress on the immune system. *Immunol. Today* 11:170–75.

Kilian, P. L., K. L. Kaffka, A. S. Stern, et al. 1986. Interleukin 1α and interleukin 1β bind to the same receptor on T cells. *J. Immunol.* 136:4509–14.

Kishimoto, T. 1987. B cell stimulatory factors: Molecular structure, biological function and regulation of expression. *J. Clin. Immunol.* 7:343–55.

Kohler, P., J. Hank, R. Exten, et al. 1985. Clinical response of a patient with diffuse histiocytic lymphoma to adoptive chemoimmunotherapy using cyclophosphamide and alloactivated haploidentical lymphocytes. *Cancer* 55:552–60.

Larsen, C., A. Anderson, E. Appella, et al. 1989. The neutrophil activating protein (NAP) is also chemotactic for lymphocytes. *Science* 243:1464–66.

Le, J., and J. Vilcek. 1987. Tumor necrosis factor and interleukin-1: Cytokines with multiple overlapping biological activities. *Lab Invest.* 56:234–48.

Lindahl-Kiessling, K., and R. D. Petersen. 1969. Mechanism of phytohemagglutinin action: Effect of certain enzymes and sugars. *Exp. Cell Res.* 55:81–84.

Lomedico, P. T., U. Gubler, C. P. Hellman, et. al. 1984. Cloning and expression of murine interleukin 1 cDNA in *Escherichia coli. Nature* 312:458–62.

Lotz, M., B. Zurau, D. Carson, and R. Jirik. 1989. Hepatocytes produce IL-6. *Ann. N. Y. Acad. Sci.* 557:509–17.

Lotze, M., L. Frann, S. Sharrow, et al. 1985. In vivo administration of purified human interleukin 2. *J. Immunol.* 134:157–66.

Luger, T. A., T. Schwarz, J. Krutmann, et al. 1989. Interleukin 6 is produced by epidermal cells and plays an important role in the activation of human T lymphocytes and natural killer cells. *Ann. N.Y. Acad. Sci.* 557:405–14.

MacNeil, I., T. Suda, K. Moore, et al. 1990. IL-10, a novel growth cofactor for mature and immature T cells. *J. Immunol.* 145:4167–73.

May, L. T., U. Santhanam, S. B. Tatter, et al. 1989. Multiple forms of IL-6, phosphoglycoproteins secreted by many different tissues. *Ann. N.Y. Acad. Sci.* 557:114–19.

McGillis, J. P., M. L. Organist, and D. G. Payan. 1987. Substance P and immunoregulation. *Fed. Proc.* 45:196–99.

Melmon, K. L., R. E. Rocklin, and R. P. Rogenkranz. 1981. Autocoids as mediators of inflammatory and immune responses. *Am. J. Med.* 71:100–105.

Michell, R. H., and D. Allen. 1975. Inositol cyclic phosphates as a product of phosophoinositol breakdown by phospholipase C. *FEBS Lett.* 53:302–12.

Miedema, F., J. Van Oostveen, R. Sauerwein, et al. 1985. Induction of immunoglobulin synthesis by interleukin 2 is T4$^+$/T8$^+$ cell dependent. *Eur. J. Immunol.* 15:107–12.

Mitchell, L. C., L. S. Davis, and P. E. Lipsky, 1989. Promotion of human T lymphocyte proliferation by IL-4. *J. Immunol.* 142:1548–57.

Mizel, S. B. 1989. The interleukins. *FASEB J.* 3:2379–88.

Moore, M. 1988. Interleukin 3: An overview. *Lymphokines* 15:219–80.

Moran, N. C., B. Uunaxs, and B. Westerholm. 1962. Release of 5-HT and histamine from rat mast cells. *Acta. Physiol. Scand.* 56:26–41.

Morrissey, P. J., R. G. Goodwin, R. P. Nordan, et al. 1989. Recombinant interleukin 7, pre-B cell growth factor, has costimulatory activity on purified mature T cells. *J. Exp. Med.* 169:707–16.

Mosmann, T. R. 1991. Cytokines: Is there biological meaning? *Curr. Opin. Immunol.* 3:311–15.

Mosmann, T. R., M. W. Bond, R. L. Coffman, et al. 1986. T cell and mast cell lines respond to B cell stimulatory factors-1. *Proc. Natl. Acad. Sci. U.S.A.* 83:5654–58.

Muraguchi, A., J. H. Kehrl, J. L. Butler, and A. S. Fauci. 1987. Regulation of human B cell activation, proliferation, and differentiation by soluble factors. *J. Clin. Immunol.* 4:337–47.

Naitoh, Y., J. Fukata, T. Tominaga, et al. 1988. Interleukin 6 stimulates the release of adrenocorticotropic hormone in conscious freely moving rats. *Biochem. Biophys. Res. Commun.* 155:1459–65.

Nakajima, K., T. Hirano, F. Takatsuki, et al. 1985. Physiochemical and functional properties of murine B cell derived B cell growth factor II. *J. Immunol.* 135:1207–10.

Navarro, S., N. Debili, J. Bernaudin, et al. 1989. Regulation of the expression of IL-6 in human monocytes. *J. Immunol.* 142:4339–45.

Nedwin, G., L. Svedersky, T. Bringman, et al. 1985. Effect of interleukin 2, interferon-gamma and mitogens on the production of tumor necrosis factor. *J. Immunol.* 135:2492–97.

Nel, A. E., M. W. Wooten, and R. M. Galbraith, 1987. Molecular signaling mechanisms in T-lymphocyte activation pathways. *Clin. Immunol. Immunopathol.* 44:167–86.

O'Dorisio, M. S., C. L. Wood, and T. M. O'Dorisio. 1985. Vasoactive intestinal peptide and neuropeptide modulation of the immune response. *J. Immunol.* 135:792s–95s.

O'Flaherty, J. T., J. R. Surles, J. Redman, et al. 1986. Binding and metabolism of platelet activating factor by human neutrophils. *J. Clin. Invest.* 78:381–88.

Okusawa, S., J. A. Gelfand, T. Ikejima, et al. 1988. Interleukin 1 induces a shock like response in rabbits. *J. Clin. Invest.* 81:1162–72.

Olson, N. C., P. B. Joyce, and L. N. Fleisher. 1990. Mono-hydroxyeicosatetraenoic acids during porcine endotoxemia. Effect of platelet-activating factor receptor antagonist. *Lab. Invest.* 63:221–32.

Oppenheim, J. J., E. J. Kovacs, and K. Matsushima. 1986. There is more than one interleukin 1. *Immunol. Today.* 7:45–56.

Paganelli, K. A., A. S. Stern, and P. L. Kilian. 1987. Detergent solubilization of the Interleukin 1 receptor. *J. Immunol.* 138:2249–53.

Park, L., D. Friend, S. Gillis, and D. Urdal. 1986. Characterization of the cell surface receptor for a multi-lineage colony stimulating factor (CSF-2a). *J. Biol. Chem.* 261:205–10.

Paul, N. L. and N. H. Ruddle. 1988. Lymphotoxin. *Annu. Rev. Immunol.* 6:407–38.

Paul, W. E. and J. Ohara. 1987. B cell stimulatory factors/interleukin 4. *Annu. Rev. Immunol.* 5:429–59.

Pauwels, R., H. Bazan, B. Platteau, and M. van der Straeten. 1980. Influence of adrenergic drugs on IgE production. *Int. Arch. Allergy Appl. Immunol.* 61:347–51.

Peschel, C., I. Green, and W. E. Paul. 1989. Preferential proliferation of immature B lineage cells in long-term stromal cell-dependent cultures with IL-4. *J. Immunol.* 142:1558–68.

Pimental, E. 1990. Colony stimulating factors. *Ann. Clin. Lab. Sci.* 20:36–55.

Pizza, G., G. Severini, D. Menniti, et al. 1984. Tumor regression after intralesional injection of IL-2 in bladder cancer. *Int. J. Cancer* 34:359–67.

Quastel, M. B., and J. G. Kaplan. 1970. Early stimulation of potassium uptake in lymphocytes stimulated with PHA. *Exp. Cell Res.* 63:230–33.

Rappaport, R. S., and G. R. Dodge. 1982. Prostaglandin E inhibits the production of human interleukin 2. *J. Exp. Med.* 155:943–48.

Reilly, F., R. McCuskey, and H. Meineke. 1976. Studies of the hematopoietic environment. VII: Adrenergic and cholinergic innervation of the murine spleen. *Anat. Rec.* 185:109–18.

Reinhardt, D., and U. Borchard. 1982. H_1 receptor antagonists: Comparative pharmacology and clinical use. *Klin. Wochenschr.* 60:983–90.

Rittenhouse-Simmons, L., and D. Deykin. 1978. Activation by calcium of platelet phospholipase A. *Biochem. Biophys. Acta.* 543:409–22.

Roehm, N. W., J. Liebson, and A. Zlotnick. 1984. Interleukin 4 induces increase in Ia expression by normal mouse B cells. *J. Exp. Med.* 160:679–94.

Sanderson, C. J., H. D. Campbell, and I. G. Young. 1988. Molecular and cellular biology of eosinophil differention factor (interleukin-5) and its effects on human amd mouse B cells. *Immunol. Rev.* 102:29–50.

Sauder, D. N. 1989. Interleukin 1. *Arch. Dermatol.* 125:679–82.

Schayer, R. W. 1963. Histidine decarboxylase in man. *Ann. N.Y. Acad. Sci.* 103:164–78.

Schrader, J., F. Battye, and R. Scollay. 1982. Expression of Thy-1 antigen is not limited to T cells in cultures of mouse hematopoietic cells. *Proc. Natl. Acad. Sci. U.S.A.* 79:4161–65.

Schulman, E. S., A. Kagey-Sobotka, and I. W. MacGlashen. 1983. Heterogeneity of human mast cells. *J. Immunol.* 131:1936–41.

Schwartz, L. B., and K. F. Austen. 1984. Structure and function of the chemical mediators of mast cells. *Prog. Allergy.* 34:271–321.

Schwartz, L. B., and K. F. Austen. 1988. The mast cell and mediators of immediate hypersensitivity. In *Immunological Diseases*, 4th ed., ed. M. Samter, D. W. Talmage, M. M. Frank, et al. pp. 157–517. Boston: Little, Brown.

Sehgal, P., D. Helfgott, U. Santhanam, et al. 1988. Regulation of the acute phase and immune responses in viral disease. *J. Exp. Med.* 167:1951–56.

Shackelford, I. A., and I. A. Trowbridge. 1984. Induction and expression of phosphorylation of the human IL-2 receptor by a phorbol diester. *J. Biol. Chem.* 259:11706–12.

Simms, J. E., C. J. March, D. Cosmna, et al. 1988. cDNA expression cloning of the IL-1 receptor, a member of the super immunoglobulin family. *Science* 241:585–89.

Smith, E. M., M. Phan, T. Kruger, et al. 1983. Human lymphocyte production of immunoreactive thyrotropin. *Proc. Natl. Acad. Sci. U.S.A.* 80:6010–13.

Smith, J. W., A. C. Steiner, W. M. Newberry, and C. W. Parker. 1971. cAMP in human lymphocytes—alterations after PHA stimulation. *J. Clin. Invest.* 50:432–41.

Stein, M. 1989. Stress, depression and the immune sytem. *J. Clin. Psychiatry* 50(55):35–40.

Streb, H., R. F. Irvine, M. J. Berridge, and I. Schulz. 1983. Release of calcium from nonmitochondrial intracellular stores in pancreatic acinar cells by inositol-1,4,5-triphosphate. *Nature* 306:67–69.

Streiter, R. M., S. W. Chensue, M. A. Basha, et al. 1990. Human alveolar macrophage gene expression of interleukin-8 by TNF-α and IL-1β. *Am. J. Respir. Cell. Mol. Biol.* 2:321–26.

Streiter, R. M., S. L. Kunkel, H. J. Showell, et al. 1989. Endothelial cell gene expression of a neutrophil chemotactic factor by TNF-α, LPS, and IL-1β. *Science* 243:1467–69.

Streiter, R. M., S. H. Phan, H. J. Showell, et al. 1989. Monokine-induced neutrophil chemotactic factor gene expression in human fibroblasts. *J. Biol. Chem.* 264:10621–26.

Suda, J., T. Suda, K. Kubota, et al. 1986. Purified IL-3 and erythropoietin support the terminal differentiation of hematopoietic progenitors in serum free culture. *Blood* 67:1002–6.

Suda, T., A. O'Garra, I. MacNeil, et al. 1990. Identification of a novel thymocyte growth promoting factor derived from B cell lymphomas. *Cell. Immunol.* 129:228–40.

Takatsu, K., Y. Kikuchi, T. Takahashi, et al. 1987. Interleukin 5, a T cell derived B cell differentiation factor also induces cytotoxic T lymphocytes. *Proc. Natl. Acad. Sci.* 84:4234–38.

Takatsuki, F., A. Okano, C. Suzuki, et al. 1988. Human recombinant IL-6/B stimulatory factor 2 augments murine antigen specific antibody responses in vitro and in vivo. *J. Immunol.* 141:3072–77.

Tanamoto, K., U. Schade, and E. T. Rietschel. 1989. Sensitization of alveolar macrophages to lipopolysaccharide-induced prostaglandin synthesis by exogenous prostaglandins. *Biochem. Biophys. Res. Commun.* 165:526–32.

Tsien, R. Y., T. Pozzan, and T. J. Rink. 1982. T cell mitogens cause early changes in cytoplasmic free calcium and membrane potential in lymphocytes. *Nature* 295:68–71.

Turnball, L. W., D. P. Evans, and A. B. Kay. 1977. Human eosinophils, acidic tetrapeptides and histamine. *Immunology* 32:57–64.

Ulich, T., J. Del Castillo, and K. Guo. 1989. In vivo hematologic effects of recombinant interleukin 6 on hematopoiesis and circulating numbers of RBCs and WBCs. *Blood* 73:108–110.

Uvnas, B., C. G. Aborg, and A. Bergendoff. 1970. Evidence for an ionic binding of histamine to protein carboxyls in the granule haparin protein complex. *Acta. Physiol. Scand. [Suppl.]* 336:3–26.

Uyttenhove, C., R. J. Simpson, and J. van Svick. 1988. Functional and structural characterization of P40, a mouse glycoprotein with T cell growth factor activity. *Proc. Natl. Acad. Sci. U.S.A.* 85:6934–38.

Valone, F. H., and E. J. Goetzl. 1983. Selective binding by human polymorphonuclear leukocytes of the immunological mediator 1-o-hexadecyl/octadecyl-2-acetyl-SN-glyceryl-3-phosphoryl-chlorine. *Immunology* 48:141–49.

Van Damme, J., M. DeLey, G. Opdenakke, et al. 1985. Homogeneous interferon inducing 22 kdal factor is related to endogenous pyrogen and IL-1. *Nature* 314:266–68.

Van Damme, J., M. DeLey, J. Van Snick, et al. 1987. The role of interferon-β, and the 26-kdal protein as mediators of the antiviral effect of interleukin 1 and TNF. *J. Immunol.* 139:1867–72.

Vitetta, E. S., J. Ohara, C. Myers, et al. 1985. Serological, biochemical and functional identity of B-cell stimulatory factor 1 and B-cell differentiation factor for IgG$_1$. *J. Exp. Med.* 162:1726–31.

Watson, M. L., G. P. Lewis, and J. Westwick. 1988. Neutrophil stimulation by recombinant cytokines and a factor produced by IL-1-treated synovial cell culture. *Immunology* 65:567.

Waxal, M. J. 1983. Membrane methylation and early biochemical reactions in the mitogenic action of lymphocytes. In *Advances in Immunopharmacology*, ed. J. W. Hadden, pp. 81–86. Oxford: Pergamon Press.

Weigert, D. A., and E. Blalock, 1987. Interaction between the neuroendocrine and immune system: Common hormones and receptors. *Immunol. Rev.* 100:79–102.

Whitefield, J. F., J. P. MacManus, A. L. Boynton, et al. 1974. Con A and the initiation of the thymic lymphoblast DNA synthesis and proliferation by calcium dependent increases in cGMP levels. *J. Cell Physiol.* 84:445–58.

Williams, L., R. Petersen, P. Shea, et al. 1981. Sympathetic innervation of murine thymus and spleen—evidence for a functional link between the nervous and immune systems. *Brain Res. Bull.* 6:83–94.

Williams, L., R. Snyderman, and R. Lefkowitz. 1976. Identification of beta adrenergic receptors in human lymphocytes by alprenolol binding. *J. Clin. Invest.* 57:149–55.

Woloski, B., E. M. Smith, W. J. Meyer, et al. 1985. Corticotropin releasing activity of monokines. *Science* 230:1035–38.

Wolvekamp, C., and R. Marquet. 1990. Interleukin 6: Historical background, genetics and biological significance. *Immunol. Lett.* 24:1–10.

Wong, G. G., and S. C. Clark. 1988. Multiple actions of interleukin 6 within a cytokine network. *Immunol. Today.* 9:137–39.

Yamasaki, K., T. Taga, T. Matsuda, et al. 1989. Interleukin 6 and its receptor. In *Lymphokine Receptor Interactions*, ed. D. Fradelizi and J. Bertoglio, pp. 143–50. London: John Libbey Eurotext.

Zhang, X., B. Klein, and R. Gataille. 1989. Interleukin 6 is a potent myeloma cell growth factor in patients with aggressive multiple myeloma. *Blood* 74:11–13.

Zhang, Y., J. Lin, Y. Yip, and J. Vilcek. 1989. Stimulation of interleukin 6 mRNA levels by tumor necrosis factor and interleukin 1. *Ann. N.Y. Acad. Sci.* 557:548–49.

Zilberstein, A., R. Ruggieri, J. H. Kohrn, and M. Revel. 1986. Structure and expression of cDNA and genes for human interferon-beta-2, a distinct species inducible by growth stimulatory cytokines. *EMBO J.* 5:2529–37.

Zilberstein, A., R. Ruggieri, and M. Revel, 1985. In *The Interferon System*, ed. R. Rossi and F. Dianzani, pp. 77–83. New York: Raven Press.

Zoon, K., Y. Karasaki, D. zur Nedden, et al. 1987. Modulation of epidermal growth factor receptors by human α interferon. *Proc. Natl. Acad. Sci. U.S.A.* 83:8226–30.

Zucali, J., G. Elfenheim, K. Barth, and C. Dinarello. 1987. Effects of human IL-1 and TNF on human T lymphocyte colony formation. *J. Clin. Invest.* 80:772–77.

5

Effector Mechanisms: Expression of Immunity

A. INTRODUCTION

Much of modern immunology has been concerned with the induction or afferent phase of the immune response, including those facets involved in antigen recognition, processing, and presentation as well as characteristics of developing immunologic diversity. This and the preceding chapter are concerned with events subsequent to induction and focus on mechanisms by which recognition of foreign stimuli is translated into biological activity. The previous chapter dealt mainly with humoral mediators and the pharmacology of both afferent and efferent immune responses, whereas the present chapter is mainly concerned with cellular mediators and activities.

If the major function of the immune system is to recognize and dispose of foreign matter, it is appropriate to be concerned with how this happens. Recognition of both antigen-specific and non-antigen-specific stimuli must become translated into some sort of biological action before the immune response can really be considered complete. Both cellular and molecular mechanisms are operative and often act synergistically for optimum function. The most obvious area of concern is neutralization or disposition of the infectious/noxious agent. A second area deals with matters relating to initiation of secondary inflammatory effectors used in disposition. Immunotoxicologists become involved when the external agent interferes with either afferent or efferent phases of the immune response or when the execution of the efferent phases results in host injury. These concerns are examined in detail by considering the various means of expression of the immune response.

Although much of contemporary immunology is concerned with antigen-specific recognition of foreignness, there is increasing realization that the body has a variety of chemical means of recognizing foreignness independent of antigen-specific means. Natural killer cells seem to be able to recognize tumor or viral substances in such an independent way. There is no doubt that both the classical and alternative complement pathways may be triggered independently of antigen-antibody complexes. Macrophages, particularly Kupffer cells, are able to recognize glycoproteins bearing a high amount of mannose (a rather universal expression of lower types of organisms) and have evolved receptors for such sugars, perhaps to deal with such microbes (Stahl 1990). Other types of molecules unique to microorganisms, e.g., lipopolysaccharides (endotoxin) and peptidoglycans, also are able to excite a wide variety of inflammatory mechanisms independent of antigen recognition by the unique nature of their chemical structures. Although the means of recognition may be different, both antigen- and non-antigen-specific effector mechanisms get translated into the same types of efferent action.

B. HUMORAL MECHANISMS

Until the 1960s, most immunology began and ended with a study of antibodies. They were the first immune effectors to be discovered and are certainly the easiest to work with. Much is known about their chemical structure, the genetic basis for generating their tremendous diversity, and their synthesis. Additionally, there is an impressive technology applicable to their demonstration and measurement.

1. Humoral Antibodies

Humoral antibodies can take part in defensive immunity in four ways, summarized in Fig. 5–1: direct neutralization of molecules or particles, opsonizing particles for phagocytosis, activation of the complement system, and participation in antibody-dependent cellular cytotoxicity (ADCC). Humoral antibodies can effectively neutralize infectious substances in comparatively few ways by themselves. If the antigenic group is identical with the toxic portion of the molecule, the antibody can simply neutralize it by binding to this region before the agent becomes bound to its receptor. Alternatively, if the antibody attaches to the cellular adhesion site of an infectious particle, the agent cannot initiate infection. An

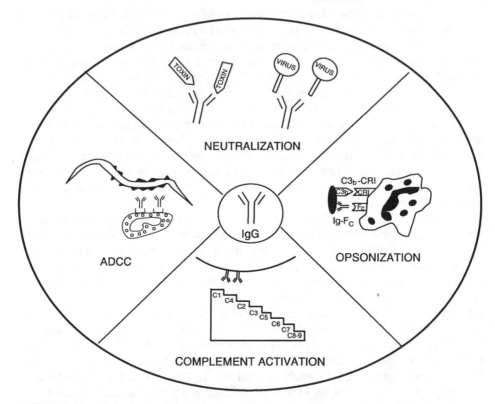

FIGURE 5–1. Major mechanisms by which humoral antibodies participate in defensive immunity. Antibodies may directly occlude or neutralize toxins or adherence receptors of infectious particles; they may opsonize particles for phagocytosis by possession of immunoglobulin Fc receptors; immune complexes may activate the complement system; and they are essential in antibody-dependent cellular cytotoxicity (ADCC).

antibody for a virus could prevent attachment, penetration, or viral uncoating, all individual steps required for completion of the viral life cycle.

On the other hand, the effect of specific humoral antibodies can be enhanced by acting synergistically with other humoral or cellular agents. One major function of antibody is to enhance engulfment by phagocytic cells, a process called opsonization. In the case of the former, antibody bound to the foreign particle becomes affixed to phagocytes by means of Fc receptors, thus greatly enhancing the cell's antigen-capturing ability. Another type of opsonization is complement dependent; this is discussed below. Antibody effectiveness is also greatly enhanced by the process of ADCC, wherein antigen-specific antibody attaches by means of Fc receptors to certain types of NK cells, macrophages, or eosinophils and other granulocytes, enabling these cells to attach intimately to the target cells and kill targets by individual means. The effect of specific humoral antibodies can also be considerably amplified by other substances. The best studied is through the cooperation of a nonspecific humoral mechanism, the complement system. Not only do complement activation products have a variety of cellular and organ inflammatory functions that can be considered defensive, but the activation system can also promote a different type of opsonization, and if the antigen is cellular, the activated complement components or fragments can cause target cell lysis. The complement system is so important in amplifying defense and inflammation that a brief examination of it follows.

2. The Complement System

Complement is not a single substance but a carefully regulated system of functionally linked proteins, many with enzymatic activities, that interact in an ordered cascade. By-products resulting from enzymatic cleavage of individual cascade components induce numerous biological effects that are responsible for many of the effector mechanisms of both specific and nonspecific immunity. Although the by-products are humoral substances, each would be impotent without its equally important cellular receptor, which functions at the cell membrane level.

Overview of Complement Activation
The individual proteins in the cascade series function as enzymes, the activation of one leading to the activation of the next in the sequence, and so on. With almost every step in the cascade (through C5), there is cleavage of a small-molecular-weight peptide (termed the *a* fragment) from the larger *b* fragment. The small peptide often has biological activity in itself. Although the larger fragment may have its own activity, it is more important in activating the next protein in the series. Each step in the cascade is subject to a number of regulating controls that either amplify, dampen, or stabilize the activation process.

There are many individual steps in the complement system, and their complexity and necessarily complicated nomenclature frighten the newcomer. To add to the complexity is the fact that there exist several pathways and several control factors. The key to understanding the complement process is to recognize that the conversion of the most abundant component, C3, by the enzyme C3 convertase is the point at which all of the paths converge and is also the main point in the cascade where even a small activation signal is greatly amplified. Two pathways, the classical and the alternative, are the routes through which foreign recognition signals result in the production of C3 convertase (see Fig. 5–2). From this point of convergence, the remaining steps are referred to as the lytic or common pathway. In addition, the positive-feedback amplification loop whereby many molecules of the activated C3 product (C3b) are produced from a small amount of convertase may also be considered a distinct pathway (Pangburn 1983).

Some sense can be gleaned from this seeming mass of confusion by concentrating on the two most important steps, the initial activating events and the amplification of the signal. The classical and alternative pathways essentially represent different ways the body has to recognize foreignness. The classical pathway (components designated by numerical terms, e.g., C1, C3) is activated primarily (but not exclusively) by antigen–antibody complexes and is the major way antibody recognition of foreignness is translated into biological action in vivo. Biological recognition of foreignness is accomplished when antigen–antibody complexes (composed of IgM, IgG$_1$, IgG$_2$, or IgG$_3$, but not IgG$_4$) react through particular portions of their constant domains with the first component of the classical pathway, a C1 complex, which then generates serine esterase activity capable of activating the next component, and so on.

The alternative pathway (components designated by letters, e.g., factor B) is the pathway in which chemical foreignness is recognized independent of anti-

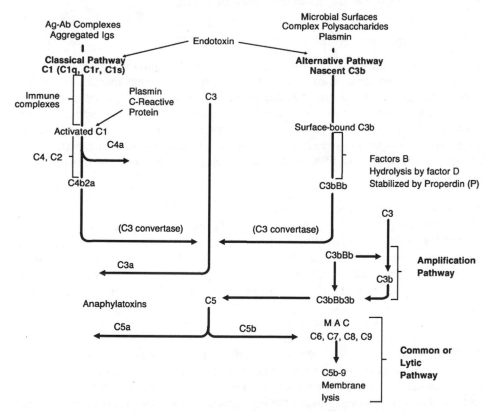

FIGURE 5–2.   An overview scheme of the complement activation pathways illustrating the key steps. The left side of the flow sheet depicts the major classical pathway steps leading to C3 convertase; the right side shows the alternative pathway. Although the lower right shows the amplification pathway by which activated C3bBb converts more C3 to activated forms, this process takes place with either pathway. The common or lytic pathway is shown in the lower right corner.

body. Such materials as highly polymerized, colloidal, or complex polysaccharide substances, i.e., products not commonly found in the body, are agents most likely to activate the alternative pathway in the absence of antibody (Osler and Sandberg 1973). Additionally, C3 convertase activation via the alternative pathway occurs on insoluble microbial cell surfaces, not on autologous host cells. In this manner, the alternative pathway functions in an antigen-independent way in defense. The C3b that has become activated by either pathway or by slow internal decay serves to make factor B a more labile substrate for proteolytic cleavage by subsequent components. This resulting protein, Bb, becomes bound to C3b, and the resulting complex is stabilized by a protein known as properdin. From here, the complex may enter the amplification loop, because in this form it is an active C3 convertase capable of generating more C3b, or, after complexing further with C3 products, it may proceed to the common pathway. In addition, the complement system is integrated with other systems; i.e., it can be activated or be the activator of the coagulation and kinin-generating systems. Certain mediators such as platelet-activating factor (PAF) also seem to be able to activate the complement system in vivo (Sun and Hsueh 1991).

Once C3b is produced and complexed, ad seriatim activation of subsequent components (C5–C9), i.e., the lytic or common pathway, is the same, regardless of the pathway by which the C3 convertase activation was initiated. This terminal sequence is lytic for bacteria, erythrocytes, and mammalian cells by inserting into the lipid bilayer of the cell and causing porous lesions that destroy normal osmotic and ionic permeability barriers (Biesecker 1983). The terminal sequence (membrane attack complex or MAC) can also attach directly to glycoprotein basement membranes (Kopp and Burrell 1982). The end result can be direct action on either the activator surface in which an immune complex is bound or on bystander surfaces.

Regulation of the Complement System

Although these individual items are considered essential for an intact host defense, it is also easy to see how unregulated amplification of such a system or direction of it to antigens present on healthy cellular membranes can lead to tissue injury. It is also easy to see in even this simple scheme how many different vulnerable points are exposed to potentially harmful substances capable of inhibiting normal function. Not only is the complement system under several different forms of regulation, but some of the activated components have regulatory effects on other components of the immune system.

Forms of complement regulation include mechanisms of enhancement, stabilization from decay, coordination of activities, amplification, and inhibition. These forms of regulation within the complement system are summarized in Table 5–1, but only the major types are discussed. One form of enhancement was mentioned previously, that of the amplification feedback loop. Many of the individual activated components are quite labile to decay, especially if they do not attach to surfaces, and some of the complexes are unstable. Mention has been made of the stabilizing role of properdin, and once bound to C3b, C3b becomes protected from decay-accelerating proteins (Factors H and I). Coordination of the overall biological effects may be seen by the nature of the sequential activation as individually activated components become available for reactivity. The process of transfer of activated components from the fluid to the solid phase helps speed up assembly and focuses the effects of activation at target sites. Some

TABLE 5–1.   Key Factors and Events in Complement Regulation

I. Enhancers: amplification
  1. Amplification feedback loop
  2. Conglutinin (anti-C3b), increases during immunization
  3. C3NeF, autoantibody for C3b,Bb
      a. Stabilizes convertase from decay
      b. Complex further activates classical pathway
  4. Interaction with other cascades, e.g., coagulation, kininogens
II. Stabilizers
  1. Properdin stabilizes C3b,Bb
  2. Bound C3b is protected from factors H and I decay
III. Control or inactivation
  1. Most activated components spontaneously decay
  2. Stochiometric inhibition
      a. C1–INH, C1 esterase inhibitor normally present
      b. C4b-binding protein
         Interferes with C3 convertase production
         Accelerates decay of C4,2
      c. Factor H, makes more susceptible to factor I, is a competitive inhibitor of factor B
         activation, dissociates Bb from C3b,Bb, augments rate of C3b inactivation
      d. S protein, competes with C5b,6,7 by binding and preventing membrane attachment
  3. Enzymatic inhibition
      a. Factor I, inactivates C3b, stopping cascade, converts to C3bi then cleaves to C3c and
         C3d, cleaves C3d on surface
      b. Nonspecific proteases inactivate fluid C3
      c. Anaphylatoxin exopeptidases
      d. Plasmin attacks activated C5,6,7
      e. Factor D can cleave C3b,Bb
  4. Membrane bound inhibitors
      a. C3b/C4b receptor (CR1), factor I cofactor, dissociates C3 and C5 convertases
      b. Decay-accelerating factor (DAF), enhances decay of C3 convertases

of the regulation is in the form of stoichiometric inhibition or molecular binding to a controlling agent. The classical pathway is in part controlled by a C1 esterase inhibitor (C1–INH) that normally helps prevent runaway activation of the classical pathway, a C4 binding protein that competitively inhibits interaction with the next pathway component (C2), and a decay-accelerating factor that acts to dampen C3 convertase production.

Factors that help regulate the alternative pathway include the interaction between two proteins, Factor H and Factor I. The former competes with the initiating Factor B for binding to available C3b and makes the C3b complexes more susceptible to Factor I proteolysis. Balancing this effect is the stabilizing action of properdin. Formation of the membrane attack complex is inhibited by various proteins, one of which (homologous restriction factor) inhibits binding of C8 to C9, the terminal complement component, and another of which blocks C7 conversion (CD59), to give two examples. Finally, various enzymes such as circulating exopeptidases and extracellular proteases help control side effects by digesting smaller cleavage fragments and any remaining unbound C3b, respectively.

Complement receptors
As with any biologically active substance, individual complement components must act by attaching to specific receptors before cell membrane perturbation can take place. In addition, many of these receptors have regulatory roles on the

complement cascade itself. One receptor, CR1 (CD35), is important in a major biological function of complement activation, immune adherence. It is found on most peripheral blood cells. Although there are a hundredfold more receptor CR1 sites on neutrophils than on erythrocytes, it should be remembered that there are far more of the latter cells. If complement is attached to a phagocyte, complement-mediated opsonization is effected independent of antibody, thus promoting phagocytosis. Often immune adherence (adsorption of immune complexes to cells) first takes place on such cells as erythrocytes, which in effect serves to increase particle size and thereby enhances the phagocytic process. The CR1 also acts as a cofactor for Factor I cleavage of C3b. This receptor is additionally found on most B cells and 15% of T cells, and it may function to help trap antigen–antibody complexes in lymph nodes.

A second receptor known as CR2 is found on 50–80% of B cells, some T cells, and certain antigen-presenting cells, where it binds C3 degradation products, helping to localize complexes to B-cell-rich areas. This attachment possibly helps facilitate antigen-driven immune responses. CR3 receptors are found principally on bone-marrow-derived cells such as monocytes, neutrophils, mast cells, and NK cells. The CR3 receptor binds breakdown products of C and is more efficient than CR1 in triggering phagocytosis and endothelial attachment of myeloid lineage cells. The less-known CR4 receptor, found on both myeloid and lymphoid elements, is related to CR3 structurally and functionally. There are other receptors for the cleavage fragments C3a, C4a, and C5a. Receptors for the first two are found on mast cells and basophils and are important in stimulating vasoactive mediator release. A C5a receptor, found on neutrophils, rapidly internalizes and recycles to cell membrane surfaces and promotes chemotaxis. Its presence on endothelial cells seems associated with regulating vascular permeability. Finally, there is an important receptor for a subcomponent of C1 (C1q), found on monocytes, B cells, and neutrophils, that is important in initial binding of activated immune complexes.

Biological Consequences of Complement Activation

Most of the well-known biological effects of complement are related to its inflammation-generating and other defensive functions, but there is a growing realization that complement products are involved in regulatory events involving other components of the immune system. Not only must one consider the biological effects of all pathway components, but the activities of activated complement receptors must be considered equally. Table 5–2 summarizes many of these effects according to the activation step in the cascade at which a particular component becomes active. Certainly in terms of its serum concentration and multiplicity of roles, C3 is the most versatile component in the cascade, and from the activation standpoint, is the hub of all activity (Lambris 1988).

One of the major functions of activated components, particularly once the common pathway is initiated, is the chemotactic effect on neutrophils. Elicitation of neutrophils is one of the major ways complement activation gets translated into cellular functions. Another way this translation is effected is through the spasmogenic and vasoactive functions of complement split products C3a and C5a. These extremely potent fragments effect local permeability increases and smooth muscle constriction and for these reasons are often called anaphylatoxins. Another major role of activated complement is through the removal of immune complexes by the processes of immune adherence and opsonization. If

TABLE 5–2.   Overview of Biological Effects of Complement Components and Receptors

Component	Biological Function
Classical pathway	
Activated C1q,r,s	Causes increased stabilization of Ag–Ab complexes[a]
C4a, kinin peptide	Causes local edema
Activated C4b	Important in virus, *Shigella* neutralization
C2a fragment	Kinin activity
CR1	C4b,C3b receptor
	Immune adherence
	Opsonization
	C3 covertase regulation
	Antigen trapping in lymph nodes
Activated C3b	Immune adherence
	Opsonization[a]
	Platelet lysis
	Alternative pathway substrate
	Target of conglutinin; enhances phagocytosis
	Chemotactic for macrophages
	Stimulates B cells to make lymphokines
	C3 important in generating 2° response
CR2	Aids in antigen trapping and presentation
C3a fragment	Vasoactive
C5a fragment	Chemotactic, vasocactive
	Potent IL-1-releasing stimulant of monocytes
Activated C567	Extremely chemotactic for PMNs[a]
C6	May be required for clotting[a]
C8	Slow membrane damage
C9	Fast membrane damage
C8–C9	Initiates prostaglandin synthesis
	Increases permeability to arachidonic acid metabolites
Alternative pathway	
Factor B	Sequence initiation
Ba fragment	Inhibits human B-cell proliferation
CR3	Important in macrophage phagocytosis and attachment to endothelium

[a]Coagulation pathways intersect with these components.

there are complement component deficiencies, or if xenobiotics interfere with this vital process, the continuous presence of circulating immune complexes could lead to deposition in vulnerable locations and cause inflammation. The beneficial effects of inflammation are enhanced at several points where the complement activation sequence interacts with other enzymatic cascades, e.g., the clotting or kinin-generating cascades (see Table 5–2). In addition, plasmin and thrombin may use C3 and C5 as substrates (and thus can activate the membrane attack sequence), and C3b can activate platelets. Finally, the end point of insertion of terminal sequences into cell membranes leads to target cell lysis, the best-known activity of complement.

Although complement activation was first discovered by studying lysis of the cholera *Vibrio* bacteria, it is doubtful that microbial lysis is a frequent or very important defense mechanism in vivo. On the other hand, complement-mediated target cell lysis of allogeneic graft cells or host cells coated with foreign antigens does represent an important means of defense. Although all of these complement-mediated mechanisms are certainly important in defense, it should be noted that nearly all of them are also inflammatory and capable of inducing host injury. These aspects of complement activation are examined in more detail in Chapter 6.

In light of all of the well-known defensive and inflammatory effects of complement, it may come as a surprise to learn that individual complement components also exert several forms of regulation on other immune effectors. To cite a few examples, C5a is a potent IL-1–releasing stimulant of monocytes, C3 fragments are involved in IL-2–dependent T-cell proliferation, and CR2 is involved in B-cell proliferation (Lambris 1988). Although C3a has been found to suppress antigen-specific antibody responses, this effect was not accomplished through suppression of lymphocyte proliferative responses (Morgan et al. 1984). Rather, the inhibitory effect depended on the stimulation of suppressor cell activity. In contrast, C5a augmented antibody responses in vitro and T-cell proliferative responses. That the alternative pathway is also involved in immunoregulation has been shown by studies in which a cleavage fragment of factor B has been found to inhibit stimulated human B-cell proliferation, whereas factor Bb enhances proliferation under similar conditions (Ambrus et al. 1990). The idea that nonantigen-specific activation can regulate B-cell responses is intriguing.

The interference of xenobiotics with the complement system is known mainly from the inflammation derived from either immune complex or nonspecific activation of the complement cascades (Chapter 6), but perhaps more attention should be focused on whether such agents could interfere with individual component activation or expression of complement receptors. At least one outside agent seems to affect the complement system in a manner inconsistent with either the alternative or classical pathway activation, and that is the infectious mononucleosis virus (Epstein–Barr virus). It may attach directly to CR2, indirectly accelerate the decay of alternative-pathway-activated C3 convertase, and affect Factor I cleavage of C3b (Lambris 1988). In this instance, interaction seems to result from similarities in amino acid sequences of agonists, but other possibilities should be examined with other agents. Microorganisms provide other insights by which chemical substances might possibly interfere with the complement system. These include microorganisms that possess substances such as sialic acid, which creates surface-related instability of the C3 convertase, enzymes that cleave complement receptors, or molecules similar to decay-accelerating factor (Cross and Kelly 1990).

C. NEUTROPHILS AND PHAGOCYTIC MECHANISMS

Neutrophil and macrophage functions are often studied in vitro because of the ease of their separation from other leukocytes and because the predominant parameters selected are usually concerned with phagocytosis. As important as phagocytosis is, in vivo functions of these cells are much more diverse, and the process is only a small part of total inflammation. Phagocytic functions can be carried out primarily by macrophages/ monocytes, neutrophils, and eosinophils. A neutrophil infiltrate or increase in peripheral blood is the main indicator of acute inflammation and is the cell type about which most of the phagocytic activity is known. The complex activities of neutrophils, including growth and maturation, are governed by a variety of mediators and cytokines. The phagocytic process is but one of these, and it can be conveniently divided into several components for discussion.

Chemotaxis

Phagocytic cells are attracted by a number of substances, and although there may be specific cytokine differences for eliciting different leukocyte types, the basic process is the same for all. Microbial cells and other foreign particles may express certain chemical structures, especially microbially derived peptides beginning with formyl-methionine sequences, that independently stimulate neutrophil chemotaxis. Neutrophils also respond to a variety of mediators such as complement-generated chemotaxins, LTB_4, a mast-cell-derived neutrophil chemotactic factor, and platelet-activating factor (PAF), as well as cytokines such as those produced by macrophages (e.g., TNF) or lymphocytes (INF-γ). Membrane signaling leads to a decrease in the negative charge of the cell membrane which affects migration as well as adhesion and receptor expression (e.g., CR3). In vivo chemotaxis must be accompanied by changes in endothelial cells to permit passage of the neutrophils into the tissue through the capillary wall (diapedesis), a process itself under the influence of many mediators, some of which may emanate from the neutrophils. The formerly random movement of the neutrophil now takes a more unidirectional path along a concentration gradient of the attractant from regions of low to high concentration (although some substances may negatively propel neutrophils).

Engulfment

Engulfment consists of attachment and ingestion phases. Attachment of unopsonized particles is determined by the surface properties of hydrophobicity and surface tension. Phagocytes can effectively phagocytize unopsonized particles with help from such substances as fibronectin or fibrin if the particle surface charge is hydrophobic and hence possesses less charge repulsion. If the cell surfaces are hydrophilic, the cells will require opsonization for optimal attachment. Opsonization can be antibody dependent via Fc receptors for heavy chains of immunoglobulins or complement dependent through various complement receptors discussed above. Actual ingestion involves invagination of the adherent particle with receptor into a membrane-bound phagosome. This is an energy-requiring process that also involves intracytoplasmic microfilament formation.

Metabolic Events

All phagocytic functions are highly energy dependent, and metabolic events are initiated with the onset of initial cell membrane signaling. Metabolic pathways undergo a strong respiratory burst resulting in increased glycolysis, an increase in hexose-monophosphate shunt activity, increased oxygen consumption, and attendant H_2O_2 and lactic acid production. Not only is energy acquired, but metabolic by-products are used in microbial killing. There is enhanced RNA transcription as well as the expected phospholipid turnover from the membrane events. The enzyme NADPH oxidase converts NADPH to NADP, which, in addition to donating electrons for energy capture, makes available a product useful in many other metabolic functions. Perhaps the most important metabolic function is involved in generating H_2O_2. The entire metabolic process is often called activation, but it must be differentiated from other types of immunologic activation.

The production of intermediate oxygen metabolites is vital to several functions of activated neutrophils and macrophages (Klebanoff 1982). An overview of the oxygen radical pathways is presented in Fig. 5-3. Superoxide anion ($O_2{}^-$) is an intermediate that, although not directly injurious, is important in generating peroxides when acted on by the enzyme superoxide dismutase. Singlet oxygen ($^1O_2$) is a metabolite with a distorted arrangement of its electrons enabling it to be more reactive. It is produced in several ways and is useful in generating toxic lipid peroxides. When formed, each molecule has a short half-life, and its energy is dissipated as light emission. This characteristic is exploited in the laboratory by the technique of chemiluminescence used to study phagocytic activation. Hydroxyl radicals are formed by the interaction of H_2O_2 and superoxide anion. It is a highly unstable intermediate reacting instantly with most organic molecules and thus is very toxic. The end product in oxygen metabolism is H_2O_2, which has microbicidal activity for organisms not capable of producing peroxidases or catalase.

Killing and Digestion Mechanisms

Once particles have been engulfed and formed into phagosomes, fusion between these and lysosomes results in direct exposure of the phagocytized elements to several killing mechanisms. Many of these are dependent on toxic oxygen intermediates and/or the enzyme myeloperoxidase (MPO). Although the oxygen metabolites are quite capable of killing microbes, their effectiveness is greatly enhanced by the basic protein MPO, the presence of halide ion, and low pH, the latter in part a result of the respiration by-product lactic acid. The combination of agents serves to bind the peroxide and halide to the target cell and to oxidize the halide ions to hypohalite ions. Among the effects generated by this peroxidative action are halogenation of bacterial membranes, decarboxylation of amino acids, and the production of toxic aldehydes and ketones.

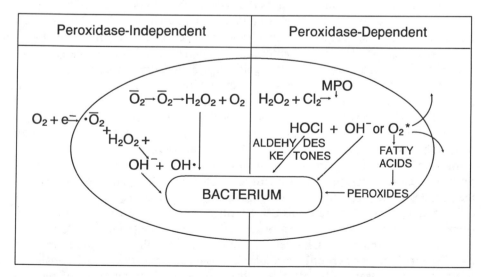

FIGURE 5-3.   The key steps in production of intermediate oxygen metabolites within phagocytes showing the major differences and modes of action of the myeloperoxidase (MPO)-dependent and -independent systems.

There are also a number of oxygen-independent means of killing microbes, mostly in the form of proteins secreted either from the granules or into the phagolysosome. Neutrophils contain a number of granules that, during activation, fuse with the phagosome and are extruded into the extracellular milieu. The contents of the granules are important in the elicitation and modulation of the immune response. A number of cationic proteins from azurophilic granules are arginine-rich molecules effective at neutral pH and are bacteriostatic or bactericidal. The granules also contain a wide variety of active materials including bactericidal proteins (Ganz, Selsted, and Szlarek 1985; Weiss, Victor, and Elsbach 1983), chemotactic factors for monocytes, and complement activators. A number of proteases, e.g., cathepsin, serine esterase, and elastase, and the peptidoglycan-digesting enzyme lysozyme are more important in digestion of engulfed bacteria than in actual killing. Lactoferrin is an iron-binding molecule that serves several functions: it increases the production of hydroxyl radicals, may inhibit the release of colony-stimulating factor from monocytes (Broxmeyer et al. 1980), and may also chelate iron necessary for the growth of most bacteria.

In addition to the antimicrobial mechanisms detailed above, it should be noted that these same mechanisms can lead to inflammation and host injury. Neutrophils in vivo can also elicit such mediators as PAF, which has a number of inflammatory reactions in tissue (see Chapter 6).

D. MACROPHAGES

The role of monocytes/macrophages in antigen presentation and in immune regulation has been discussed elsewhere, but their role in primary defense in both antigen–specific and nonspecific mechanisms needs to be examined. One of the major characteristics concerning macrophage chemotaxis and adhesion is that such functions can largely be in response to T-cell-derived cytokines, particularly IFN-γ, as well as to foreign matter acting independently. Thus, macrophage activation can be antigen-specific or nonspecific. In antigen–specific situations, the T cell provides the recognition, and the macrophages the effector functions. Monocytes/macrophages in turn secrete cytokines that stimulate neutrophil infiltration. They possess Fc, CR1, CR3, and C5a receptors and thus are very responsive to complement activation signals. They also have receptors for sugars typically found on many microorganisms, e.g., mannose, L-fucose, galactose, N-acetylmuramic acid. The life span of mononuclear phagocytes is considerably longer than that of neutrophils, and their lysosomal development is more complicated. Lysosomal enzymes assume more of a role in digestive functions and tissue injury, and there is more production of toxic lipid peroxides. Also, macrophages have more secretory products than neutrophils, which account for many additional functions.

Macrophages are more important against intracellular infections. They cannot physically engulf such protected microbes, but protein antigens recycled to cell membranes (i.e., presentation) can stimulate T-cell responses that in turn elicit other macrophages. Infected cells can be killed in inflammatory bystander reactions or, if a part of chronic infections, continuously activate macrophages in an adjuvant-like manner (see Chapter 8). Continuous stimulation of macrophages by IFN-γ may produce chronic, granulomatous inflammatory changes consisting of giant multinucleate cells with the ability to produce high amounts of proteolytic enzymes, fibroblast infiltration, and collagen deposition. In this manner, chronic macrophage activity is important in wound repair and fibrosis. Finally,

macrophages are important as scavengers of various substances such as by pha-
gocytizing effete and worn-out blood cells or removing cholesterol-rich low-
density lipoproteins from the circulation. Macrophages are also a source of many
of the complement components and thus can replenish chemotactic stimuli.

E. T-CYTOTOXIC AND NK CELLS

Several lymphocyte subsets possess efferent, cytolytic functions against target
cells expressing antigens associated with either infectious agents, alloantigens (on
transplanted cells), or tumors (see Fig. 5–4). Although CD4$^+$ T cells are mainly
important in afferent responses, they may function in defensive ways by producing cytokines that activate and expand other cell populations. CD8$^+$ T$_c$ lymphocytes (cytotoxic lymphocytes or CTL) act directly on target cells independent of
other means, although their activity may be enhanced by IFN-γ. Natural killer
cells also kill on direct contact, but the means of target recognition is different.

The major role of CD4$^+$ T cells in delayed-type hypersensitivity is to recognize
antigen presented in a MHC class II context, to activate and expand their own
population via IL-2 secretion, and to produce effector function by recruiting and
activating additional mononuclear cells. CD4$^+$ cells accomplish these functions
by cytokine secretion, primarily by IFN-γ and TNF. Cell populations other than
macrophages may also be activated. For example, eosinophil recruitment is modulated by IL-5, and IL-2 also activates NK cells. One cytokine, lymphotoxin
(TNF-β), is capable of lysing cells independently of direct attachment between
effector and target cell. It also mediates neutrophil–endothelial cell interaction.

CD8$^+$ T cells (CTL) recognize antigen on target cells in a MHC class I context
with their antigen–specific T-cell receptors (TCR). They undergo selection and

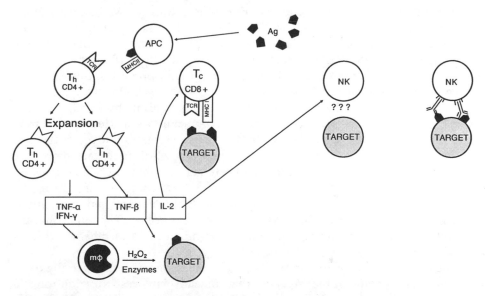

FIGURE 5–4.   Summary of killing mechanisms by various lymphocyte subsets. CD4$^+$ T$_h$ cells
proliferate on antigen presentation and produce various mediators that primarily function by
activating macrophages but to a lesser extent also act directly on the target cell. CD8$^+$ T$_c$ cells
become activated when recognizing presented antigen in an MHC class I context. The NK cells
primarily kill target cells by direct contact through an unknown recognition factor(s) as well as
participate in ADCC by attaching immunoglobulins to their Fc receptors.

maturation in the thymus but differentiate into functionally lytic CTLs when they bind to antigen and receive cytokine stimulation from CD4$^+$ cells, primarily IL-2. Thus, in order to be fully effective, both CD4$^+$ and CD8$^+$ cells must be activated by antigen. When the CD3–TCR complexes on CTL membranes become cross-linked, cell signaling begins, and the cell becomes functionally activated to be lytic.

Human NK cells are a distinct subset of lymphocytes bearing a finely granular cytoplasm (Jondal 1987). They do not require thymic maturation and do not express typical T- or B-cell markers or TCR–CD3 complexes, although they do possess IL-2 receptors. They require intimate contact with target cells before lysis can take place, but there are two means of achieving this attachment. One distinctive marker, CD16, is the NK Fc receptor for IgG. If target cells become coated with enough antigen–specific antibody, direct attachment by NK cells may be achieved through ADCC. However, most attachment is accomplished through an as yet unknown chemical means that seems to recognize certain viral or tumor-associated markers. Other than for the antibody associated with ADCC reactions, NK function and number are not affected by prior antigen contact, although they do respond to IL-2 and certain other environmental stimuli. Although there is no doubt that there is a morphologically and functionally definable NK cell that comprises the bulk of cells lysing targets in this manner, there also appears to be at least another cell population in both mice and humans capable of lysing target cells in a non-MHC-restricted manner (Lanier et al. 1986). That these are T-cytotoxic cells adds to the confusion of terms.

Thus, although T-cytotoxic cells and NK cells kill primarily by direct contact with living cells, only the former are considered to do so in an antigen–specific, MHC class I context. However, this statement needs further examination. T cells recognize antigenic epitopes presented within the folding of MHC class I molecules, and NK cells do not function in this manner. However, MHC class I molecules also seem to be important in NK-cell recognition in a very different way. In these cases, it is speculated that the MHC class I molecules normally obscure hypothetical self-recognition structures on cell membranes. If the MHC molecules become displaced or altered by infection or tumor processes, thus exposing these recognition groups, they will be subject to NK attack (Janeway 1991).

At the present time there are two recognized mechanisms by which both NK and T$_c$ cell types kill target cells after intimate contact between effector and target cells has been initiated (Berke 1991). One postulated mechanism involves the production and secretion of a cytolytic protein, perforin, which functions to produce transmembrane channels with an influx of external calcium ions, which, together with secreted lytic granules and serine proteases, leads to porous membrane lesions and cytolysis. When activated by attachment, polymerization of monomeric precursors located in cytoplasmic granules of NK cells occurs. The cell membrane activation causes the granules to mobilize toward point of attachment and leads to perforin production (Podack 1985).

The other proposed cytolytic mechanism involves lymphocyte triggering of an internal disintegration of the target cell that somehow involves redistribution and linkage of target cell membrane receptors and accumulation of intracellular calcium ions. DNA fragmentation, protease production, and massive permeability changes result.

When first described, lymphokine-activated cells (LAK) were NK cells that had been isolated and expanded in vitro under laboratory conditions. They were obtained by in vitro activation with IL-2, and their function was defined by their ability to kill autologous tumor cells in short-term (4–hr) assays (Herberman et al. 1987). Whereas the LAK cytotoxicity for normal cells is <5%, it may be as high as 92% for limited types of autologous tumor cells, e.g., melanoma and renal cell carcinomas (Grimm et al. 1982). It has been reported that LAK cells, in combination with IL-2 therapy, induced marked regression in certain tumors (Rosenberg et al. 1987). Similar results have been reported in murine tumor models (Rosenberg 1985). In addition to the NK-cell method of killing, these cells produce significant amounts of TNF-α and IFN-γ. If LAK cells are capable of being produced in vivo, it might take place in graft-versus-host disease, where mature, competent lymphocytes are transplanted into an immunologically incompetent recipient. The transplanted lymphocytes recognize their new host as foreign, expand, and become activated (i.e., become LAK cells) in a host who cannot respond and control their expansion.

F. MAST CELLS AND BASOPHILS

Basophils and mast cells are considered to be the major effector cells of allergy and inflammation but have important defensive functions as well. Although they are best known for allergic types of function, they most likely have beneficial effects as well, e.g., promotion of wound healing and repair, tumor angiogenesis, and participation in defense against helminthic (parasitic worm) infections. Both have superficially similar morphology and function but differ in several important respects, particularly in the types of mediators released (Schleimer et al. 1984). Basophils are circulating granulocytes that constitute less than 1% of the total white blood cell population but may occasionally infiltrate tissues in certain types of immune injury. Mast cells are heterogeneous populations localized in the skin and respiratory and intestinal tracts. Mast cells are fundamentally of two basic types, mucosal and connective tissue, based on morphological, physiological, and ontogenetic differences (Irani and Schwartz 1989). Characteristics of these two types of mast cells and basophils are compared in Table 5–3. The basic-

TABLE 5–3.   Comparison of Basophils and Mast Cells

	Basophils	Mast Cells	
		Connective Tissue	Mucosal
Location	Peripheral circulation	Ubiquitous, perivascular	Gut and lung predominantly
T-cell dependency		Independent	Dependent
Lipid mediators	Low amounts only	PAF	LTC$_4$
		TxB$_2$	LTB$_4$
		LTD$_2$	
Cytoplasmic IgE	+	−	+
Staining	Conventional	Conventional	Requires special fixation/ staining
Neutral protease content		Tryptase–chymase	Tryptase
Theophylline	Sensitive	Sensitive	Refractory
Disodium cromoglycate	Sensitive	Sensitive	Refractory

staining connective tissue mast cell, itself very heterogeneous, is the one for which most studies have been conducted. Sometimes referred to as type T mast cells (tryptase positive, chymase negative) in humans, they are found mostly around blood vessels in submucosa, skin, connective tissue, and serosal surfaces. Mucosal mast cells or type TC cells (tryptase positive, chymase positive) are not seen in normally stained sections, as they are very formaldehyde sensitive and require special staining techniques. They are mostly confined to the mucosa of the midgut and lung.

Basophils and connective tissue mast cells have preformed cytoplasmic granules containing pharmacologically active mediators of inflammatory reactions. These basic-staining granules are rich in histamine, heparin, leukotrienes, and eosinophil chemotactic factor A (ECF-A). Human mast cells produce much larger amounts of arachidonic acid metabolites than do basophils, particularly PGD_2 in mucosal mast cells, thromboxane (a potent platelet stimulator), and LTC_4 in connective tissue mast cells. The latter, formerly called slow reactive substance, is a powerful bronchoconstrictive agent and stimulator of mucous hypersecretion, but unlike the immediate effect of histamine, LTC_4 action induces delayed responses in the lung. Also, human lung mast cells are much more potent producers of PAF and contain four times more histamine than basophils.

Another class of important mediators released by these cells are families of kinin-generating enzymes, the kallikreins. Kallikreins are a group of mildly proteolytic serine proteases found in different forms in tissue and plasma that release peptides, or kinins, from circulating kininogen precursors in the plasma. Kallikrein activation and kininogen are essential for activation of factor XII of the intrinsic blood coagulation pathway. The kinins affect smooth muscle contraction, chemotaxis, dilatation of peripheral arterioles, and increased capillary permeability. One member, bradykinin, is present in all inflammation and, in addition to the physiological aspects, is also responsible for the burning pain. The kinins have the ability to initiate prostaglandin synthesis, which may exert some of the effects attributed to kinins or modulate their activity.

Finally, activated murine mast cells are also an important source of a variety of cytokines. For example, the cells are dependent on autocrine-produced IL-3 and IL-4 as growth factors.

Preformed and newly synthesized mediators are released on cross-linking of cell membrane receptors by various agents. These cells possess high-affinity, ϵ-chain-specific Fc receptors ($Fc_\epsilon RI$) (Metzger 1991). Specific antigen, anti-IgE, a wide variety of mediators, or certain lectins may stimulate the receptors to initiate the cell-signaling process. This reflects the variety of individual receptors, other than the $Fc_\epsilon RI$, that are also present on basophil cell membranes (Marone 1989). The anatomic site of antigen stimulation and type of cells present affect the type of organ reaction observed. For example, lung mast-cell-derived LTC_4 is responsible for most of the bronchoconstriction and mucus hypersecretion of allergic diseases of the airways (Schleimer et al. 1984).

G. EOSINOPHILS

Eosinophils are acid-staining granulocytes of the peripheral blood that normally appear in low concentration (0.5–4%). Eosinophil production in the bone marrow is dependent on T-cell cytokines IL-3, IL-5, and GM-CSF. At least some eosinophil function is also T-cell-dependent (Frew and Kay 1990). Their increase in the circulation is T-cell modulated and is regarded as evidence of an IgE-mediated allergic reaction, a parasitic worm infection, or certain clinical diseases such as atopic dermatitis. T-cell influence is also important in the activation and survival of eosinophils in the generation of an allergic reaction known as the late-phase response (see Chapter 6).

There is a bewildering array of mediators produced by eosinophils in the various types of intracytoplasmic granules (Samter and Gleich 1988). They possess receptors for IgG, IgE, C3b, and C5a. The characteristic feature of an eosinophil is the inclusion of primary granules associated with the cell membranes, called Charcot–Leyden crystals, which consist largely of lysophospholipase. Secondary granules feature several distinctive proteins, major basic protein (MBP), peroxidase, and eosinophil-derived neurotoxin among others. The MBP has both inflammatory and anti-inflammatory functions, depending on concentration. It causes histamine release from mast cells and basophils additionally. It is also inflammatory in a number of hypersensitivity diseases. For example, it is highly toxic for bronchial epithelium and is considered to be a major effector cell in the initiation of bronchial asthma (Frigas and Gleich 1986). Although without much effect against bacteria, MBP is highly toxic to helminths. Eosinophil peroxidase catalyzes the H_2O_2 oxidation of substances in microbes as well as host tissue. Eosinophil-derived neurotoxin produces a characteristic syndrome of neuromuscular incoordination and weakness when injected intrathecally into animals. Unlike neutrophils, which primarily release LTB_4, the predominant leukotrienes released by eosinophils seem to be LTC_4 and LTD_4. Eosinophils also produce large amounts of (as well as respond to) PAF.

These important cells have many functions, some inflammatory and some antiinfectious. This diversity may be related in part to their great heterogeneity in density and chemical content. Their defensive role against parasitic infections is accomplished through their ability to participate in ADCC reactions that allow them to attach (via specific IgE attached to their cell membrane Fc receptors) directly to parasites much too large to be phagocytized. Once attached, they release toxic granule proteins and oxygen metabolites. Previously, it had been thought that eosinophils were largely anti-inflammatory in allergic reactions by releasing mediators and enzymes that counteracted basophil-derived mediators. This was partly because of observations such as that the biological activity of LTD_4 and LTC_4 was reported to be inhibited by the eosinophil products arylsulfatase and peroxidase, respectively. Inactivation of these mediators would reduce both bronchoconstriction and mucus secretion. However, many of these studies have been critically reexamined, and the data have failed to be reconfirmed (Samter and Gleich 1988).

There is a growing awareness that eosinophils are prime contributors to local tissue damage (Hoidal 1990). With asthma, the cell is now regarded as a potent proinflammatory cell with tissue-injuring capabilities, and its mediators, particularly MBP, are instrumental in inducing epithelial injury and bronchial hyperreactivity (Gleich 1990). The cells are also thought to contribute to the injury of lower airway diseases such as hypersensitivity pneumonitis, idiopathic pulmonary fibrosis, interstitial diseases associated with drug-induced disorders, and adult respiratory distress syndrome (Davis et al. 1984), all of which may also have immunotoxicologic components. When compared to neutrophils in an in vitro cytotoxicity assay, activated human eosinophils were much more cytotoxic and therefore could be considered potentially more damaging to host tissue (Roberts et al. 1991). Eosinophil-derived mediators such as neutrophil chemotactic factor (NCF) and/or LTC$_4$ also attract polymorphonuclear leukocytes into the inflamed areas, but these are more characteristic of late-phase reactions (see Chapter 6).

H. PLATELETS

Platelets are not usually considered in the armamentarium of immunologic weapons, but they are important sources of mediators. Platelets are actually small cytoplasmic fragments derived from megakaryocytes. Their roles in promotion of coagulation has long been appreciated, and among other things, they are a source of supply for factors V and VIII, fibrinogen, and thrombospondin. They have receptors for thrombin, and their surfaces are important in procoagulant production. The coagulation mechanism can be considered an important defensive mechanism preventing bleeding by adhering to damaged endothelium and producing hemostatic platelet plugs in injured capillaries well before clot formation can take place. The mechanism also plays a role in inflammation in that fibrin deposition aids in walling off infectious substances, preventing their dissemination. They have remarkable adherent properties to extracellular surfaces and molecules such as collagen. Moreover, they also can produce fibronectin, which further aids adherence processes. Thromboembolus formation in capillaries is a feature of certain types of immune injury.

Platelets are an important source of vasoactive amines, particularly serotonin and platelet factor 4, key products in regulating vascular permeability and promoting chemotaxis of monocytes and neutrophils. Platelets were the first cells described as targets of what we now know to be PAF (Benveniste, Henson, and Cochrane 1977), and they also produce this multifunctional substance, which contributes to the vasoactivity. Platelets have a variety of receptors and respond to signals from other sources. Thromboxane A$_2$ activates platelets, whereas PGI$_2$ and PGE$_1$ inhibit platelet function through stimulation of adenylate cyclase. They have the complement receptors CR1, which are important in aiding in removing immune complexes by phagocytic processes.

I. ENDOTHELIAL CELLS

Until quite recently, endothelial cells lining the capillaries of the vasculature were only thought of as targets of injury, but consideration of their functions combined with recent discoveries concerning their definition strongly suggest they should be included in any list of immunologic accessory cells. Endothelial cells might be considered the gatekeepers between the vasculature and the interstitial tissues, carefully controlling cells and molecules that pass between the two tissues. Changes in endothelial permeability are subject to many influences, including local arteriolar blood pressure and dilatation, osmotic balance, changes in endothelial adhesive properties and microtubular structure, and the formation of intraendothelial gaps and intracellular vesicles. Normal endothelium of most capillaries consists of a continuous, unbroken layer of cells with closely adnexed junctions. Passage of electrolytes and water is permitted, but subject to the balance between interstitial and plasma osmotic pressures and between vascular and tissue hydrostatic pressures. As arterioles dilate a pooling or stasis of blood takes place that may be accompanied by an increase in local hemodynamic pressure.

If the integrity of the endothelial barrier is compromised at such times, there is an outward flow of fluid with a high protein concentration, which results in an excessive osmotic pressure in the interstitium and an impairment of fluid return to the capillaries. The resulting edema is a basic feature of inflammation and causes little problem when it takes place in the skin but may be a dangerous situation if it occurs in certain vulnerable organs such as the lung.

In addition to the effects of arteriolar contraction, neutrophil interaction with endothelial cells also contributes to the permeability change (Wedmore and Williams 1981). As slowing and stagnation of blood flow take place, leukocytes settle out of the main flow and rest on the capillary walls. Following this margination process, physiological changes in activated leukocytes induce adhesive interactions with the endothelial cells. This process involves expression of a complex family of leukocyte receptors called integrins and various corresponding endothelial adhesion molecules (Wardlaw 1990). Comparison of their molecular structures reveals that these endothelial adhesins belong to the immunoglobulin superfamily. This process should prove to be of increasing interest to immunotoxicologists in that xenobiotics can promote or interfere with this process either directly on the endothelium or indirectly through cytokine stimulation of other cells. Bacterial endotoxin is such a substance.

As the changes in surface expression of adhesion molecules are taking place, changes are also occurring in the cytoskeletal structure of the endothelial cells that contribute further to the increase in permeability. The distribution of contractile elements (actin, myosin, etc.) or stress fibers is concentrated near the junctional tips of the cells and becomes activated on cell signaling and calcium ion influx (Grega 1986). The contraction of these elements greatly determines cell retractability and widening of the interendothelial gaps.

Cells and molecules may emigrate from the capillaries in two ways, through the endothelial gaps or directly through endothelial cell cytoplasm. Leukocytes, mainly neutrophils at first and then monocytes, migrate through the widened gaps in the capillary walls created by the retracted cells. This occurs mainly in certain postcapillary venules called high-endothelial venules (because they are lined with tall, metabolically active cells), which are particularly susceptible to leukocyte adhesion. Lymphocytes can migrate through the endothelial cytoplasm as well as through the gaps (Weiss 1972). Another morphological change in the endothelial cells that contributes to edema formation is the appearance of increased numbers of pinocytotic vesicles, which transport fluids and small molecules across the barrier.

In such a critical position, endothelial cells are highly responsive to a number of mediators, including PAF, histamine, and oxidant injury. They are also a source of mediators and substances important in defense and repair, e.g., prostaglandins, factor VIII, plasminogen activator, and collagen. They respond to TNF-α and IL-1 to produce their own mediators such as neutrophil chemotactic factor (Strieter et al. 1989) and a substance (CD11/CD18) that enhances neutrophil adhesion (Pohlman et al. 1986). γ-Interferon not only enhances the activities of other cytokines but promotes attachment of lymphocytes to endothelial cells. They can produce IL-1 and PAF, which participate in neutrophil adhesion (Brevario et al. 1988). Another consequence of TNF-α stimulation of endothelial cells is to up-regulate the expression of MHC class I but not class II molecules (Collins et al. 1986).

J. INTEGRATION

The foregoing discussion is limited in that it has been dissected into individual component parts but fails to give an overall impression of how all work together in a regulated system. Cellular and molecular immunologists necessarily work with isolated systems and define such a bewildering array of stimuli, responses, and isolated factors that providing an integrated view of the process is a formidable task. Regardless of the mechanism of foreign recognition, a number of means of translation into an effector response is available. In many instances, such translation results in inflammation. This highly complicated process is well-known and exists in a number of varieties. In addition, several efferent immune mechanisms are constantly being stimulated and are effective without our ever knowing of their presence.

The exact type of response is governed by the physical and chemical nature of the stimulus, prior history of exposure to that same stimulus (or other mediator/cytokine-generating stimuli that may be occurring simultaneously), the genetic make-up of the individual, and numerous environmental factors present at the time of contact. If the stimulus is a living agent, its biological make-up, dose, route of infection, and degree of virulence also greatly influence the nature of the response. The point is that there is no one special type of immune response for a given antigen and that multicapability has insured our survival. Through its tremendous reserve, redundant mechanisms, and intricate regulation, the immune system is buffered against changes in antigen expression or mechanisms of virulence by rapidly reproducing and evolving microbes.

1. Infectious Disease

The competition of even the most primitive invertebrates and vertebrates against microorganisms is evolutionarily so old, and there are so many different types of potential pathogens, that it is reasonable to expect a wide variety of overlapping defenses to have evolved. Immediately after the discovery of bacterial causes of infectious disease by Koch and Pasteur, the science of immunology was born and grew up together with microbiology. Consequently, most of what is known about the effector mechanisms of immune responses has been learned from the study of infectious processes.

It is important to bear in mind the large number of non-antigen-specific mechanisms available that no doubt evolved first. The very process of inflammation exists in virtually every multicellular phylum. Perhaps the first humoral defenses to evolve were primitive proteins surviving today as acute-phase reactants that react against a wide spectrum of similar structures. C-reactive protein might be considered in that light as it reacts with a variety of microbially derived polysaccharides. Other types of microbial products, e.g., bacterial endotoxin, are potentially so dangerous to survival that numerous simultaneously induced inflammatory cell and cytokine responses have evolved (Morrison and Ryan 1987). Since the diversity of microbial pathogens or competitors is so extreme, it follows that a diverse spectrum of both antigen-specific and non-antigen-specific responses have evolved. These mechanisms have proven so effective and so redundant that in many cases the immune response to the microbe has resulted in major injury to the innocent bystander host that is often more severe than the initial infectious process (see Chapter 6). Much of the pathology against agents such as tubercle bacilli or schistosomes is immunologically mediated. Moreover, overproduction of cytokines in response to microbial products is a major factor in the pathogenesis of septic shock (Morrison and Ryan 1987).

Specific immune responses are primarily (but not exclusively) vertebrate phenomena. Absence of immunoglobulins is related to repeated infections with extracellular Gram-positive bacteria. This indicates that antibodies are primarily effective in neutralizing protein exotoxins or eliminating infectious particles that can be easily phagocytized. Any microorganism that circulates for any appreciable length of time in the blood is vulnerable to any antibody- or complement-dependent mechanism. It is important to keep in mind that antibody mediation frequently entails processes involving cooperation with other cells, e.g., ADCC and opsonization. Protein exotoxins, cell wall components (e.g., peptidoglycans and lipopolysaccharides), and surface structures (e.g., capsules, flagella, adhesins, and pili) are all excellent antigens and, under the right conditions, represent points of immune attack.

Although most antibodies are directed toward specific antigens produced by a limited number of B-cell clones, an interesting exception occurs against what have been termed superantigens. Superantigens are largely protein exotoxins that stimulate extraordinary numbers of CD4$^+$ T cells bearing genes for a variable region of the TCR-β chain TCR (reviewed by Misfeldt 1990). In this sense they resemble nonspecific mitogens except that they require antigen presentation in an MHC class II context. Perhaps this is another example of an evolutionary method of overkill to insure protection against a large number of potentially very dangerous substances.

Cellular mechanisms of immunity are most effective against intracellular infections, i.e., those caused by viruses and many types of Gram-negative bacteria. It is the cytotoxic mechanisms that clear the body of cells expressing foreign antigens on their cell membranes. Some microorganisms, e.g., *Listeria*, certain fungi, and the tubercle bacillus, have evolved mechanisms for surviving within macrophages. Consequently, mechanisms of defense against these agents are more complicated. Since these agents are not cleared as rapidly, and since they are composed of substances resistant to rapid degradation (peptidoglycan and lipopolysaccharide), they tend to form chronic infections, i.e., those in which numerous host–parasite interactions take place over a longer period of time.

The most important means of defense against such microbes is via CD4$^+$ T-cell evocation of macrophage responses. As the microbe has developed cell wall components that insure survival under adverse conditions (e.g., muramyl dipeptide, MDP), the host defense system has been simultaneously evolving with the result that MDP induces enhanced macrophage activity; i.e., it is an adjuvant (see Chapter 8). Not only do activated macrophages possess more intracellular killing abilities, they also produce increased amounts of cytokines (e.g., IL-1, TNF-α, IFN-γ).

Some intracellular infections stimulate the production of IFN-γ and IFN-β, which offer a primitive form of non-antigen-specific immunity in that they prevent superinfection by more viruses and inhibit replication. The CTLs and NK cells are also effective against cells intracellularly infected, particularly with viruses, if viral antigen is expressed on target cell membranes. In addition to ADCC, NK cells also seem to be able to recognize virally infected cells by an antigen-independent mechanism. Cells not expressing external viral antigen can be lysed as bystanders by cytokines such as TNF-α and lymphotoxin.

A number of special mechanisms of immunity have evolved to deal with parasitic worm infections and even ticks and mite larvae, organisms much too large to be phagocytized. Chief among these are IgE-mediated reactions in concert with eosinophil action. As antibody becomes attached to sites on these target parasites, eosinophils may attach via Fc receptors (ADCC) and produce eosinophil-derived toxins, e.g., major basic proteins. Not only are these mechanisms directly toxic to both larval and adult stages of the helminths, they also retard egg maturation and exhibit anti-tick-feeding properties as well (Samter and Gleich 1988). Although this text has not discussed organ functions as means of defense (e.g., sneezing, coughing, blinking), one aspect of IgE effector-cell antigen-induced inflammation may fit into this category. Some regard the diarrhea caused by the extreme water exudation of the intestinal epithelia into the lumen and intestinal smooth muscle contraction as essentially defensive functions to rid the gut of parasitic contents.

2. Tumors

The other beneficial value of the immune response is towards tumors, but here the evidence is not nearly so impressive as with infectious disease, especially in humans. On the one hand, it is known that certain types of tumors appear more commonly in immunosuppressed individuals and that certain tumors respond to immunotherapeutic strategies, but most of the evidence has been obtained from manipulation of transplantable tumors in experimental animals or working with tumor cell lines in vitro, and even in these, knowledge as detailed as that available for immune defenses against infectious agents is lacking. Yet, teleologically, an intact immune response must be important in insuring survival against the emergence of at least certain types of neoplastic processes.

Humoral immune responses against tumors are confined to reacting with a limited number of protein tumor-specific antigens associated with the cell membrane. Some laboratory evidence exists that antibodies in the presence of complement may lyse tumor cells expressing these antigens and that they can participate in arming macrophages or NK cells for ADCC killing. Whether these mechanisms actually are of benefit in vivo to the host with a spontaneously arising tumor is unknown. There is even the possibility that humoral antibodies directed toward tumor cells may act in an enhancing manner by preventing target cell attachment of T-cytotoxic cells or by forming immune complexes that block antigen receptors on T-cytotoxic cells. In the presence of complement, the latter could even be destroyed. Another disadvantage of a humoral response is that antigen expression by tumor cells can even be repressed in the presence of antibody, a process called antigenic modulation, which also occurs with certain infectious agents.

The evidence for the benefit of intact effectors of cellular immunity is better. MHC class I-restricted CTLs have been shown to be of benefit against virus-induced or -associated tumors. Tumor-infiltrating lymphocytes have been described in specific human carcinomas. These cells as well as peripheral CTLs obtained from patients lyse tumor cells explanted from the same patient. As stated previously, NK cells activated and expanded with IL-2 (LAK cells) are also effective against a limited number of tumor types. The epidemiologic evidence linking adequate NK number and function with the presence or absence of tumors is more impressive. Another host defense factor that *ought* to be effective in vivo is TNF, which is produced mainly by activated monocytes. As the original name indicated, TNF causes necrosis of a variety of tumor cells in vitro. It not only is effective directly on target cells but also is a cytokine that enhances or activates many other effector components.

If immune responses are effective in preventing the establishment of tumors or in helping the host spontaneously recover, the question might be asked, why then do we get tumors? Considering only those tumors in which there might be an effective immune component operating, tumors can be examined for various escape mechanisms or virulence factors. If the tumor cells are coated with a non-antigenic protective layer, e.g., sialic acid, protection against effectors would be afforded. Some tumors produce immunosuppressive prostaglandins, e.g., PGE_2. Melanoma cells shed vesicles that inhibit expression and/or induction of macrophage MHC class I antigens (Poutsiaka et al. 1985). Certain virus infections might also be able to induce a similar effect. Another possibility is induction of excessive amounts of transforming growth factor β, a down-regulating cytokine that inhibits T-cell proliferation, cytoxic reactions, and many proinflammatory functions.

References

Ambrus, J. L., Jr., M. G. Peters, A. S. Fauci, and E. J. Brown. 1990. The Ba fragment of complement factor B inhibits human B lymphocyte proliferation. *J. Immunol.* 144:1549–53.

Benveniste, J., P. M. Henson, and C. Cochrane. 1977. Leukocyte-dependent release from rabbit platelets: The role of IgE, basophils and platelet-activating factor. *J. Exp. Med.* 136:1356–77.

Berke, G. 1991. T-cell mediated cytotoxicity. *Curr. Opin. Immunol.* 3:320–26.

Biesecker, G. 1983. Membrane attack complex of complement as a pathologic mediator. *Lab. Invest.* 49:237–49.

Brevario, F., F. Bertocchi, E. Dejana, and F. Bussolino. 1988. IL-1–induced adhesion of polymorphonuclear leukocytes to cultured human endothelial cells. Role of platelet-activating factor. *J. Immunol.* 141:3391–97.

Broxmeyer, H. E., M. De Sousa, A. Smithyman, et al. 1980. Specificity and modulation of the action of lactoferrin, a negative feedback regulator for myelopoiesis. *Blood* 55:324–33.

Collins, T., L. A. LaPierre, W. Fiers, et al. 1986. Recombinant human tumor necrosis factor increases mRNA levels and surface expression on HLA-A,B antigens in vascular endothelial cells and dermal fibroblasts in vitro. *Proc. Natl. Acad. Sci. U.S.A.* 83:446–50.

Cross, A. S., and N. M. Kelly. 1990. Bacteria–phagocyte interactions: Emerging tactics in an ancient rivalry. *FEMS Microbiol. Immunol.* 64:245–58.

Davis, W. B., G. A. Fels, X. H. Sun, et al. 1984. Eosinophil-mediated injury in lung parenchymal cells and interstitial matrix. A possible role for eosinophils in chronic inflammatory disorders of the lower respiratory tract. *J. Clin. Invest.* 74:269–78.

Frew, A. J., and A. B. Kay. 1990. Eosinophils and T-lymphocytes in late-phase allergic reactions. *J. Allergy Clin. Immunol.* 85:533–39.

Frigas, E., and G. J. Gleich. 1986. The eosinophil and the pathophysiology of asthma. *J. Allergy Clin. Immunol.* 77:527–37.

Ganz, T., M. E. Selsted, and M. E. Szlarek. 1985. Defensins: Natural peptide antibiotics of human neutrophils. *J. Clin. Invest.* 76:1427–35.

Gleich, G. J. 1990. The eosinophil and bronchial asthma: Current understanding. *J. Allergy Clin. Immunol.* 85:422–36.

Grega, G. J. 1986. Contractile elements in endothelial cells as potential targets for drug action. *Trends. Pharmacol. Sci.* 7:452–57.

Grimm, E. A., A. Mazumder, H. Z. Zhang, and S. A. Rosenberg. 1982. Lymphocyte activated killer cell phenomenon: Lysis of natural killer cell-resistant fresh solid tumor cells by interleukin 2 activated autologous human peripheral blood lymphocytes. *J. Exp. Med.* 155:1823–41.

Herberman, R. B., J. Hiserodt, N. Vusanovic, et al. 1987. Lymphokine-activated killer cell activity. Characteristics of effector cells and their progenitors in blood and spleen. *Immunol. Today* 8:178–81.

Hoidal, J. R. 1990. The eosinophil and acute lung injury. *Am. Rev. Respir. Dis.* 142:1245–46.

Irani, A.-M. A., and L. B. Schwartz. 1989. Mast cell heterogeneity. *Clin. Exp. Allergy* 19:143–55.

Janeway, C. A., Jr. 1991. To thine own self be true. *Curr. Opin. Biol.* 1:239–41.

Jondal, M. 1987. The human NK cell—a short over-view and a hypothesis on NK cell recognition. *Clin. Exp. Immunol.* 70:255–62.

Klebanoff, S. J. 1982. Oxygen-dependent cytotoxic mechanisms of phagocytes. In *Advances in Host Defense Mechanisms*, Vol. 1, ed. J. I. Gallin and A. S. Fauci, pp. 111–46. New York: Raven Press.

Kopp, W. C., and R. Burrell. 1982. Evidence for antibody-dependent binding of the terminal complement component to alveolar basement membrane. *Clin. Immunol. Immunopathol.* 23:10–21.

Lambris, J. D. 1988. The multifunctional role of C3, the third component of complement. *Immunol. Today* 9:387–93.

Lanier, L. L., J. H. Phillips, J. Hackett, Jr., et al. 1986. Natural killer cells: Definition of a cell type rather than a function. *J. Immunol.* 137:2735–39.

Marone, G. 1989. The role of the mast cell and basophil activation in human allergic reactions. *Eur. Resp. J.* 2(Suppl. 6):446s-55s.

Metzger, H. 1991. The high affinity receptor for IgE on mast cells. *Clin. Exp. Allergy* 21:269–79.

Misfeldt, M. L. 1990. Microbial "superantigens." *Infect. Immun.* 58:2409–13.

Morgan, E. L., W. O. Weigle, and T. E. Hugli. 1984. Anaphylatoxin-mediated regulation of human and murine immune responses. *Fed. Proc.* 43:2543–47.

Morrison, D. C. and J. L. Ryan. 1987. Endotoxins and disease mechanisms. *Annu. Rev. Med.* 38:417–32.

Osler, A. G., and A. L. Sandberg. 1973. Alternate complement pathways. *Prog. Allergy* 17:51–92.

Pangburn, M. K. 1983. Activation of complement via the alternative pathway. *Fed. Proc.* 42:139–43.

Podack, E. R. 1985. The molecular mechanism of lymphocyte-mediated tumor cell lysis. *Immunol. Today* 6:21–27.

Pohlman, T. H., K. A. Stanness, P. G. Beatty, et al. 1986. An endothelial cell surface factor(s) induced in vitro by lipopolysaccharide, interleukin 1, and tumor necrosis factor-α increases neutrophil adherence by a CDw18–dependent mechanism. *J. Immunol.* 136:4548–53.

Poutsiaka, D. D., D. D. Taylor, E. M. Levy, and P. H. Black. 1985. Inhibition of recombinant interferon-γ-induced Ia antigen expression by shed B16 F10 melanoma cell membrane vesicles. *J. Immunol.* 134:145–50.

Roberts, R. L., B. J. Ank, and E. R. Stiehm. 1991. Human eosinophils are much more toxic than neutrophils in antibody-independent killing. *J. Allergy. Clin. Immunol.* 87:1105–15.

Rosenberg, S. A. 1985. Lymphokine-activated killer cells: A new approach to the immunotherapy of cancer. *J. Natl. Cancer Inst.* 75:595–603.

Rosenberg, S. A., M. T. Lotze, L. M. Muul, et al. 1987. A progress report on the treatment of 157 patients with advanced cancer using lymphokine activated killer cells and interleukin-2 or interleukin-2 alone. *N. Engl. J. Med.* 316:889–97.

Samter, M., and G. J. Gleich. 1988. The eosinophil. In *Immunological Diseases*, 4th ed., ed. M. Samter, D. W. Talmage, M. M. Frank, et al., pp. 279–300. Boston: Little, Brown.

Schleimer, R. P., D. W. MacClashan, Jr., S. P. Peters, et al. 1984. Inflammatory mediators and mechanisms of release from purified human basophils and mast cells. *J. Allergy Clin. Immunol.* 74:473–81.

Stahl, P. D. 1990. The macrophage mannose receptor: Current status. *Am. J. Respir. Cell Mol. Biol.* 2:317–19.

Strieter, R. M., S. L. Kunkel, H. J. Showell, et al. 1989. Endothelial cell gene expression of a neutrophil chemotactic factor by TNF-α, LPS, and IL-1β. *Science* 243:1467–69.

Sun, X., and W. Hsueh. 1991. Platelet-activating factor produces shock, in vivo complement activation, and tissue injury in mice. *J. Immunol.* 147:509–14.

Wardlaw, A. 1990. Leukocyte adhesion to endothelium. *Clin. Exp. Allergy* 20:619–26.

Wedmore, C. V., and T. J. Williams. 1981. Control of vascular permeability by polymorphonuclear leukocytes in inflammation. *Nature* 289:646–50.

Weiss, J., M. Victor, and P. Elsbach. 1983. Role of charge and hydrophobic interactions of the bactericidal/permeability protein of neutrophils on gram negative bacteria. *J. Clin. Invest.* 71:540–49.

Weiss, L. 1972. *The Cells and Tissues of the Immune System*, p. 45. Englewood Cliffs: Prentice Hall.

6

Mechanisms of Injury by the Immune System

A. INTRODUCTION

There are several semantic pitfalls that can be encountered in any discussion of immune injury. When a foreign material elicits an adverse reaction in an individual, it is tempting to conclude the victim suffers an "allergy," but this overused term is often chosen carelessly and without foundation. Immunologists and toxicologists use the term "hypersensitivity" in different ways. The former use it in an antigen-specific sense, regarding it synonomously with "allergy." However, many toxicologists consider hypersensitivity the exaggerated response of a certain minority of the population at the lower end of any dose–response curve (Pratt 1990). We use the term in this text in the immunologic sense. To confuse the matter further, the term "hypersensitivity" has been used in several other contexts, e.g., hypersensitivity pneumonitis and multiple chemical hypersensitivity, which deviate from the usage as defined here. These specialized usages are discussed in turn.

It is important to determine and confirm the mechanism involved in immunologic hypersensitivity. Immunologic hypersensitivity implies that (1) the biology of the host has been irreversibly altered; (2) the host will respond to lower concentrations of the sensitizing agent than normal subjects; and (3) subsequent reactions in sensitized subjects may be injurious and even fatal. Obviously, human immunologic hypersensitivity is a serious medical/legal and industrial hygiene problem. Sensitized people may be forced to change life styles or occupations. Conversely, irritant or nonspecific reactions do not involve biological alterations in the host with long-term untoward health effects. When the causative agent is removed, the problem abates, whereas progressive sequelae often ensue from antigen-initiated immune injury.

It will also be important at the outset to distinguish immunologic hypersensitivity from true toxicity or damage to the immune system. Even though these two types of responses may superficially resemble each other, it is important to draw a distinction between them because the two have very different mechanisms and are discussed individually in separate chapters. People exposed to environmental agents may be adversely affected in either case.

B. DIFFERENTIATION OF HYPERSENSITIVITY FROM TOXICITY

There are three general guidelines that may be useful in distinguishing hypersensitivity from toxicity. First, the matter of dose may be helpful. Although some toxicants in the natural world are extremely potent, capable of exerting their effects in nanogram ranges, these extreme examples do not exist outside of infectious disease. Normally a poison is defined as something that has a lethal dose (LD_{50}) of 50 mg/kg body weight or less (Ottoboni 1984). Even if we consider that many things are toxic in smaller concentrations, allergens tend to be effective in even much greater dilutions, provided that they are affecting a presensitized, allergic individual. This brings up the second consideration, that of the requirement of presensitization. True allergens have no effect on nonimmune individuals on the first encounter. People who have never been out of Europe may safely rub their skin with American poison ivy, but only once! They simply would have had no prior sensitization experience. Unfortunately, one can become sensitized to substances (e.g., penicillin or papain) unknowingly, because such materials are or have been used commonly in many consumer products, and ample opportunity exists for presensitization. A final distinction between hypersensitivity and toxicity may be made by observing the incidence of those affected. True toxins adversely affect nearly all members of a population to the same extent within a given dose range. However, allergies are by definition idiosyncratic—not everyone exposed to allergens, e.g., ragweed pollen or egg white, develops a hypersensitivity—and only sporadic incidence of signs and symptoms among those exposed is presumptive evidence of a hypersensitivity. Other mechanisms of idiosyncratic reactions to xenobiotics are discussed in Chapter 10.

There remains the matter of distinguishing among the many different types of immune or immune-like injuries. In 1963, different types of hypersensitivity were classified by the Coombs and Gell system. This system, although heuristic at the time and in use for many years, does not go far enough in light of modern knowledge. It is oversimplified and often unhelpful in that in nature, these forms seldom appear individually but rather as mixed components. Most importantly, the system only deals with host injury *by* the immune system and not to damage done *to* it. Although the original four classes persist, the lines between them are not nearly so distinct, and many additional considerations must be made.

C. IgE-MEDIATED HYPERSENSITIVITY

The term hypersensitivity usually refers to that dependent on the special immunoglobulin class IgE (Coombs and Gell, type I). It has also been synonymously referred to as immediate-type hypersensitivity because of the rapid appearance of a wheal and flare skin response immediately after skin testing with antigen. This term has lost its usefulness because of the fact that not all IgE-mediated reactions induce such immediate-in-time responses.

1. Immediate Reactions

Immediate hypersensitivity may develop within families as a result of genetic propensity. Because of the genetic abnormality, there may be defects in the function of regulatory cell subsets or isotypic switching in B cells. The result is that, on initial exposure to allergen, B cells synthesize and secrete copious amounts of IgE. The concentration of IgE in serum of normal individuals is very low, on the order of <50–300 ng/ml, but higher levels are stimulated by certain parasitic infections or are associated with certain clinical states of atopy. Although the specificity of IgE molecules can be shown to be directed to a variety of antigens unrelated to the parasites, the bulk of it in allergic states is directed toward offending allergens.

When one compares the ubiquity of IgE with the comparatively low incidence of IgE-mediated disease, the question has long been considered to be what the function of IgE is in normal health. The IgE heavy chains attach to Fc receptors for the ϵ chains (Fc$_\epsilon$) on various cells. There are two types of these receptors for IgE (see Table 6-1 for a comparison). The high-affinity receptor (Fc$_\epsilon$RI) is found on basophils and mast cells, whereas the low-affinity receptor (Fc$_\epsilon$RII) is the same as the CD marker CD23, which has a wide distribution on potential antigen-presenting cells including B cells. It has been proposed that in addition to its pathology-promoting role, IgE also serves a positive function interacting with Fc$_\epsilon$RII receptors that might play a significant role in antigen capture and potentiating induced immune responses (Mudde et al. 1990). The IgE also participates in defense against parasitic worms by attaching to Fc$_\epsilon$RII receptors on eosinophils and neutrophils by the mechanisms of antibody-dependent cellular cytotoxicity (ADCC).

There can be from 5,000 to 27,000 Fc$_\epsilon$RI receptor sites for IgE heavy chains per basophil and up to 40,000 in atopic individuals. When two or more sites are cross-linked by any means, especially by affixed IgE reacting with specific antigen, a complex energy-dependent transduction of signals through the cell membrane stimulates the release of several mediators from cytoplasmic granules (Fig. 6-1). These mediators have powerful pharmacological properties and account for the major signs and symptoms of common allergies. The prototype of these mediators is histamine, whose mode of action (smooth muscle contraction, capillary dilatation, and increase in permeability) is brought about within seconds to minutes after release, leading to the once popular term, immediate-type hypersensitivity. If released in the major airways of the lung, histamine contracts bronchial smooth muscle and also stimulates mucus secretion, narrowing the airway lumina. Because of the reduced airway diameter, there is difficulty in moving air in and out of the lung. Mediators such as trytpase, chymase, and bradykinin-generating enzymes may, in some species, accelerate bronchoconstriction. Within minutes of granule release, the primary effector cells begin to synthesize additional mediators from cell membrane perturbation using the arachidonic acid and other pathways.

If the skin is the target organ, histamine and other products dilate venules and

TABLE 6-1.   Comparison of IgE High- and Low-Affinity Receptors

	Fc$_\epsilon$RI	Fc$_\epsilon$RII
Distribution	All mast cells and basophils	30% B cells 1% T cells 2% monocytes (Seasonal increase in atopics) Most eosinophils Platelets
Affinity	$K_d = 1 \times 10^{-9}$ M	$K_d = 1 \times 10^{-7}$ M
Number/cell	10^4 (basophils) 10^6 (mast cells)	1,000 (platelets) 5×10^5 (monocytes)
Function	Mediator release	Mediator release Antigen presentation IgE regulation

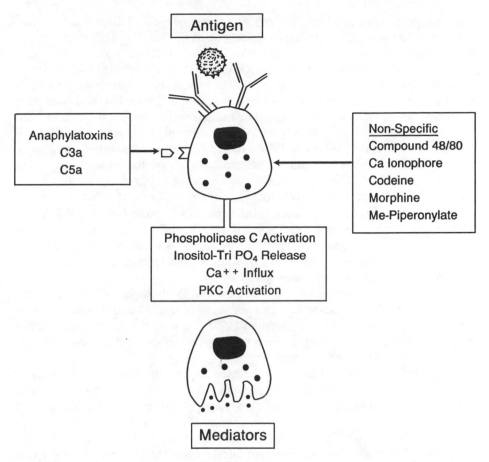

FIGURE 6–1.   Activation of mast cells/basophils. When two or more IgE receptor sites are cross-linked by any means, specifically by membrane-bound IgE reacting with antigen or nonspecifically by various activators, transduction of signals through the cell membrane stimulates the release of mediators from the cytoplasmic granules.

affect endothelial cells in such a way as to cause dilatation of superficial venules, contraction of endothelial cells, and a resultant increase in vascular permeability. Cutaneous sensory neurons are also stimulated, the afferent fibers of which originate near blood vessels and mast cells. One effect of this stimulation is a local pruritus. Efferent fibers bearing the impulses are carried back in the same branches and release the neuropeptide substance P, which causes a flare. The result is the "wheal-and-flare" reaction, a large area of vasodilatation yielding swelling (the wheal) and a redness (flare) that is considerably wider than that over which histamine could diffuse. Heparin may potentiate the reaction by preventing clotting of blood in the allergic site. Observation of this reaction is the basis for assessment of human IgE-mediated allergies carried out by scratch testing. In addition, specifically synthesized mediators alter the trafficking of eosinophils. Eosinophil chemotactic factor (ECF-A) and inflammatory factor of anaphylaxis (INF-A) stimulate the release of cells from the bone marrow, resulting in increased percentages of this special class of granulocytes in the peripheral blood. Increased numbers of eosinophils in the peripheral blood are considered to be a hallmark of allergic reactions, and many of them marginate in capillaries of the allergic site.

Laboratory tests can be used to support a tentative medical diagnosis of immediate hypersensitivity. The primary clinical means of detecting IgE-mediated hypersensitivity remains with the skin test (scratch test), in which the skin is superficially abraded with a small, sharp instrument and small doses of suspected allergen are applied to the abraded areas. The appearance and size of the wheal-and-flare response occurring within minutes, compared to saline and histamine controls, can be considered positive. The radioallergosorbent test (RAST) is an in vitro radioisotopic method often used to document the presence of allergen-specific IgE in serum (Adkinson 1974). Basically, suspected antigen, coupled to a solid-phase support (e.g., cellulose acetate disks), is incubated with serum and washed before the addition of radiolabeled antihuman IgE. After further washing, the disk is placed in a suitable isotope counter. Although this is a very objective test, the presence of circulating IgE correlates with symptoms at only about 70% (Berg and Johansson 1974). One may exhibit positive skin sensitivity without showing clinical signs and symptoms of allergy on natural exposure to the same agent, but skin reactions are regarded by most allergists as having a higher correlation with clinical state than RAST testing.

Although technically more difficult to perform, the basophil histamine release assay gives a better correlation between release of mediators and symptoms. Here the correlation exceeds 90% (Siraganian 1975). Because the assay measures the release of histamine following interactions between cell-bound IgE and allergen, this high correlation is not unexpected.

Predicting the ability of agents to be used in humans to induce immediate-type hypersensitivity is a much more difficult matter. Not only is there no good, inexpensive animal model for human atopy, there are so many individual genetic and environmental reasons unrelated to the antigen that people develop such allergies (see Chapter 10). One exception is in the evaluation of products that might be contacted by inhalation exposure. An intratracheal test (IT test) was validated by the Procter and Gamble Company as a means of evaluating large-molecular-weight xenobiotics (e.g., detergent enzymes) for their ability to induce an immediate hypersensitivity response in the respiratory tracts of workers involved in the manufacture of the product (Ritz and Bond 1986; Sarlo and Clark 1992). In this test, guinea pigs are dosed intratracheally with the xenobiotic weekly for 10 weeks. During this period of exposure, the guinea pigs have a chance to develop an immediate hypersensitity response to the agent. The response is measured by quantitating the circulating level of antibody and the gross respiratory responses (changes in the respiration rate) of the animals immediately following challenge. Antibody level is assessed using the passive cutaneous anaphylaxis assay and is related to the allergic potency of the xenobiotic being tested. This procedure is an in vivo skin test technique that takes advantage of guinea pig antibodies' ability to passively fix to mast cells/basophils, allowing release of mediators on antigen challenge. Questions have been raised in the past about the appropriateness of intratracheal dosing versus inhalation exposure, but comparisons of the intratracheal and inhalation routes indicated that the appearance of antibodies and onset of respiratory symptoms were similar regardless of method (Ritz and Bond 1986).

To use these data for risk assessment purposes, the response of the animals to the new enzyme or other large-molecular-weight xenobiotic is compared to that to other materials that have a documented history of safe use in consumer and occupational settings. If the responses of the two materials are the same, then consumer and occupational exposures to the new material are set at the same level as those for the historical ones. If the responses are different, then adjustments in exposure are made accordingly.

2. Late-Phase Reactions

If sensitized human subjects are subjected to pulmonary function testing following bronchoprovocation testing with offending antigen, two distinct types of reactions, based on time after inhalation as measured by the forced expiratory volume in 1 sec method (FEV_1), may be encountered, and indeed both forms may even be seen in the same patient (Pepys 1969). Both early and late types are IgE dependent but evolve into distinctly separate pharmocological reactions. In the first or immediate type, there is a rapid decline in FEV_1 within 15 min that rapidly reverses to near-normal levels. It is indicative of the immediate release and activity of histamine-type mediators released from lung mast cells. It is primarily a bronchoconstrictive response.

The second type of lowered FEV_1 response occurs 6–8 hr afterwards and can be more severe than the first but recovers within 12–24 hr. This reaction has been termed the late-phase reaction (LPR). This response is primarily one of increased mucus secretion and airway edema in addition to bronchoconstriction. Late-phase reactions also may occur in the skin, where they follow a similar time course as the pulmonary reactions. Instead of a wheal-and-flare reaction, LPR skin reactions may take on the appearance of a large subcutaneous swelling that is very painful. Immediate histamine release appears to be of prime importance in the early reaction, whereas cyclooxygenase and lipoxygenase products are more important in LPR skin reactions (Reshef et al. 1989).

In addition, a family of cytokines known as histamine-releasing factors are currently being recognized as essential in devlopment of the LPR. These factors are released from a variety of cells (e.g., B and T lymphocytes, platelets, alveolar macrophages, and vascular endothelial cells) and act primarily on basophils primed with a certain type of IgE known as IgE^+ (MacDonald and Lichtenstein 1990). There is the view that the LPR may be a more appropriate model of allergic inflammation than the traditional acute response to antigen (MacDonald and Lichtenstein 1990).

Although not all additional details of the development of the LPR are agreed on, it appears that mast-cell-derived mediators such as neutrophil chemotactic factor, LTB_4, and platelet-activating factor (PAF) also contribute to the reaction by attracting neutrophils and eosinophils to the allergic site (Henderson 1988). A comparison of classical immediate reactions and LPRs may be found in Fig. 6–2. There is also evidence that T cells accumulate in both skin and lung LPRs and may influence the tissue response by producing cytokines that promote activation and survival of eosinophils, promote MHC II expression on antigen-presenting cells, and prime mast cells/basophils for mediator release (Frew and Kay 1990). Although the neutrophils may function positively by ingesting and removing cellular debris, they may also contribute to the local tissue damage by means of metabolic production of hydrogen peroxide, which interacts with the myeloperoxidase system. The products of this system are injurious to basement membranes and epithelial cells. In addition, elastase and collagenase are released, which can also damage structural elements of tissue, and these become important

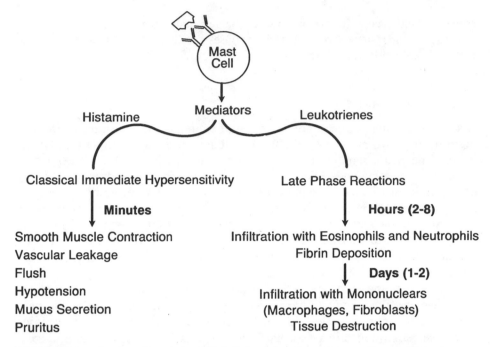

FIGURE 6–2.   A comparison of classical, IgE-dependent, immediate reactions and late-phase reactions (LPR) initated by activation of membrane-bound IgE on mast cells and basophils.

if the condition is a chronic one. Release of PAF may also contribute directly to the vasoactive and dynamic alterations of airway function.

3. Bronchial Asthma

One of the major clinical forms of immune injury triggered by exposure to xeno-biotics (in terms of morbidity) is bronchial asthma. Asthma is clinically defined as reversible obstruction of the airways and is caused by their hyperresponsiveness. Much of this hyperresponsiveness may be explained by underlying inflammation, which induces these tissues to acquire greater reactivity to stimuli, but part may also be explained by genetic predisposition (see Chapter 10). A variety of cells produce an array of mediators that interact in a number of ways to contribute to the bronchial hyperresponsiveness that underlies the clinical aspects of asthma (Barnes 1989).

In normal subjects, important pulmonary functions such as bronchoconstriction, pulmonary vessel dilation, and mucus secretion are stimulated by cholinergic release of acetylcholine on muscarinic receptors in the respective target organs. Conversely, relaxation of smooth muscle, decreased capillary dilatation, and decreased goblet cell secretion are the results of stimulation of the β-adrenergic receptors in target cells and tissues. This stimulation activates adenylate cyclase with the attendant production and accumulation of cAMP. The synergistic action of these two opposing neuropharmacological systems may simplistically be viewed as resulting in the necessary tone required to carry out normal function, and any upset in β-adrenergic stimulation or excess cholinergic function will change the balance and lead to asthma (Szentivanyi 1968). One possible type of asthma may then be viewed as blockade of the β-adrenergic functions. A possible insight into how such a blockade might occur is afforded by the observation that autoantibodies to β_2-adrenergic receptors have been associated in some individuals with abnormal autonomic responsiveness (Fraser, Venter, and Kaliner 1981).

As useful as the Szentivanyi theory has been, it does not fully explain all of the observations. It does not consider the possible cholinergic modulating effects of α_1- and α_2-adrenergic stimulation. The theory predicts that β-blockade in normal subjects would lead to unopposed cholinergic bronchoconstriction, but this is mainly seen in only those suffering from moderate to severe asthma; i.e., something identifies the asthmatic victim other than mere imbalance of this system. Most importantly, the theory was formulated long before the discovery of neuropeptide transmitters that also affect these same functions. Noncholinergic excitatory functions can also be stimulated by peptides such as substance P, and nonadrenergic inhibitory functions can be stimulated by peptides such as VIP (vasoactive intestinal peptide) (Barnes 1987). One can make a similar case for asthma induction via an imbalance of these peptides. Inflammation could lead to release of excitatory peptides or result in enzymatic degradation of the inhibitory peptides; either way the balance would be upset in favor of hyperresponsiveness. But again, an additional host factor must be necessary, because VIP or substance P produces bronchodilation or bronchoconstriction, respectively, only in asthmatics but not in normal subjects (Cavanah and Casale 1990).

It is essential first to realize that not all bronchial asthma is allergy induced. Indeed, asthma is a heterogeneous disease, no doubt with separate etiologies. Because of the intimate relationship between control of bronchial secretion and smooth muscle function by autonomic neurotransmitters and mast cell secretion of mediators affecting the production of these transmitters, it is obvious that asthma is a complicated disease, and only some of it may be IgE induced. Nonspecific irritants, certain drugs, and both physical and psychological stress can trigger asthmatic attacks in the pharmacologically predisposed. Childhood asthma is usually IgE mediated, and positive skin tests can be demonstrated to responsible allergens. It is estimated that a proven antigenic component can be associated with asthma only 35–55% of the time (McFadden 1984). When asthma develops after 40 years of age, there is a poor correlation with skin test sensitivity, and there is often evidence of prior bronchial irritation.

Occupational Asthma

An important respiratory disease in industrial health is occupational asthma, a disease that differs from IgE-mediated atopic asthma in several respects. The disease may develop in people who are not necessarily clinically atopic, and it often requires longer periods of exposure before sensitization and before it leads to the development of signs and symptoms (Seaton 1984). Clinically, patients suffering from occupational asthma may present a spectrum of asthmatic responses following exposure or challenge; i.e., early, late-phase, dual, or even repetitive responses may be evoked. A reaction consisting of wheezing and coughing may occur soon after exposure and last for about an hour, or, more typically, it may not begin until several hours after exposure and last for a day or more. Although occupational asthma has a complex pathophysiology not well understood, many of the components are physiological manifestations of late-phase reactions. The response to the larger-molecular-weight inducers of this disease is largely IgE mediated, but poorly understood pharmacological mechanisms not necessarily dependent on IgE mediation are responsible for reactions to the smaller-molecular-weight substances (discussed in more detail in Chapter 11).

Animal Models of Asthma

There has been much interest in using animal models of asthma, but they remain subject to many drawbacks. The main problem is that spontaneous disease resembling human bronchial asthma occurs rarely in animals and there are so many important interspecies differences in immunologic, anatomic, and pharmacological parameters among them. Yet, well-chosen animal models are useful in several other respects (Wanner et al. 1990). They enable the use of invasive techniques in vivo, provide easy access to tissues for in vitro studies, and provide several important ways to perform preclinical trials for human drugs. Most of all, several strains from different species can be genetically manipulated to produce hybrids with characteristics remarkably similar to selected human asthmatic parameters. Ideally, animal models for asthma should mimic the pathophysiology and immunopathology of the human disease in that (1) airway hyperreactivity should be demonstrable either before or following antigenic challenge; (2) pulmonary function changes elicited by challenge with allergen should be consistent with reversible airway obstructive disease; and (3) the presence of allergen-specific IgE should be documented by serological assays or appropriate in vivo methods. In addition, treatment modalities effective in man should be effective in the animal models.

Models have been implemented to study immediate allergic lung responses to large-molecular-weight allergens or parasitic extracts. Many studies are performed in the cross-bred Basenji–Greyhound (BG) dog, rat, or mouse. Hybrids between Greyhounds and Basenji dogs generate offspring with nonspecific airway hyperreactivity. The BG dog responds to a wide range of therapeutic bronchoconstrictors including histamine and methacholine. The dogs can be sensitized with extracts of *Ascaris suum*. When they are challenged with this antigen, the pulmonary function changes are consistent with the pathophysiology of human asthma (Hirschman, Malley, and Downes 1980; Peters, Hirschman, and Malley 1982). Moreover, sensitivity can be passively transferred to normal dogs via serum exchanges, skin test reactivity is demonstrable, and propranolol treatment increases airway resistance and response to bronchodilators in a manner similar to humans.

Some strains of Sprague–Dawley rats have genetically determined airway hyperreactivity that can be evoked by classical bronchoconstrictors, and allergic responses consistent with the definition of human asthma have been reported. The allergic response can be modulated by common inhibitors of mast cell degranulation (e.g., cromolyn) and phosphodiesterase activity (e.g., theophylline). Unlike the case in humans, the primary physiological response is mediated by serotonin.

Airway hyperreactivity can be induced in normal sheep by immunization with *Ascaris* antigens. Pulmonary challenge results in immediate bronchoconstriction followed by a classical late asthmatic response. Airway hyperreactivity to a variety of stimuli is demonstrable following resolution of both the immediate and late reactions. Data suggest that histamine and leukotrienes may play roles in the pathophysiology of the early and late responses (Abraham et al. 1983; Lemanski and Kaliner 1988).

The rabbit has been used as a model for both the early and late asthmatic reactions. As in the sheep, the early response is mediated by histamine and other pharmacologically active mediators (Larsen 1985). The late response is characterized by infiltration of neutrophils in both the large and small airways, which release platelet-activating factor. This mediator in turn stimulates other cells to participate in the response.

The lack of suitable reagents has hampered the development of models to study the allergic reactions induced by low-molecular-weight chemicals. Hapten-protein conjugates may be required for both the sensitization and challenge phases. The reagents are also necessary for laboratory studies to document the presence of hapten-specific IgE antibodies in serum but must meet certain criteria. The hapten must be covalently linked to protein with a high molar substitution ratio (hapten:protein) without altering the allergenic characteristics of the hapten. In addition, the newly synthesized conjugate must be soluble under physiological conditions and easily aerosolized by conventional means. With the exception of highly reactive haptens, it is often difficult to synthesize conjugates meeting all of these criteria.

Asthma induced by low-molecular-weight chemicals has been modeled in several species including primates. The guinea pig has been used in studies of toluene diisocyanate (TDI)-induced asthma. Although no underlying bronchial hyperreactivity has been demonstrated in the guinea pig, it is well documented that bronchoconstriction can be initiated in this species by IgE-like release of mediators from mast cells and basophils (Kallos and Kallos 1934). The principal mediators of allergic reactions in the guinea pig may be leukotrienes. The TDI reaction in guinea pigs involves cytophilic antibody and the release of pharmacological mediators (Karol et al. 1980; Tse, Chen, and Bernstein 1979). However, the relevance of the model to the human experience is unclear in that there is very poor correlation of clinical sensitivity and the presence of immune effectors in humans. This is discussed in more detail below and in Chapter 11.

The rabbit has been used to study hypersensitivity reactions to plicatic acid, the agent responsible for red cedar asthma in exposed workers (Chan et al. 1987). Specific IgG and IgE were demonstrable in serum of immunized animals. When challenged with the acid, the rabbits responded with increases in respiratory frequency and pulmonary resistance.

Although the strengths of these animal models outweigh their weaknesses, their limitations should be considered in the interpretation of data (Wanner et al. 1990). The direction for further development of additional models is clear. There is a critical need to develop rapid, cost-effective in vivo or in vitro models that predict whether chemicals can induce immediate hypersensitivity reactions in the lung or skin. The chemical and pharmaceutical industries could use these models to screen commercial candidates at an early stage of development. Potentially allergenic compounds would be dropped from consideration. The result would be cost savings, reduced animal utilization, and safer consumer products.

D. CYTOTOXIC ANTIBODIES

Injury by cytotoxic antibodies (class II, Coombs and Gell) refers to cellular lysis or other damage brought about by antibodies of immunoglobulin classes other than IgE, reacting directly with antigens on the cell. The antibody could be directed toward (1) a foreign (extrinsic) antigen that had a similar chemical structure to an intrinsic antigen on a cell membrane, (2) a biologically important receptor on the cell membrane, (3) an extrinsic antigen that has become nonspecifically adsorbed to a cell membrane, or (4) an intrinsic antigen normally shielded from immune effectors that becomes exposed by a xenobiotic or disease process (Fig. 6–3). Most knowledge concerning cytotoxic antibodies has been learned from studies of infectious disease, where microbes induce responses against antigens that cross-react with epitopes on host tissue, i.e., autoimmunity. The etiology of rheumatic fever has been associated with previous infections of β-hemolytic, group A hemolytic streptococci. Although several theories of pathogenesis exist, all involve the induction of streptococcal antibodies that share cross-reactivity with important tissue antigens in the myocardium. Whether such antibody responses to nonmicrobial xenobiotics can similarly cross-react with host tissue antigens remains an interesting but largely unproven question.

The latter case is of concern in immunotoxicology because there are certain drugs (e.g., apronalide [Sedormid] or quinine derivatives) that are haptenic in inducing antibodies, and when these combine with the drug, the complexes have a high affinity for attaching to platelet CR receptors. If the substance is haptenic and stimulates an antibody response, the result could be a diminution of platelets from either lysis or enhanced phagocytosis, resulting in the syndrome of idiopathic thrombocytopenic purpura, a bleeding disorder (Karpatkin 1988). In some instances, drug-dependent antibodies have even led to a disseminated intravascular coagulation (Spearing et al. 1990). Erythrocytes can be targeted similarly as innocent bystanders when certain drugs or drug–antibody immune complexes become adsorbed to membrane surfaces. Subsequent coating with IgG and complement may lead to an acquired hemolytic anemia. The case with α-methyldopa is distinctively different. Somehow the drug leads to an alteration of immunoregulation that produces excessive antibodies with an Rh specificity (Worlledge, Carstairs, and Dacie 1966). Drug-induced agranulocytosis must be looked at more carefully because in addition to the possibility of similar immune complex adsorption mechanisms, some drugs (e.g., chloramphenicol) may induce direct bone marrow toxicity. In either event, such drugs can be considered immunotoxic by our definition. The list of agents known to induce these types of damage to platelets, erythrocytes, and granulocytes is extensive, and a few well-known examples of each appear in Table 6–2.

Another form of cytotoxic damage to normal host tissue by antibody is through the intermediary of antibody-dependent cellular cytotoxicity (ADCC).

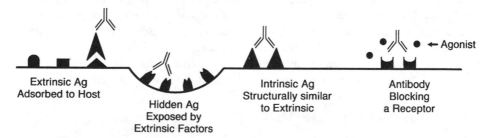

FIGURE 6–3.   Examples of different modes of action of cytotoxic antibodies. Beginning from the left, antibodies are shown reacting with an extrinsic antigen physically adsorbed to host cells. The next depicts the exposure of an intrinsic antigen normally shielded from immune effectors, now capable of reacting with antibodies. The third example shows antibodies reacting with a host antigen with a similar chemical structure. The example on the far right shows antibodies blocking a biologically important receptor on a cell membrane.

TABLE 6-2.   Some Agents Leading to Hematological Immunotoxicity

Immunologic thrombocytopenic purpura	Autoimmune hemolytic anemia	Idiosyncratic neutropenia
Sedormid (apronalide)	α-Methyldopa	Indomethacin
Quinine	Penicillin	p-Aminophenol deriva-
Quinidine	Quinidine	tives
Heparin	Stibophen	Pyrazolon derivatives
Gold salts	Chlorpromazine	Chloramphenicol
Sulfonamides	Sulfonamides	Penicillins
Sulfa derivatives	Cephalothin	Phenothiazines
p-Aminosalicylic acid	Procainamide	Phenytoins
Phenytoin	Isoniazid	Sulfonamides
Heroin	Diclofenac	
Indomethacin and aspirin		
Toluene diisocyanate		
Vinyl chloride		

Antibody that attaches to Fc receptors of NK cells, neutrophils, or eosinophils will destroy any cell to which specific antigen is attached. Another question and possible shortcoming of the Coombs and Gell system in light of modern knowledge is where to place the cytotoxic activity of NK cells that attach to host tissue by other means: IL-2–activated NK cells (lymphokine-activated killer [LAK] cells) increase their adhesion and cytotoxicity for endothelial cells and may account for the toxicity associated with LAK use in cancer treatment (Aronson et al. 1988).

Antibodies specific for hormone or neurotransmitter receptors on cellular membranes certainly can lead to well-characterized autoimmune disorders. Four such disorders have been described in detail: Graves' disease (anti-thyroid-stimulating hormone-receptors), myasthenia gravis (anti-nicotinic-acteylcholine-receptors), type B insulin-resistant diabetes (anti-insulin-receptors), and allergic respiratory disease (anti-β_2-adrenergic-receptors) (Fraser and Venter 1984). The perplexing question about antibodies with such specificities is how to explain their origin. The possibility of coincidental cross-reactivity with environmental stimulants is largely conjectural with one exception. It is possible that receptor-specific antibodies arise by forming antiidiotypic antibodies against antibodies directed to external ligands. By definition, an antiidiotypic antibody is an antiantibody and is considered the internal image of the original antigen (Jerne 1974), and if that is true, the antiidiotypic antibody ought to possess similar biological functions as the original antigen. In fact, spectacular proof of this has been demonstrated with idiotypic antibodies obtained from animals immunized with antibodies against insulin or β blockers, which not only compete with the original hormone antigens for receptor sites but also mimic some of the forms of agonist activity of those hormones (Schreiber et al. 1980; Shechter et al. 1982).

A variation of this form occurs when antibody is directed against a noncellular structure (e.g., against glomerular or alveolar basement membrane) or a biologically important molecule (e.g., anti-vitamin-B$_{12}$-intrinsic-factor). Subsequent reaction certainly could lead to altered function, although not strictly cytotoxic in nature. Some studies have shown that certain lectins and cationic proteins can become "planted" in the complex structure of the glomerular basement membrane and, as antigens, elicit antibody responses that can be harmful. In these cases the antibody is specific for antigens extrinsic to the host (Golbus and Wilson 1979; Border et al. 1982). It has been speculated that membrane alteration can occur by natural means to noninfectious environmental agents. Daniell, Couser, and Rosentstock (1988) reported on a worker exposed to organic solvents with this type of glomerulonephritis and have reviewed the epidemiologic literature for workers similarly associated with these types of agents.

When antibodies become bound to such biologically critical membranes, they fix complement, cleaving off chemotactic peptides. Neutrophils become attracted early and are activated at the site, causing local tissue injury by production of toxic oxygen radicals and proteolytic enzymes. If the condition persists, macrophages accumulate at the site and can produce injury by secretion of cytokines such as TNF-α (Hruby et al. 1991). The possibility also exists that membranes can be damaged directly by terminal complement components (Kopp and Burrell 1982). When kidney sections from this type of glomerulonephritis are stained with fluorescent-labeled antiimmunoglobulin, the pattern results in a fine, continuous pattern outlining the basement membrane; i.e., all of the membrane is stained.

E. IMMUNE COMPLEX DISEASE

Immune complex disease (Coombs and Gell, type III) is a distinct type of injury resulting from the deposition of soluble antigen–antibody complexes in key anatomic locations, e.g., capillary beds in the skin or glomerular tufts in the kidney. Complement is an important part of the development of this form as well as in immune cytotoxic injury. Immune complexes deposited at the critical tissue sites activate the complement cascade, thereby attracting inflammatory cells.

Traditionally, two prototype diseases (serum sickness and the Arthus reaction) have been offered to illustrate immune complex diseases in humans, but neither is a very good example. Some but not all of the manifestations of serum sickness are traceable to immune complexes, although the syndrome has an IgE component as well. The disease was formerly common at a time when horse antisera and antitoxins were used to treat pneumococcal pneumonia, diphtheria, and tetanus, among others. Serum sickness was basically brought about through the induction of humoral antibody responses to the large amount of foreign antigen injected (horse proteins). The disease became manifest by various combinations of onset of fever, malaise, pruritic rash, lymphadenopathy, nausea, vomiting, mild proteinuria, vasculitis, and arthralgia. Precipitating antibody presumably reacted with undegraded horse antigens still present, formed immune complexes, and deposited in the vascular bed in certain target organs leading to inflammation. Despite the advent of antibiotics and replacement of heterologous serum treatment with immunoglobulins of human origin, serum sickness remains of interest because of the similarity of signs, symptoms, and lesions induced by various drug-induced immune reactions.

The second prototype traditionally given for immune complex disease has been the Arthus reaction, long a laboratory curiosity. The reaction is produced in rabbits repeatedly given intradermal injections of a protein antigen. After eleven or twelve injections given every other day, there will appear within 48 hr an intense inflammatory reaction at the site of the last injection so severe as to lead to necrosis. It is thought that the immune complexes localize on blood vessel walls, activate complement, and attract neutrophils followed later by monocytes and aggregated platelets. Products of activated inflammatory cells and thromboemboli then destroy the vessel wall. It is doubtful if such a necrotic dermal reaction occurs in humans. Humans do not produce precipitins nearly as well as the Arthus-prone rabbit, and secondly there is just no occasion to immunize humans in such an artificial manner. The edematous subcutaneous skin reaction occasionally seen in humans following intradermal skin test antigens is now considered to be mediated by the late-phase reaction sequence.

Formerly, the disease hypersensitivity pneumonitis was believed to be a pulmonary form of an Arthus reaction in which the presence of circulating precipitating antibodies was thought to react with inhaled protein antigens, leading to an immune-complex-mediated inflammation of the alveolar interstitium (Pepys 1969). Although precipitins often accompany overt clinical disease, their presence is now considered evidence of antigenic contact only, rather than as an indicator of pathogenesis (Burrell and Rylander 1981).

The modern prototype of immune complex disease replacing serum sickness and the Arthus reaction is immune-complex-mediated glomerulonephritis. This form, distinct from the anti-glomerular-basement-membrane type of injury discussed earlier can be produced experimentally in rabbits by intravenously injecting large amounts of foreign protein. As antibody production to the foreign proteins accelerates, constant interaction of antibody with the continuously present antigen leads to circulating immune complex formation. The biological properties of the resultant complexes are dependent on their size, charge, and antigen:antibody ratios. Most complexes are rapidly removed from circulation by normal phagocytic processes, but those with high ratios resist clearance and are deposited in various anatomically vulnerable sites such as in the renal glomeruli (Barnett 1986). As they lodge in the renal glomerular capillaries, complement is fixed, and inflammatory cells are activated. Toxic oxygen radicals and proteolytic enzymes from inflammatory cells degrade endothelial cells and basement membrane such that immune complexes move through the capillary wall toward the tubule lumina. Their deposition is thus random throughout the glomerular walls, and when stained by fluorescent-labeled antiglobulin, the deposits take on a discontinuous, granular appearance ("lumpy-dumpy" deposits). The majority of immune-induced glomerulonephritis in humans is produced in this manner, and although the offending antigen is often traceable to antigens of infectious microorganisms or autoantigens, it is conceivable that the immune reactions are to extrinsic antigens of environmental importance.

Several diseases are associated with large amounts of circulating immune complexes, but only in a few is their pathogenic significance clear. Immune complexes are associated with various autoimmune diseases, appear following certain infectious diseases, and are frequently found in malignancy (Barnett 1986). Although their role in immunotoxicity has not been adequately assessed, their appearance could be taken to mean a profound antibody response to a large amount or a continuing supply of antigen and, in addition to glomerulonephritis and vasculitis, could be indirectly responsible for such immunotoxic sequelae as reduced phagocytosis (Starkebaum, Jiminez, and Arend 1982) or inhibition of B-cell antibody production by simultaneously interacting with Fc and antigen receptors (Taylor 1982).

Several laboratory methods are available for detection of immune complexes in serum or tissue. Comparison of results from fluorescent antibody studies with conjugate specificities for immunoglobulins, C1q, and C3b indicates the deposition of immune complexes in situ. Additional sensitivity may be provided by using polyclonal rheumatoid factor, an antiimmunoglobulin that utilizes exposed Fc determinants on the complexes (McDougal et al. 1982). Analytical ultracentrifugation data may be useful in indicating the presence of immune complexes because uncomplexed IgG and IgM have distinctive sedimentation coefficients and patterns, but this is not a procedure widely available in diagnostic settings. Various techniques of precipitation of complexes with polyethylene glycol (PEG) have also been described (Hudson and Hay 1989). Because PEG precipitates proteins in relation to their molecular size, differential precipitation of the larger complexes can be accomplished by varying the PEG concentration used. Other techniques take advantage of the fact that serum immune complexes will react with or consume precise amounts of such added reactants as C1q, rheumatoid factor (an anti-IgM), or anti-C3. Finally, use may be made of the Raji cell assay, which employs a B-lymphoblastoid cell line that possesses Fc and C receptors on its cell membranes but no expression of innate immunoglobulins (Theofilopoulos and Dixon 1976).

F. NON-SPECIFIC COMPLEMENT ACTIVATION

Although complement can be effectively activated by IgG_1, IgG_3, and IgM (and to a lesser extent by IgG_2) after reacting with homologous antigen, complement may also be activated in the absence of antibody, usually via the alternative pathway. A variety of large-molecular-weight molecules that tend to be colloidal or finely dispersed in physical state, highly polymerized such as polysaccharides, or certain proteolytic enzymes like thrombin can activate the alternative pathway. Some important inflammatory materials, e.g., bacterial endotoxin, can activate either complement pathway independently (Morrison and Kline 1977). Their importance is that inflammation can be induced without the requirement of prior antigen-specific sensitization. Although a number of substances can be shown to exhibit this property under appropriate in vitro conditions, to incriminate this pathway as a mechanism in immunotoxicity requires that an additional host defect must also be present to explain idiosyncrasy. Why would such a mechanism occur only in certain individuals of a population, all of whom might be exposed to the given agent? Possibly the possession of an unusually labile complement component or a genetic lack of one of the important control substances is also necessary (Berrens, Guikers, and van Dijk 1974).

Many substances, especially inhalants, have been shown to activate complement in vitro (see Table 6–3), but great care must be taken in extrapolating results obtained from such studies to realistic in vivo situations. Far fewer studies are available that have subjected test animals to in vivo testing to determine if these substances actually incite injurious complement-dependent reactions. One approach is to measure peripheral complement levels following exposure, but such levels are not usually affected unless the challenge dose is very high. A second approach is to pretreat an animal with cobra venom factor, which, when done properly, activates and consumes most of the C3 in vivo. The animal is then exposed to the suspected agent, and appropriate responses are compared with untreated controls. Another problem is in the choice of animal species. Guinea pigs have such a high reserve of complement that it may be difficult to show that any of the total hemolytic activity has been reduced. Hence, one must look for the appearance of various activated components or split fragments.

TABLE 6–3.   Occupational Materials Known to Activate Complement Non-specifically
In Vitro

Cereal grain extracts
Chrysotile asbestos fibers
Cotton dust
Cuprophane hemodialyzer membranes
Fungal extracts
Pigeon dropping extracts
Radiocontrast media
Rye dust
Silage
Spring wheat dust
Sugar cane polysaccharide
Volcanic ash

Inhaled cell wall components of bacteria and fungi, e.g., peptidoglycan (Smith et al. 1980) and bacterial lipopolysaccharide (Lantz et al. 1985; Burrell, Lantz, and Hinton 1988) have been shown to activate the alternative complement pathway and to result in physiological and pathological alterations in pulmonary function and structure. The disease hypersensitivity pneumonitis may be initiated by complement activation leading to inflammation after inhalation of moldy vegetable dusts (Olenchock and Burrell 1976). Such activation may occur in the absence of antigen-specific immunization and cannot be induced in complement-deficient or cobra-venom-treated animals (Burrell and Pokorney 1977). Although the pathogenesis of this disease is complicated and involves many other factors (Richerson 1983), this type of evidence indicates that the initial inflammation may be mediated by nonspecific complement activation.

At least two iatrogenic (physician-induced) reactions involve nonspecific complement activation, although the extent to which these factors participate in pathogenesis is uncertain. These reactions are the anaphylactoid shock syndrome produced in certain people by injection of water-soluble iodinated radiocontrast media used in radiologic evaluations (Arroyave, Schatz, and Simon 1979) and that which sometimes occurs immediately following initiation of extracorporeal renal hemodialysis (Craddock et al. 1977). Both syndromes involve complement alterations in the absence of specific antibody, although the etiology of each reaction is far more complicated and requires interaction with other immunologic components (see Chapter 11). The density of the radiocontrast medium and the polymeric nature and high degree of surface area of the filter membranes of the dialyzer are thought to be the responsible initiators.

The question of whether complement may be activated following ingestion of antigen has been addressed with uncertain conclusions. Aspirin- and sodium-salicylate-associated bronchospasm in certain asthmatics has been reported, and depressed peripheral complement levels have been demonstrated in a portion of these (Arroyave et al. 1977), although negative results have been reported as well (Pleskow et al. 1982). At best, complement activation may only be an accompanying phenomenon, not an inciting factor. This may be the case with many types of inflammation in which complement activation has been reported. Numerous studies have been conducted on various types of pulmonary inflammation, especially that initiated by contact with bacterial endotoxin, and although much evidence exists for complement activation, the collective thinking is that it is unnecessary for inflammation.

A slightly different immune-like reaction may occur in byssinosis, a disease found in handlers and processors of raw cotton. The raw cotton is grossly contaminated with many biologically active materials, most of them from the plant parts surrounding the bolls known as bracts (Nichols 1991). One of the materials associated with cotton bract dust is a tetrahydroxyflavan polymer known to react nonspecifically with the Fc portion of immunoglobulin molecules (Edwards and Jones 1973). Whether this reaction activates complement is unknown, but the presence of this precipitated protein may possibly be inflammatory. In this case immunoglobulin is involved, but not in its usual well-known capacity. Such examples as these further illustrate the limitations of the original Coombs and Gell system in addressing all of the many forms of immune injury.

G. DELAYED-TYPE REACTIONS

The final category in the original Coombs and Gell system, type IV, is the most obsolete in light of modern knowledge. Originally it referred to damage mediated by cytotoxic lymphocytes occurring 48–72 hr after contact with antigen. Formerly there was a greatly oversimplified distinction between immediate and delayed-type hypersensitivities, wherein the former was thought to be a humoral allergy and the latter cellular. In fact, both of these types possess elements of each. For example, T-cell modulation clearly controls IgE responses and the pathogenesis of immediate types of disease (Sustiel and Rocklin 1989) whereas IgE has been found to be important in the elicitation of the effector cells for the delayed type (Ptak, Geba, and Askenase 1991). There has even been the suggestion that since both eosinophils and T lymphocytes are involved in LPR as well as classical delayed-type reactions, the main difference is in the kinetics of response of the indicated cell populations (Gaga et al. 1991).

The antigen can be viewed either as an intrinsic part of living cells or as an extrinsic one adsorbed to host tissue. It exists in the form of two basic prototypes having a common immunologic basis. One, emanating from the study of infectious disease, is the tuberculin skin reaction used to detect immunologic contact with the tubercle bacillus. The skin is injected with a small amount of the purified protein tuberculin derivative (PPD), and if the injected person has had immunologic contact with the protein in the past, presumably through infection, an inflammatory response will appear within 24–72 hr at the injection site. For this reason, this form of hypersensitivity has been classically referred to as delayed-type hypersensitivity (DTH), in contrast to the immediate type discussed above. The reaction is characterized by redness (erythema) and a solid swelling (induration) that may last for several days and be so severe as to desquamate the skin and become necrotic. Since the prototype was associated with infectious disease, and since it may be seen with several other types of infection, this form is sometimes also called "allergy of infection." This is an unfortunate choice of terms because, as we shall see, disposition of infectious agents can be accomplished by different cell-mediated mechanisms, and the same immunologic mechanism is also responsible for immune reactions to many inanimate xenobiotics.

Of more immunotoxicologic relevance is the other prototype, a result of skin contact with a variety of extrinsic antigens leading to the expression of allergic contact dermatitis, of which poison ivy is the best-known American example.

This lymphocyte-mediated event doubtless involves many mediators, and in nature, allergic contact dermatitis may coexist with IgE-mediated sensitivity to the same antigen. In fact, 5–hydroxytryptamine, usually considered a mediator of immediate-type reactions, and small amounts of antigen-specific IgE have been found to be important in *initiating* elicitation of the T cells responsible for the effector mechanisms of delayed-type contact dermatitis in mice (Ptak, Geba, and Askenase 1991).

1. Mechanisms

Contemporary immunology recognizes two forms of antigen-specific, cell-mediated responses. Delayed-type hypersensitivity, i.e., tuberculin-type reactivity, results from antigen-activated $CD4^+$ T cells secreting various lymphokines, which in turn nonspecifically summon or cause subsequent inflammatory events. Chief among these inflammatory mediators are activated macrophages, which then become the major effector cells of DTH in the efferent phase of the immune response (see Fig. 5–4 in Chapter 5). It is these activated macrophages that attempt to resolve or dispose of the infectious agents inciting the original response. It will be recalled that $CD4^+$ cells require presentation of antigen peptides in MHC class II context in the afferent phase. It is this form that is responsible for tuberculin-type DTH and contact dermatitis.

This is in contrast to the other major form of antigen-specific cell-mediated immunity, that of cytotoxic T lymphocytes (T_c cells, or CTLs), where antigens via T_h cells help to activate $CD8^+$ lymphocytes to differentiate into cytotoxic effector cells capable of lysing target cells expressing antigen in a MHC class I context. Damage is done by direct contact with target cells and subsequent lysis. Occasionally reference is made to a T_{dth} cell unique to these kinds of reactions, and there is some evidence that a particular subset of T-helper cells, T_h1, may be more efficient in the induction process in mice (Cher and Mossman 1987), but such a subset has not been documented in humans. After antigen-specific sensitization, provocation of a positive skin test is possible with much lower doses of antigen than those required for sensitization.

These two lymphocyte-mediated prototypes also differ in certain pathological details. In allergy of infection reactions, very few lymphocytes are found infiltrating the sites of positive skin tests and even fewer are antigen-reactive ($< 0.01\%$: Meltzer and Nacy 1989). After a few hours, a perivenous infiltrate of monocytes/macrophages occurs that is accompanied by neutrophils and basophils, depending on the species. Antigen-reactive T cells release lymphokines such as macrophage migration inhibitor and tumor necrosis factor β, which alter the traffic patterns and the activation status of both monocytes and uncommitted lymphocytes. In some species, the factors also initiate the partial degranulation of mast cells with the release of serotonin and possibly other mediators. The vasoactive effect increases the vascular permeability and allows mononuclear cells to extravasate from the blood vessels. Activated macrophages possess greatly enhanced microbiocidal activity and may contribute further to the inflammation. Sensitized lymphocytes and activated macrophages occur generally throughout the system as well as locally, such that reactions may be provoked at sites distant from that of initial inflammation. The ensuing reaction may exhibit the dual effects of tissue injury and defense against infection. In regard to tissue injury, the macrophage should receive much more attention than the cytotoxic lymphocyte of the past (Meltzer and Nacy 1989). The matter of histological and physiological manifestations of DTH varies greatly with species, a matter that cannot be stressed too much. The dermal reactivity in mice is particularly different from that described above (Dvorak, Galli, and Dvorak 1986).

Occasionally under conditions of chronic stimulation, the macrophages fuse to form heterokaryotic giant cells. More frequently, the macrophages are compressed to form epithelioid cells. Lymphocytes and fibroblasts form a collar around the epithelioid cells, i.e., granuloma formation. Most granulomata resolve with time and result in little residual scarring, but some associated with infectious agents that cannot be destroyed by the immune system (i.e., tubercle bacilli) may under go further modification. Fibroblasts and their secretory products form a fibrocytic or fibroblastic barrier between the agent and host tissue. Similar granulomata may be formed in response to potentially immunotoxic materials such as silica or beryllium.

Aside from the use of skin tests used to detect exposure to infectious agents, a more important aspect of DTH is that of contact dermatitis. The pathology of allergic contact dermatitis is confined to the epidermis rather than the dermis as with the tuberculin reaction. However, the human skin reaction has several unique facets, chief of which is the vesicular, pruritic eruption characteristic of poison ivy dermatitis. In the induction of contact sensitivity to xenobiotics, some haptenic, low-molecular-weight, often lipid-soluble chemicals can penetrate into the epidermis, binding to host carrier proteins and creating neoantigens. Sensitization in the skin is then induced through presentation of these antigens by MHC class II + Langerhans cells to $CD4^+$ T cells.

Populations of sensitized T cells may be generated in two ways. In peripheral sensitization, resident skin T cells may react with antigen-bearing Langerhans cells along with the MHC class I molecules. Alternatively, the antigen-specific Langerhans cells may move from the skin to paracortical regions of the afferent lymph nodes. In both types of sensitization, the activated T cells express IL-1 receptors. The IL-1 produced by keratinocytes and other cells then stimulate lymphocytes through this receptor. The stimulated lymphocytes produce IL-2, which augments clonal expansion of other antigen-specific clones of T-effector and memory cells. In the afferent phase, the development of sensitization usually takes 7–20 days for strong sensitizers to years for less potent agents.

On antigen reexposure of the sensitized individual, monocytes synthesize and release thromboplastin and plasminogen activator, which activate the blood-clotting process through the generation of leukotactic peptides. This serves to trap activated leukocytes in a network of fibrin threads. Vesicle formation results from the release of vasoactive mediators that increase capillary permeability. Pruritus is most likely caused by degranulation of infiltrated basophils. The destruction of antigen-coated skin cells may be from interactions with sensitized cytotoxic T cells or lymphotoxins.

Retrospective diagnosis of human contact sensitivity reactions is usually made by patch testing. In this test, a nonirritating concentration of the sensitizing agent is placed in contact with unabraded skin by means of an applied patch. If antigen-specific memory cells are present in the blood, erythema and induration will be evoked within 48 hr. Almost 80% of reactions of the skin to xenobiotics are caused by irritant or toxic reactions and are not immunologic in nature, but they may be confused with antigen-induced delayed hypersensitivity reactions (Mathias 1983). The lesions are characterized as a nonsensitizing, nonimmunological local inflammatory response after the first exposure to the chemical. Almost any chemical, under selected conditions, can evoke such an irritant response. These conditions may include concentration, length of exposure, and the presence of confounding factors such as heat and sunlight. Although the histopathology of an irritant reaction may resemble delayed hypersensitivity, the biological mechanisms active in the process vary.

Delayed-type hypersensitivity reactions can also occur in the lung. Such immune injury plays a large part in the body's reaction in such infections as tuberculosis and histoplasmosis. Moreover, T-cell-mediated reactions are part of the complicated host response to inhaled organic dusts leading to hypersensitivity pneumonitis (Richerson 1983).

2. Assessment

There are several methods used to determine the sensitization potential of chemicals. The most commonly used animal tests for contact sensitivity induction are the guinea pig maximization test (GPMT) and the Buehler test (BT). In the GPMT, three groups of animals are used, with twenty to twenty-five animals in each group. One group receives intradermal injections of Freund's complete adjuvant (FCA). The second group receives an intradermal bolus of the test material at the highest tolerated dose. The induction group is immunized with both FCA and the test material. After 7 days, the animals receive an epicutaneous application of test material in petrolatum. To promote contact with the skin, the material is covered with a surgical dressing for 48 hr. Twenty-one days after the initial exposure, the animals are challenged for 24 hr with a topical application of the test material, and the intensity and duration of the skin reactions are determined relative to controls.

Although there is an excellent correlation between individual chemicals that are known sensitizers and human sensitization, the GPMT method has several disadvantages. The method cannot adequately predict the sensitization potential of formulations. In addition, the GPMT has poor reproducibility in repetitive testing studies (Marzulli and McGuire 1982). The method also gives false-negative reactions with known human sensitizers. However, because the GPMT uses a nonspecific immunostimulant and bypasses the normal skin penetration barriers, it is generally believed that the test overestimates the risk of sensitization.

The standard BT uses twenty animals in three groups: the sensitized or induced group, a vehicle control group, and an unsensitized control group. Often a positive control group of animals sensitized with dinitrofluorobenzene (DNFB) is included in the assay. Once a week for 3 weeks, a minimally irritating dose of test material is placed on the same skin site and covered with a surgical dressing (Buehler 1985). After 2 weeks, the induced and control animals undergo a 6- to 24-hr topical patch challenge with the test material placed on a naive skin site. Reactivity is determined on the basis of intensity and the incidence of positive skin tests in the induction group. The incidence is the number of animals with skin test scores of 1 or greater. The scoring is based on a scale of 1 (mild erythema or redness) to 3 (severe erythema). The severity is defined as the sum of the skin test scores divided by the number of animals. A proposed sensitization ranking appears in Table 6-4.

With the exception of water-soluble heavy metal salts, the BT is an effective

TABLE 6-4. **Sensitization Ranking Assessed by Skin Test Positivity**

Percentage Sensitization	Sensitization Rank
0–8	Weak
29–64	Moderate
65–80	Strong
81–100	Extreme

Source: From Gilman (1982).

screen for sensitization induced by technical-grade chemicals or formulations used for human topical exposure. The test can also be used to resolve questions of threshold sensitization or potency and antigenic cross-reactivity. Although it had been suggested that the BT underestimates the risk of sensitization, recent data have suggested that the accuracy rate of the BT may be as high as 97% (Robinson et al. 1989).

To resolve problems of overestimation (GPMT) and possible underestimation (BT) of sensitization in the tests, guinea pig sensitization should be used as a preclinical screen prior to human patch testing. If human studies are not possible, then the adjuvant-based tests should be undertaken with confirmation in an epicutaneous open or patch test method (Anderson and Maibach 1985).

The guinea pig testing protocols have limitations. Both require numerous animals and large amounts of test material. The test dose is usually the minimum irritating dose. This may be several hundred times higher than the concentration used by consumers. In addition, the qualitative nature of the endpoint (erythema and induration), coexisting irritant reactions, and the use of colored test materials may adversely influence the data interpretation.

Alternative animal methods for predicting skin sensitization have been developed. The purpose of the new models was to ascertain more objective, biologically relevant endpoints and to reduce the use of animals. In the mouse ear-swelling test (MEST), the highest nonirritating dose of test material is used in the assay. After topical application of the test material in solvent, test material in FCA is injected intradermally. Following repeated topical applications, the animals are rested for a period of time. After the test material is applied to the dorsal side of the ear, the ear thickness is measured relative to the control ear (Gad et al. 1986). Correlation of data shows that the test accurately predicts sensitization when compared to the GPMT. A refinement of the test is the murine local lymph node (MLLN) assay. In this assay, test material is repeatedly administered to the ear (Kimber, Mitchell, and Griffin 1986). After challenge, contact sensitization is measured as a function of tritiated thymidine incorporation in proliferating lymphocytes within the draining lymph node. For strong and selected weak sensitizers, the correlation between MLLN and guinea pig data was excellent (Kimber 1989).

In addition, contact sensitization of chemicals has also been attempted by in vitro animal assays. Primary generation of antigen-specific helper T cells has been achieved using hapten-modified syngeneic Langerhans cells. Cells recovered from the assays can be rested and rechallenged with the sensitizing material. If antigen-specific T cells are present, they will undergo a rapid proliferative cycle. The proliferation can be measured by the incorporation of tritiated thymidine. This method has several advantages: only small numbers of animals are required for the assay; large numbers of chemicals can be tested with a relatively short turn-around time; the endpoint is objective and quantifiable. The major disadvantage of the system is that the role of skin metabolism is circumvented. Hence, sensitizers arising as a consequence of metabolic processes would be missed in the assay. When strong sensitizers were used in the in vitro assays, there was a strong correlation between in vivo and in vitro sensitization. A comparison of sensitization induced by moderate and weak sensitizers is in progress (Hauser and Katz 1988).

Before these alternative assays may become widely implemented, they must be acceptable to the federal regulatory agencies for use in the registration of consumer products. Since the agencies have a 30- to 40–year data base on guinea pig assay systems, conversion to new assay systems may be difficult.

As attractive as animal and in vitro predictive assays are, there remain a number of problems. Animal methods of predicting immune-based reactions cannot take into account such important human features as the importance of the MHC complex, the genetic polymorphism that regulates IgE levels and basophil degranulation, and the metabolic pathways of xenobiotics in affecting adverse reactions (Sanner and Higgins 1991). Predicting idiosyncratic reactions to new materials is even more difficult if such reactions are not immune in origin.

More direct and meaningful methods of assay are performed on panels of human volunteers. The human repeat-insult patch test (HRIPT) is usually performed to confirm product safety under exaggerated conditions relative to consumer use levels (Stotts 1980). In addition to consumer use levels, the concentration of test material is determined by data from other human and guinea pig studies. The test concentration is usually tenfold less than the guinea pig sensitizing dose. Also, the induction dose may have minimum irritating potential as determined in human irritancy testing.

During the induction phase, approximately one hundred normal subjects are topically exposed to the chemical on the upper arm (Draize, Woodward, and Calvery 1944; Shelanski and Shelanski 1953). Using a 5–day test week, subjects are patch tested three times a week for 3 weeks. Patches are held in place for 24 hr, and all test sites are visually scored before and after application. After 14–17 days, subjects are challenged by patch testing at the induction site and the alternate arm. The reaction is scored at 24, 48, and 72 hr. To confirm sensitization, the positive subjects can be rechallenged at a later date. The skin reactions are scored on a 0 (no visible reaction) to 5 scale. A severe reaction with erythema, edema, induration, and/or blisters is considered a grade 5 reaction.

In a limited data survey, only a small proportion of test chemicals are demonstrable human sensitizers. However, over 50% of the chemicals gave a positive reaction in guinea pig assays. Hence, there may be a great propensity for false-positive reactions in the animal assays. Only one false-negative reaction occurred in the guinea pig assays (Robinson et al. 1989).

Because of the possible sensitization to test chemicals, there has been a reluctance to implement HRIPT protocols. Although some sensitization may occur as a consequence of testing, the reactions are confined to the test site and resolve quickly (Robinson et al. 1989). Moreover, sensitized subjects are able to use the sensitizing chemical under normal conditions (Weaver, Cardin, and Naibach 1985; Weaver and Herrmann 1981) without recurrence of skin reactions.

In addition to subjectively measured human skin tests, in vitro assays utilizing human donor cells can be used to assess DTH. The extent of antigen-specific lymphocyte proliferation can be quantitated by measuring tritiated thymidine up-take in stimulated cultures after exposure to appropriate antigen. This lymphocyte transformation assay is an excellent correlate of DTH reactions (Rocklin, Myers, and David 1970). Data have suggested that free haptens need not be covalently bound to protein to stimulate lymphocyte proliferation in such assays to diagnose drug-related occupational allergies (Stejskal, Olin, and Forsbeck 1986). The lymphocyte transformation test is popular among cellular immunologists because the endpoint is objective and quantifiable, it is comparatively easy to carry out, and the data obtained can be semiautomated (in radioisotope counters).

3. Other Forms of Delayed-in-Time Reactions

Although it has long been thought that this type of hypersensitivity is cell-mediated and not antibody mediated, and that there was a great distinction of time between antigen contact and skin reaction, these former distinctions are becoming blurred with the acquisition of new knowledge. For example, cellular and antibody-mediated types may and often do coexist in the same individual. One of the classic contact sensitins is the especially potent DNFB, a compound that universally sensitizes all humans or lab animals that come in sufficient contact with it. Elicitation of delayed-type reactions in mice is measured by changes in tissue thickness of the foot pad or ear by means of a constant-pressure spring-loaded caliper. However, this same parameter can be induced in mice with DNFB-specific monoclonal IgE (Ray et al. 1983). Thus, either DTH reactions are comprised of mixed components, DNFB sensitivity is not what we think it is, or the common model of human DTH is invalid. Most likely, elements of both IgE-mediated and cell-mediated responses occur simultaneously in mice (Mekori and Galli 1990).

Moreover, there are other types of delayed-in-time reactions to extrinsic agents. One of these, formerly called the Jones–Mote reaction, is called cutaneous basophil sensitivity (CBH) and was most often studied in guinea pigs being immunized with antigens in Freund's-type adjuvants. Histologically similar reactions can also be induced in rabbits and chickens. The CBH requires five to ten times greater doses of antigen for sensitization and elicitation. It is a transient skin reaction following antigen contact that appears as early as 8 hr after contact, accompanied by a local increase in histamine and many infiltrating basophils (Askenase 1979). The reactions are transient in another sense; i.e., such reactivity may occur early in the course of an immunization and then later disappear through prolonged immunization.

It is thought that a T cell reacting with antigen liberates a lymphokine that is chemotactic for basophils, the degranulation products of which produce the inflammation (Dvorak, Galli, and Dvorak 1986). Infiltrating basophils comprise a substantial portion of cells found at the site but comprise only 0.5% of circulating leukocytes. The reactions are poorly circumscribed and indurated, which is explainable by the paucity of interstitial fibrin deposits (Dvorak, Galli, and Dvorak 1986). The CBH reactivity is passively transferable not only by lymphoid cells but also, curiously, by immune serum (Askenase 1973). The significance of this latter finding is uncertain except that these reactions are clearly not classically DTH mediated. Although humans are not immunized in the manner used to elicit this laboratory curiosity, basophils are part of the infiltrating cells that take part in the complex DTH skin reactions, albeit to a smaller extent than guinea pig CBH.

Another example of a delayed-in-time reaction is the late-phase reaction discussed above. It can occur within the skin, on the conjunctiva, or as a pulmonary response to an inhaled substance (Henderson 1988). Manifestations may begin as early as 2–4 hr after contact, peak between 6 and 12 hr, and resolve by 24 hr. Although it an IgE-dependent reaction, the pharmacological mediators are different. Since basophil production and function are T-cell-dependent processes, and basophilic products are responsible for subsequent inflammatory events, there is a suspicion that antigen-T-cell interaction is the first step in this complicated reaction. Part of the time differential is related to the attraction of inflammatory cells to the area by chemotactic factors resulting from antigen reacting with IgE bound to a variety of cells including macrophages, eosinophils, and platelets as well as basophils (Frew and Kay 1990). Hence, the late-phase reaction may be mediated by an IgE-mediated release of mediators leading to a classical inflammatory response.

H. HYPERPLASIA

Other results of immune injury may be stimulation of receptors, changes in cell types, or increased cellular division of a specific cell type. These changes may result from either acute or chronic stimulation. Long-acting thyroid stimulator (LATS), originally thought to be a thyroid-stimulating hormone associated with Graves' disease, is an antibody specific for thyroid-stimulating hormone receptor that stimulates DNA synthesis and/or adenylate cyclase activity in thyroid tissue (Fraser and Venter 1984). This results in a prolonged stimulatory effect on the thyroid.

Chronic asthma leads to the formation of nasal polyps, bronchial smooth muscle hypertrophy, and mucus metaplasia in which there is replacement of ciliated epithelium with goblet cells (Callerame et al. 1971). In chronic fibrotic diseases (e.g., coalworkers' pneumoconioses) anti-connective-tissue antibodies occurring over a long period of time result in interalveolar septal thickening (Burrell et al. 1974) and may contribute to pulmonary fibrosis (Lewis and Burrell 1976).

I. HYPERSENSITIVITY-LIKE REACTIONS

There are several interactions of xenobiotics and host factors that *appear* to be allergic in nature but, when examined closely, have been found to involve other mechanisms. In this sense, the reactions could more likely be viewed as classical toxic reactions except that the confusing matter of individual idiosyncrasy is often involved; i.e., not everyone exposed to the agent reacts adversely. Idiosyncrasies often are found to have a genetic or environmental basis. Good examples are infants born with the inability to produce the intestinal enzyme lactase (Van Dyke 1989). For such infants, ordinary lactose-containing milk is quite troublesome and resists absorption, resulting in a gastrointestinal disturbance once blamed on hypersensitivity. In fact, a genetic propensity must be present in order for the agent to induce its harm. Celiac sprue is another food intolerance mimicking hypersensitivity involving wheat. In this condition, the soluble protein of wheat flour, α-gliadin, induces a damaging inflammatory reaction in the epithelial layer of the gut, leading to a malabsorption syndrome (Trier 1989). Although it was once believed to be caused by another enzyme deficiency, growing evidence indicates that the gliadin shares a significant structural homology with an adenovirus (Cole and Kagnoff 1985). As a result of earlier presensitization to the adenovirus protein, epithelial lymphocytes respond to the gliadin with subsequent adverse inflammatory effects. Now there is evidence of an immune etiology; however, in this case the immune response is a normal one. It is only that the timing of two unrelated environmental exposures is unfortunate, and one response (to the adenovirus) sets up the other (to the gliadin).

Immunoglobulins may react nonspecifically with foreign agents. Staphylococcal protein A, an infectious disease substance, is well known to react with the Fc portion of certain immunoglobulin isotypes, and this occurs with at least one other environmental substance as well, the tetrahydroxyflavan polymer associated with cotton bracts referred to previously (Edwards and Jones 1973). Whether this latter reaction leads to inflammation is unknown.

A large and varied number of agents are also known to cause the nonspecific release of histamine from mast cells (Lagunoff, Martin, and Read 1983). They include cytotoxic enzymes, polysaccharides, plant lectins, complement anaphylatoxins, polybasic compounds (e.g., compound 48/80), certain kinins and other polypeptides, calcium, and methyl piperonylate, a component of cotton dust. Some compounds act directly on mast cells (e.g., methyl piperonylate, plant lectins, compound 48/80), whereas other compounds initiate histamine release through the intermediary of nonspecific complement activation, e.g., inhaled *Aspergillus* spores (Burrell and Pokorney 1977).

Finally, the most "immune-like" injury of all occurs through the interference of mediator production by the autonomic nervous system. Toluene diisocyanate (TDI) is a widely used manufacturing substance capable of acting as an irritant at higher concentrations (0.5 ppm), but at extremely low concentrations (0.02 ppm or lower) it can induce occupational asthma. However, only 15% of TDI asthmatics possess antigen-specific IgE antibodies (Butcher et al. 1980). The agent apparently induces its effect by blocking β-adrenergic stimulation of production of cAMP, a mediator responsible for smooth muscle relaxation and inhibition of bronchial secretion (Van Ert and Battigelli 1975; Davies et al. 1977). This results in unopposed α-adrenergic or cholinergic stimulation of cell receptors, resulting in bronchconstrictive and mucous-secreting effects and giving the same appearance as an IgE-mediated event.

Another way of simulating a true IgE-mediated event would be by direct overstimulation of cholinergic fibers. Organophosphate pesticides have such a cholinergic-stimulating effect by inhibiting acetylcholinesterase normally responsible for degrading the cholinergic agonist (Murphy 1986). Superficially, the clinical results of these types of exposure range from bronchial asthma to anaphylactoid signs, and symptoms would resemble an "allergy."

J. AUTOIMMUNITY

Although immunology is usually defined as the study of the body's reaction to nonself, occasionally the body becomes autoreactive to self antigens as a result of a combination of genetic and pathological mechanisms. Any type of antigen-specific immune response directed at one's own molecular, cellular, or tissue antigens is termed autoimmunization and results when the immune system is either "tricked" into recognizing self antigens as foreign or produces immune effectors against normal, self antigens in sufficient quantities to produce injury. This can be brought about by a variety of etiologies, summarized in Table 6–5. A xenobiotic or infectious agent may alter the native molecule, creating a new antigen. When recognized as foreign, the antigen induces an immune response that may cross-react with the native material, thus breaking tolerance to self. Another recognized mechanism occurs when a substance triggers the release of native materials ordinarily not in contact with the immune system (sequestered antigens, e.g., those associated with the ocular lens). Apparently, such sequestered antigens develop embryologically without interactions with the immune system when self-reactive clones are being deleted from what will become the individual's immunologic repertoire.

One well-studied example from infectious disease is the matter of coincidental specificity between an extrinsic antigen and intrinsic, host material. The best-known example of this is the cross-reacting antibodies for group A streptococcal cell membranes and human myocardial sarcolemmal antigen (Kaplan and Meyeserian 1962; Van de Rijn, Zabriskie, and McCarty 1977). In a different type of pathway, host tissue may be coupled to an extrinsic antigen such that subsequent immune effectors reacting with that antigen damage the cell (or immune complexes involving that antigen are adsorbed to a cell, rendering it vulnerable to inflammatory disposition). This was described above as the mechanism for thrombocytopenic purpura because of the immune complexes being adsorbed to platelets. The theoretical possibility that autoimmune reactions could arise by the inhibition of T-suppressor cells for a particular host antigen must also be considered as an additional mechanism. Finally, evidence exists that in some autoimmune disorders, a substance triggers a reaction in hosts genetically predisposed to develop this form of immunity.

One of the most remarkable discoveries relating immune function to infectious microorganisms has been the definition of heat shock proteins. These proteins with highly conserved amino acid sequences and functions are produced not only

TABLE 6–5.   Hypothetical Etiologic Mechanisms to Explain Autoimmunity

Type	Examples	Proposed Mechanism
Antireceptor	Graves' disease	Antiidiotype
	Myasthenia gravis	Aberrant clone
	Type B insulin-resistant diabetes	
Sequestered Ag	Goodpasture's nephritis	Abnormal release of Ag from site
	Ocular phacoanaphylaxis	developed lacking contact with
	Hashimoto's thyroiditis	developing thymus
Antibody-mediated	Rheumatic fever	Antibody to extrinsic agent with
	Glomerulonephritis	coincidental self-reactivity
T-cell-mediated	Multiple sclerosis	Aberrant clone or response to unknown Ag with cross-reactivity to self
	Allergic encephalomyelitis	
	Rheumatoid arthritis	
Autoimmune complexes	Systemic lupus erythematosus	Defect in C-dependent removal of complexes
	Glomerulonephritis	

Source: Adapted from Lachman (1990).

by a wide range of microorganisms but by many types of eukaryotic cells as well (Kaufmann 1990). Some of these proteins play a major role in the folding and unfolding as well as assembly of polypeptides. One important type participates in immunoglobulin assembly, for example. Another role these proteins play is in accelerating the removal of denatured proteins unable to be reassembled or folded. These substances are constitutively present in all cells but undergo enhanced production when a cell is confronted with an environmental stress such as a sudden change in temperature or an encounter with toxic oxygen metabolites. Parasitic microorganisms may produce these proteins when stressed by sudden changes in temperature encountered during transmission from an invertebrate vector to a mammalian host or when encountering inflammatory stress incited by phagocytes. At the same time, mammalian cells under stress from infectious agents may produce similar proteins. If host immune responses are directed against these types of proteins produced by pathogenic microbes, the effectors could conceivably cross-react with the highly conserved sequences in the host's own tissue with resulting autoimmunity.

Autoimmune diseases may be tissue specific (e.g., autoimmune diseases of the central nervous system or thyroid) or nonspecific, where signs and symptoms may be referable to many organs (e.g., rheumatoid arthritis or systemic lupus erythematosus). The injury produced in autoimmune disorders can involve many of the above mechanisms of inducing allergic disease. Cytotoxic injury to cardiac tissue is involved in rheumatic fever; i.e., a straightforward immune response to an extrinsic antigen is really responsible for this classical autoimmune disease. The disease idiopathic thrombocytopenic purpura is self-destructive by immune means, but again the antigen is really extrinsic to the individual.

In contrast, people with a disease known as systemic lupus erythematosus (SLE) produce numerous antibodies to a variety of their own soluble antigens (because of an unknown stimulus, although a genetic predisposition is very important), and when the two components react in appreciable numbers, the complexes localize in the kidney and lead to glomerulonephritis. Those with a homozygous deficiency of complement components C1 or C4 are extremely prone to develop SLE, and it has been proposed that lacking such critical complement components may mean that normally circulating immune complexes are not phagocytized by fixed macrophages in the liver sinusoids, and the continued presence of circulating complexes acts as a positive feedback mechanism for inciting more antibody production (Lachman 1990). There is a view that autoimmunity is really a normal process going on continuously in all people, but disease results when there is a *quantitative* excess and continued presence of either an effector stem cell, its products, or, as in this case, immune complexes (Smith and Steinberg 1983).

Cell-mediated immunity is often the major effector mechanism in autoimmune tissue damage. Formerly, one of the major drawbacks to using rabies vaccines made from phenolized suspensions of rabid animal brains (the original Pasteur vaccine) was that its administration often induced cell-mediated immunity against the neural proteins also present in the vaccine, which could subsequently react with host tissue, leading to a postvaccinal demyelinating encephalitis (Patterson 1986).

Autoimmunity as a separate immunologic subdiscipline no longer has the same interest in America as it does in Europe. Through the 1960s, the topic received considerable investigative effort, as many diseases of unknown etiopathogenesis

TABLE 6-6.   **Substances Known to Be Associated with Autoimmune Responses**

Antihypertensive agents	Miscellaneous drugs
Hydralazine	Penicillamines
Methyldopa	Chlorpromazine
Antiarrhythmic agents	Propylthiouracil
Procainamide	Chlorthalidone
Practolol	Griseofulvin
Quinidine	Oxyphenisatin
Anticonvulsant drugs	Metals
Phenytoin	Lithium
Ethosuximide	Gold
Primidone	Mercury
Antimicrobials	Cadmium
Penicillin	Miscellaneous
Sulfonamides	Solvents
Isoniazid	Vinyl chloride
Nitrofurantoin	Methylcholanthrene

Source: Adapted from Bigazzi (1985).

were studied from this aspect. From these studies, a relatively few entities from clinical medicine were shown to have a major autoimmune component in explaining their pathology, and these have been well characterized. However, there is a growing new concern that autoimmunization is occasionally found to be an unexpected complication of exposure to drugs or environmental agents. For example, a milder form of lupus without the renal involvement may develop on treatment with certain drugs such as hydralazine, procainamide, and many other chemically unrelated compounds (Hess 1981). Exactly how the use of the drug leads to this disease is uncertain. This relatively rare incident may perhaps first be triggered by oxidative metabolism of phagocytes, which leads to an acetylation of the drug to metabolites that induce immune dysregulation (Rubin and Burlingame 1991), but this hypothesis fails to explain the idiosyncratic nature of the disease. In only certain individuals, activated B cells responding with a variety of antitissue antibodies when complexed with native nucleohistone antigen lead to systemic immune complex disease. The evidence indicates that the reaction is clearly not related to similarities of drug structures.

Autoimmune aberrations are well known in several of the pneumoconioses, i.e., pulmonary diseases incited by the chronic inhalation of environmental dusts (Burrell and Lapp 1992). Although the consequences of the production of such autoimmune effectors is not always easy to assess, a number of such agents known to induce autoimmune markers are presented in Table 6-6. Some of these agents do in fact induce clinical changes in humans, as in the frequent case of methyldopa-induced erythrocyte antibodies, which occasionally lead to an acquired hemolytic anemia (Schreiber and Frank 1988). Most importantly, some of the substances listed induce only laboratory abnormalities, and others have only been shown to induce changes in animal studies.

References

Abraham, W. M., J. C. Delehunt, L. Yerger, and B. Marchette. 1983. Characterization of a late pulmonary response after antigenic challenge in allergic sheep. *Am. Rev. Respir. Dis.* 128:839–44.

Adkinson, N. F. 1974. Measurement of total serum IgE and allergen specific immunogloblin E antibody. In *Manual of Clinical Immunology*, ed. N. R. Rose and H. Friedman, pp. 591–602. Washington: American Society for Microbiology.

Anderson, K. E., and H. I. Maibach. 1985. Guinea pig sensitization assays. *Curr. Prob. Dermatol.* 14:263–90.

Aronson, F. R., P. Libby, E. P. Brandon, et al. 1988. IL-2 rapidly induces natural killer cell adhesion to human endothelial cells. A potential mechanism for endothelial injury. *J. Immunol.* 141:158–63.

Arroyave, C. M., M. Schatz, and R. A. Simon. 1979. Activation of complement system by radiocontrast medium: Studies in vivo and in vitro. *J. Allergy Clin. Immunol.* 63:276–80.

Arroyave, C. M., D. D. Stevenson, J. H. Vaughn, and E. M. Tan. 1977. Plasma complement changes during bronchospasm provoked in asthmatic patients. *Clin. Allergy* 7:173–82.

Askenase, P. 1973. Cutaneous basophil hypersensitivity in contact sensitized guinea pigs. *J. Exp. Med.* 138:1144–55.

Askenase, P. 1979. Basophil arrival and function in tissue hypersensitivity reactions. *J. Allergy Clin. Immunol.* 64:79–89.

Barnes, P. J. 1987. Neuropeptides in the lung: Localization, function, and pathologic implications. *J. Allergy Clin. Immunol.* 79:285–95.

Barnes, P. J. 1989. New concepts in the pathogenesis of bronchial hyperresponsiveness and asthma. *J. Allergy Clin. Immunol.* 83:1013–26.

Barnett, E. V. 1986. Circulating immune complexes: Their biologic and clinical significance. *J. Allergy Clin. Immunol.* 78:1089–96.

Berg, T. L. O., and S. G. O. Johansson. 1974. Allergy diagnosis with the radioallergosorbent test. A comparison with the results of skin and provocation sites in an unselected group of children with asthma and hay fever. *J. Allergy Clin. Immunol.* 54:207–21.

Berrens, L., C. L. H. Guikers, and A. van Dijk. 1974. The antigens in pigeon-breeders' disease and their interactions with complement. *Ann. N.Y. Acad. Sci.* 221:153–62.

Bigazzi, P. E. 1985. Mechanisms of chemical-induced autoimmunity. In *Immunotoxicology and Immunopharmacology*, ed. J. H. Dean, M. I. Luster, A. E. Munson, and H. Amos, pp. 277–90. New York: Raven Press.

Border, W. A., H. J. Ward, E. S. Kamil, et al. 1982. Induction of membranous nephpopathy in rabbits by administration of an exogenous cationic protein. *J. Clin. Invest.* 69:451–61.

Buehler, E. V. 1985. A rationale for the selection of occlusion to induce and elicit contact hypersensitivity in the guinea pig. *Curr. Prob. Dermatol.* 14:39–58.

Burrell, R., D. K. Flaherty, P. B. DeNee, et al. 1974. The effect of lung antibody on normal lung structure and function. *Am. Rev. Resp. Dis.* 109:106–13.

Burrell, R., R. C. Lantz, and D. E. Hinton. 1988. Mediators of pulmonary injury induced by inhalation of bacterial endotoxin. *Am. Rev. Respir. Dis.* 137:100–105.

Burrell, R., and Lapp, N. L. 1992. The immunology of the mineral pneumoconioses. In *Immunology and Allergy Clinics of North America*, ed. D. Banks, pp. 379–400. Philadelphia: W. B. Saunders.

Burrell, R., and D. Pokorney. 1977. Mediators of experimental hypersensitivity pneumonitis, *Int. Arch. Allergy Appl. Immunol.* 55:161–69.

Burrell, R., and R. Rylander. 1981. A critical review of the role of precipitins in hypersensitivity pneumonitis. *Eur. J. Respir. Dis.* 62:332–43.

Butcher, B. T., C. E. O'Niel, N. A. Reed, and J. E. Salvaggio. 1980. Radioallerosorbent testing of toluene diisocyaniate-reactive individuals using p-tolyl diisocyanate antigen. *J. Allergy. Clin. Immunol.* 66:213–16.

Callerame, M. L., J. J. Condemi, M. G. Bohrod, and J. H. Vaughn. 1971. Immunologic reactions of bronchial tissue in asthma. *N. Engl. J. Med.* 284:459–64.

Cavanah, D. K., and T. B. Casale. 1990. Neurophysiologic regulatory factors in asthma. *Insights Allergy* 5(5):1–5.

Chan, H., K. S. Tse, J. Van Oostdam, et al. 1987. A rabbit model of hypersensitivity to plicatic acid, the agent responsible for red cedar asthma. *J. Allergy Clin. Immunol.* 79:762–67.

Cher, D. J., and T. R. Mossman. 1987. Two types of murine helper T cell clone. II. Delayed type hypersensitivity is mediated by T_H1 clones. *J. Immunol.* 138:3688–94.

Cole, S. G., and M. F. Kagnoff 1985. Celiac disease. *Annu. Rev. Nutr.* 5:241–66.

Coombs, R. R. A., and P. G. H. Gell. 1963. Classification of allergic reactions underlying disease. In *Clinical Aspects of Immunology*, ed., P. G. H. Gell and R. R. A. Coombs, pp. 317–337. Philadelphia: F.A. Davis.

Craddock, R. P., G. Fehr, K. L. Brigham, et al. 1977. Complement and leukocyte-mediated pulmonary dysfunction in hemodialysis. *N. Engl. J. Med.* 296:769–74.

Daniell, W. E., W. G. Couser, and L. Rosentstock. 1988. Occupational solvent exposure and glomerulonephritis. A case report and review of the literature. *JAMA* 259:2280–83.

Davies, R. J., B. T. Butcher, C. E. O'Neil, and J. E. Salvaggio. 1975. The in vivo effect of toluene dissocyanyte on lymphocyte adenosine monophosphate production by isoproterenol prostaglandin histamine. *J. Allergy Clin. Immunol.* 60:223–29.

Draize, J. H., G. Woodard, and H. D. Calvery. 1944. Methods for the study of irritation and toxicity of substances applied topically to the skin and mucus membranes. *J. Pharmacol. Exp. Ther.* 83:337–90.

Dvorak, H. F., S. J. Galli, and A. M. Dvorak. 1986. Cellular and vascular manifestations of cell-mediated immunity. *Hum. Pathol.* 17:122–37.

Edwards, J. H, and B. M. Jones. 1973. Pseudoimmune precipitation by the isolated byssinosis "antigen." *J. Immunol.* 110:498–501.

Fraser, C. M., and J. C. Venter. 1984. Anti-receptor antibodies in human disease. *J. Allergy Clin. Immunol.* 74:661–73.

Fraser, C. M., J. C. Venter, and M. Kaliner. 1981. Autonomic abnormalities and autoantibodies to β-adrenergic receptors. *N. Engl. J. Med.* 305:1165–70.

Frew, A. J., and A. B. Kay. 1990. Eosinophils and T-lymphocytes in late-phase allergic reactions. *J. Allergy Clin. Immunol.* 85:533–39.

Gad, S., B. J. Dunn, D. W. Dobbs, et al. 1986. Development and validation of an alternative dermal sensitization test: The mouse ear swelling test (MEST). *Toxicol. Appl. Pharmacol.* 84:93–114.

Gaga, M., A. J. Frew, V. A. Varney, and A. B. Kay. 1991. Eosinophil activation and T lymphocyte infiltration in allergen-induced late phase skin reactions and classical delayed-type hypersensitivity. *J. Immunol.* 147:816–22.

Gilman, N. R. 1982. Skin and eye testing in animals. In *Principles and Methods of Toxicology*, 2nd ed., ed. A. W. Hayes, pp. 209–22. New York: Raven Press.

Golbus, S. M., and C. B. Wilson. 1979. Experimental glomerulonephritis induced by in situ formation of immune complexes in glomerular capillary wall. *Kidney Int.* 16:148–57.

Hauser, C., and S. I. Katz. 1988. Activation and expansion of hapten- and protein-specific T helper cells from nonsensitized mice. *Proc. Natl. Acad. Sci. U.S.A.* 85:5625–28.

Henderson, W. R., Jr. 1988. Role of neutrophils in allergic inflammation. *Insights Allergy* 3(6):1–5.

Hess, E. V. 1981. Introduction to drug-related lupus. *Arthritis Rheum.* 24:6–9.

Hirschman, C. A., A. Malley, and H. Downes. 1980. Basenji–Greyhound dog model of asthma: Reactivity to *Ascaris suum,* citric acid and methacholine. *J. Appl. Physiol.* 49:953–57.

Hruby, Z. W., K. Shirota, S. Jothy, and R. P. Lowry. 1991. Antiserum against tumor necrosis factor-alpha and a protease inhibitor reduce immune glomerular injury. *Kidney Int.* 40:43–51.

Hudson, L., and F. C. Hay. 1989. *Practical Immunology,* pp. 455–56. Oxford: Blackwell.

Jerne, N. K. 1974. Idiotypic networks and other preconceived ideas. *Immunol. Rev.* 79:5–24.

Kallos, P., and L. Kallos. 1934. Experimental asthma in the guinea pig. *Int. Arch. Allergy Appl. Immunol.* 73:77–85.

Kaplan, M. H., and M. Meyeserian. 1962. An immunological cross-reaction between group-A streptococcal cells and heart tissue. *Lancet* 1:706–10.

Karol, M. H., C. Dixon, M. Brady, and Y. Alarie. 1980. Immunological sensitization and pulmonary hypersensitivity by repeated inhalation of aromatic isocyanates. *Toxicol. Appl. Pharmacol.* 53:260–70.

Karpatkin, S. 1988. Immunological platelet disorders. In *Immunological Diseases*, 4th ed., ed. M. Samter, D. W. Talmage, M. M. Frank, et al., pp. 1631–62. Boston: Little, Brown.

Kaufmann, S. H. E. 1990. Heat shock proteins and the immune response. *Immunol. Today* 11:129–36.

Kimber, I. 1989. Aspects of the immune response to contact allergens: Opportunities for the development and modification of predictive test methods. *Fund. Chem. Toxicol.* 27:755–62.

Kimber, I., J. A. Mitchell, and A. C. Griffin. 1986. Development of a murine local lymph node assay for the determination of sensitizing potential. *Fund. Chem. Toxicol.* 24:585–86.

Kopp, W. C., and R. Burrell. 1982. Evidence for antibody-dependent binding of the terminal complement component to alveolar basement membrane. *Clin. Immunol. Immunopathol. 23:10–21.*

Lachman, P. J. 1990. Complement deficiency and the pathogenesis of autoimmune complex disease. *Chem. Immunol.* 49:245–63.

Lagunoff, D., T. W. Martin, and G. Read. 1983. Agents that release histamine from mast cells. *Annu. Rev. Pharmacol. Toxicol.* 23:331–51.

Lantz, R. C., K. Birch, D. E. Hinton, and R. Burrell. 1985. Morphometric changes of the lung induced by inhaled bacterial endotoxin. *Exp. Mol. Pathol.* 43:305–32.

Larsen, G. L. 1985. The rabbit model of the late asthmatic reaction. *Chest* 87:184(s)–88(s).

Lemanski, R. F., and M. Kaliner. 1988. Late phase IgE mediated reactions. *J. Clin. Immunol.* 8:1–13.

Lewis, D. M., and R. Burrell. 1976. Induction of fibrogenesis by lung antibody-treated macrophages. *Br. J. Ind. Med.* 33:25–28.

MacDonald, S. M., and L. M. Lichtenstein. 1990. Histamine-releasing factors and heterogeneity of IgE. *Spring. Sem. Immunopathol.* 12:415–28.

Marzulli, F., J. McGuire. 1982. Usefulness and limitations of various guinea-pig test methods in detecting human skin sensitizers—validation of guinea-pig tests for skin hypersensitivity. *Fund. Chem. Toxic.* 20:67–74.

Mathias, C. G. T. 1983. Clinical and experimental aspects of cutaneous irritation. In *Dermatology*, 2nd ed., ed. F. N. Marzulli and H. I. Maibach, pp. 167–168. Washington: McGraw–Hill.

McDougal, J. S., M. Hubbard, F. C. McDuffie, et al. 1982. Comparison of five assays for immune complexes in the rheumatic diseases. *Arthritis Rheum.* 25:1156–66.

McFadden, E. R., Jr. 1984. Pathogenesis of asthma. *J. Allergy Clin. Immunol.* 73:413–24.

Mekori, Y. A., and S. J. Galli. 1990. [^{125}I]Fibrin deposition occurs at both early and late intervals of IgE-dependent or contact sensitivity reactions elicited in mouse skin. *J. Immunol.* 145:3719–27.

Meltzer, M. S., and C. A. Nacy. 1989. Delayed-type hypersensitivity and the induction of activated, cytotoxic macrophages. In *Fundamental Immunology*, 2nd ed., ed. W. E. Paul, pp. 765–77. New York: Raven Press.

Morrison, D. C., and L. F. Kline. 1977. Activation of the classical and properdin pathways of complement by bacterial lipopolysaccharides (LPS). *J. Immunol.* 118:362–68.

Mudde, G. C., T. T. Hansel, F. C. von Reijsen, et al. 1990. IgE—An immunoglobulin specialized in antigen capture. *Immunol. Today* 11:440–43.

Murphy, S. D. 1986. Toxic effects of pesticides. In *Casarett and Doull's Toxicology. The Basic Science of Poisons*, 3rd ed., ed. C. D. Klaassen, M. O. Amdur, and J. Doull, pp. 519–81. New York: Macmillan.

Nichols, P. J. 1991. The search for the etiologic agents and pathogenic mechanisms of byssinosis: In vivo studies. *Proc. Cotton Dust Res. Conf.* 15:307–20.

Ottoboni, M. A. 1984. *The Dose Makes the Poison*. Berkeley: Vincente Books.

Patterson, P. Y. 1986. Microbe-induced autoreactive host responses and autoimmune disease. In *The Biologic and Clinical Basis of Infectious Disease*, 3rd ed., ed. G. P. Youmans, P. Y. Patterson, and H. M. Sommers, pp. 81–88. Philadelphia: W. B. Saunders.

Pepys, J. 1969. Hypersensitivity diseases of the lungs due to fungi and organic dusts. *Monogr. Allergy*, 4:1–147.

Peters, J. E., C. A. Hirshman, and A. Mislley. 1982. The Basenji–Greyhound dog model of asthma: leukocyte histamine release, serum ISE and airway response to inhislex antigen. *J. Immunol.* 129:1245–49.

Pleskow, W. W., D. E. Chenoweth, R. A. Simon, et al. 1982. The absence of detectable complement activation in aspirin-sensitive asthmatic patients during aspirin challenge. *J. Allergy Clin. Immunol.* 72:462–68.

Pratt, W. B. 1990. Drug allergy. In *Principles of Drug Action. The Basis of Pharmacology*, 3rd ed., ed. W. B. Pratt and P. Taylor, pp. 533–64. New York: Churchill Livingstone.

Ptak, W., G. P. Geba, and P. W. Askenase. 1991. Initiation of delayed-type hypersensitivity by low doses of monclonal IgE antibody. *J. Immunol.* 146:3929–36.

Ray, M. C., M. D. Tharp, T. J. Sullivan, and R. E. Tigelaar. 1983. Contact hypersensitivity reactions to dinitrofluorobenzene by monoclonal IgE anti-DNP antibodies. *J. Immunol.* 131:1096–1102.

Reshef, A., A. Kagey-Sobotka, N. F. Adkinson, Jr., et al. 1989. The pattern and kinetics in human skin of erythema and mediators during the acute and late-phase response (LPR). *J. Allergy Clin. Immunol.* 84:678–87.

Richerson, H. B. 1983. Hypersensitivity pneumonitis—pathology and pathogenesis. *Clin. Rev. Allergy* 1:469–83.

Ritz, H. L., and Bond, G. G. 1986. Respiratory and immunological responses of guinea pigs to repeated intratracheal administration of enzyme-detergent solutions: A comparison of intratracheal and inhalation modes of exposure. *Toxicologist* 6:138.

Robinson, M. K., J. Stotts, P. J. Danneman, and T. L. Nusair. 1989. A risk assessment process for allergic sensitization. *Fund. Chem. Toxicol.* 27:479–89.

Rocklin, R. E., O. L. Myers, and J. R. David. 1970. An in vitro assay for cellular hypersensitivity in man. *J. Immunol.* 104:95–102.

Rubin, R. L., and R. W. Burlingame. 1991. Biochemical mechanisms in autoimmunity. *Biochem. Soc. Trans.* 19:153–59.

Sanner, M. A., and T. J. Higgins. 1991. Chemical basis for immune mediated idiosyncratic drug hypersensitivity. *Annu. Rep. Clin. Med.* 26:181–90.

Sarlo, K., and E. D. Clark. 1992. A tier approach for evaluating respiratory allergenicity of molecular weight chemicals. *Fund. Appl. Toxicol.* 18:107–14.

Schreiber, A. B., P. O. Couraud, C. Andre, et al. 1980. Antialprenolol anti-idiotypic antibodies bind to β-adrenergic receptors and modulate catecholamine-sensitive adenylate cyclase. *Proc. Natl. Acad. Sci. U.S.A.* 77:7385–89.

Schreiber, A. D., and M. M. Frank. 1988. Autoimmune hemolytic anemia. In *Immunological Diseases*, 4th ed., ed. M. Samter, D. W. Talmage, M. M. Frank, et al., pp. 1609–30. Boston: Little, Brown.

Seaton, A. 1984. Occupational asthma. In *Occupational Lung Diseases*, ed. W. K. C. Morgan and A. Seaton, pp. 498–520. Philadelphia: W. B. Saunders.

Shechter, Y., R. Maron, D. Elias, and I. R. Cohen. 1982. Auto-antibodies to insulin receptor develop simultaneously as anti-idiotypes in mice immunized with insulin. *Science* 216:542–45.

Shelanski, H. A., and M. V. Shelanski. 1953. A new technique of human patch tests. *Proc. Sci. Sect. Toilet Goods Assoc.* 19:46–49.

Siraganian, R. P. 1975. Automated histamine release. A method for in vitro allergy diagnosis. *Int. Arch. Allergy Appl. Immunol.* 49:108–10.

Smith, H. R., and A. D. Steinberg. 1983. Autoimmunity—a perspective. *Annu. Rev. Immunol.* 1:175–210.

Smith, S. M., I. S. Snyder, and R. Burrell. 1980. Mitogenic response to *Micropolyspora faeni* cell walls. *J. Allergy Clin. Immunol.* 65:298–304.

Spearing, R. L., C. M. Hickton, P. Sizeland, et al. 1990. Quinine-induced disseminated intravascular coagulation. *Lancet* 336:1535–37.

Starkebaum, G., R. A. H. Jimenez, and W. P. Arend. 1982. Effect of immune complexes on human neutrophil phagocytic function. *J. Immunol.* 128:141–47.

Stejskal, V. D. M., R. G. Olin, and M. Forsbeck. 1986. The lymphocyte transformation test for diagnosis of drug-induced occupational allergy. *J. Allergy Clin. Immunol.* 77:411–26.

Stotts, J. 1980. Planning, conduct, and interpretation of human predictive sensitization patch tests. In: *Current Concepts in Cutaneous Toxicity*, ed. V. A. Drill and P. Lazar, pp. 41–53. New York: Academic Press.

Sustiel, A., and R. Rocklin. 1989. T cell responses in allergic rhinitis, asthma, and atopic dermatitis. *Clin. Exp. Allergy* 19:11–18.

Szentivanyi, A. 1968. The β-adrenergic theory of atopic abnormality in bronchial asthma. *J. Allergy* 42:203–42.

Taylor, R. B. 1982. Regulation of antibody responses by antibody toward the immunogen. *Immunol. Today* 3:47–51.

Theofilopoulos, A. N., and F. J. Dixon. 1976. Complement receptors on Raji cells in vitro detectors of immune complexes in human sera. In *Manual of Clinical Immunology*, ed. N. R. Rose and H. Friedman, pp. 676–81. Washington: American Society of Microbiology.

Trier, J. S. 1989. Celiac sprue. In *Gastrointestinal Disease: Pathophysiology, Diagnosis, Management,* 4th ed., ed. M. H. Sleisinger, and J. S. Fordtran, pp. 1134–52. Philadelphia: W. B. Saunders.

Tse, C. S. T., E. Chen, and I. L. Bernstein. 1979. Induction of murine reagenic antibodies by toluene diisocyanate. An animal model of immediate hypersensitivity to isocyanate. *Am. Rev. Respir. Dis.* 120: 829–36.

Van de Rijn, I., J. B. Zabriskie, and M. McCarty. 1977. Group A streptococcal antigens cross reactive with myocardium: Purification of heart-reactive antibody and isolation of the streptococcal antigen. *J. Exp. Med.* 146:579–99.

Van Dyke, R. W. 1989. Mechanics of digestion and absorption of food. In *Gastrointestinal Disease: Pathophysiology, Diagnosis, Management*, 4th ed., ed. M. H. Sleisinger, and J. S. Fordtran, pp. 1062–87. Philadelphia: W. B. Saunders.

Van Ert, M., and M. C. Battigelli. 1975. Mechanism of respiratory injury by TDI (toluene diisocyanate). *Annals of Allergy* 35:142–47.

Wanner, A., W. M. Abraham, J. S. Douglas, et al. 1990. NHLBI summary: Models of airway hyperresponsiveness. *Am. Rev. Respir. Dis.* 141:253–57.

Weaver, J. E., C. W. Cardin, and H. I. Naibach. 1985. Dose-response assessments of kathon biocide. I. Diagnostic use an diagnostic threshold patch testing with sensitized humans. *Contact Dermatitis* 12:141–45.

Weaver, J. E., and K. W. Herrmann. 1981. Evaluation of adverse reports for a new laundry product. *J. Am. Acad. Dermatol.* 4:577–84.

Worlledge, S. M., K. C. Carstairs, and J. V. Dacie. 1966. Autoimmune hemolytic anemia associated with α-methyldopa therapy. *Lancet* 2:135–39.

7

Damage to the Immune System

A. INTRODUCTION

In addition to inducing host damage *by* the immune system, environmental agents may also induce damage *to* that system. As was the case with the induction of tissue injury by the immune system, various genetic and environmental factors may also influence susceptibility to immune system damage. Indeed, much of what is known about the nature of the specific defects and of the consequences of immunodeficiency has been learned from the study of genetic or developmental abnormalities. These are known as *primary* immunodeficiencies to distinguish them from *secondary* immunodeficiencies, i.e., those brought about after a normal immune system has developed. Additional insight into how environmental agents can induce immunodeficiency has been learned from the purposeful administration of drugs to induce clinical immunosuppression, and a discussion of these may be found in Chapter 8. Finally, the specter of the most profound form of immunodeficiency, the acquired immunodeficiency syndrome (AIDS), in this case a virus, has stimulated much research into the nature of how a normal immune system may be severely compromised by an environmental agent. Immunotoxicologists are interested in determining if nonliving environmental agents can induce any kind of acquired or secondary immunodeficiency that could lead to a compromise of human health.

B. PRIMARY IMMUNOLOGIC DEFICIENCY DISEASES

Congenital or primary deficiencies become manifest early in life when repeated infections are experienced by the infant. These result from either genetic anomalies or failure of normal embryological development of critical immune system components. Although the state of primary immunodeficiency is rather common, the etiology is extremely heterogeneous, and no single entity is necessarily very common. Some syndromes have been reported in only a very few patients, whereas others such as selective IgA deficiency are fairly common, occurring in as many as one in every eight hundred individuals. Not only are there many components of the immune system, any one of which is susceptible to an anomaly, but even in one specific type of disorder there may be a range of functional defects in patients expressing such a type. Often the type of recurrent infections will suggest the nature of the immune defect (refer to Table 7-1) inasmuch as certain immune components are most effective agsinst specific pathogens. Congenital immunodeficiencies may affect either the antigen-specific or non-antigen-specific immune systems. A selected list of many of the known diseases appears in

TABLE 7-1.   The Association Between Human Immune Defects and Susceptibility to Infections

Antibody Response	Cell-Mediated Response	Neutrophil	Opsonin/ Spleen	Complement
Haemophilus	Cytomegalovirus	*Aspergillus*	Pneumococci	Staphylococci
Pneumococci	Herpes zoster	*Bacteroides*	Meningococci	Streptococci
Campylobacter	*Salmonella*	*Pseudomonas*	Streptococci	*N. meningitidis*
Echovirus	*Legionella*	*Klebsiella*	Hemophilus	*N. gonorrhoeae*
Giardia	Mycobacteria	*E. coli*		
	Coccidioides	Staphylococci		
	Histoplasma			
	Cryptococci			
	Candida			
	Toxoplasma			
	Pneumocystis			

Table 7-2. The complete list is extensive, and the reader is referred to specialized treatments for more detail (Buckley 1988; Waldman 1988).

As expected, these diseases affect nearly every immune component. Humoral immunity defects can occur at the B-cell or pre-B-cell level (resulting in hypo- or agammaglobulinemia) or may affect only those lymphocytes producing particular isotypes, e.g., IgA, IgM, or IgE. In the latter case, the defect usually leads to an excess production of that isotype. T-cell dysfunction may be brought about at several levels including failure of normal embryological development of the thymus (DiGeorge syndrome). If the defect occurs at the stem cell level, both B and T lymphocyte production are affected, as in the severe combined immunodeficiency (SCID) syndrome. There are several forms of this disease, and in one presenting with reticular dysgenesis, phagocytic function is also compromised. Many of these diseases affect more than the immune system: there are often severe metabolic defects present as well. For example, there is a deficiency of adenosine deaminase in one clinical type of SCID; the Wiskott–Aldrich syndrome, is additionally characterized by platelet deficiency and eczema; and there

TABLE 7-2.   Classification of Selected Primary Immunodeficiency Diseases

Disease	Affected Component
X-linked agammaglobulinemia	Pre-B cells
Selective IgA deficiency	IgA B lymphocyte
Selective IgM deficiency	T_h cells
IgE hyperglobulinemia	Unknown
X-linked immunoproliferative disease	B cell, possibly T cells
DiGeorge syndrome	Embryological failure to develop third and fourth branchial pouches
Nezelof's syndrome	Thymus, T cells, metabolic defects
Severe combined immunodeficiency (different types)	T cells; metabolic defects; thymic stem cells
Wiskott–Aldrich syndrome	?
Ataxia telangiectasia	T-helper cells, B cells, multisystem defects
Hereditary angioedema	Deficiency of C1 esterase inhibitor
Hereditary neutropenia	Error in myeloid differentiation
Chronic granulomatous disease	Errors in neutrophil metabolism

Source: Adapted from Buckley (1988).

is also failure of parathyroid development in the DiGeorge syndrome. Dysfunction may involve only certain types of immune response, as in those with selective IgM deficiency, thought to involve a T-helper-cell defect, or the Wiskott–Aldrich syndrome, where the patients have a pronounced inability to respond to polysaccharide antigens.

A number of phagocytic disorders are also known involving defects at several levels (Quie 1982). These include selective defects in myeloid precursors, sustained neutrophil production, chemotaxis, and killing of ingested bacteria. Abnormalities of neutrophil function also occur with other types of immunodeficiency, e.g., in SCID with reticular dysgenesis or in X-linked agammaglobulinemia. In the latter, compromised function would in part result from failure of opsonic enhancement of phagocytosis, although neutropenia is also present. Similarly, compromised phagocytic function would accompany certain of the complement component deficiencies, which would interfere with chemotactic as well as opsonic functions.

Children with certain types of impairment of the killing functions in phagocytes known as chronic granulomatous disease (of which there is more than one type) have normal antibody- and cell-mediated forms of immunity. Their phagocytes can respond normally to chemotactic stimuli, but the neutrophils lack the ability to generate peroxides, which are largely responsible for intracellular killing (Malech and Gallin 1987). Here, the genetic defect in oxidative metabolism is caused by the genetically determined absence of a cytochrome necessary for the normal transfer of electrons. Because of the impaired ability of neutrophils to form peroxide, survival advantage is shifted to bacteria that can produce peroxidase (catalase). This defect in function is manifested in an increased frequency of skin or tissue infections with catalase-positive microorganisms (Mills and Quie 1983). In addition, inflammatory processes may not be resolved, leading to extensive granuloma formation and scarring (Gallin and Buescher 1983).

Deficiencies in almost every complement component (including C1 inhibitor) in both pathways and certain of the receptors have been reported. Although some of these deficiencies result from continued complement consumption by underlying disorders, others are caused by genetic/developmental defects, but these are very rare. Many of those discovered with component deficiencies were initially thought to be in normal health, but long-term retrospective studies have shown that many of these, particularly those whose late-acting components are affected, have an unusual propensity to develop autoimmune diseases later (Frank 1988). This should serve as a warning to immunotoxicologists that long-term effects of depressed parameters may require more consideration over time. Nevertheless, many patients with complement deficiencies remain in normal health for many years. Deficiencies of alternative pathway components or C3 seem more susceptible to infections than others. Decrements in C3 function often are associated with pyogenic infections, whereas patients with a recurrent history of meningitis have reported defects in complement components C5–C9.

One interesting deficiency, known as hereditary angioedema, results from a selective deficiency of a normal inhibitor for C1 esterase and kallikrein. Minor stimuli somehow trigger excessive classical and kinin-generating pathway activation, since the normal inhibiting mechanism of these systems is absent. The result is multisystem edema caused by widespread change in capillary permeability that is often life threatening, particularly when the larynx is affected. It is of note that these minor environmental stimuli (e.g., food, dust) might be considered "immunotoxic" when in fact the basic defect is genetic.

This brief synopsis could well serve as a guide for those interested in immuno-toxicology in that selective damage to the immune system by xenobiotics might be expected to become manifest in similar manners, providing the damage is extensive enough. Should such toxicities that result in permanent or progressive damage be proved, experience with primary immunodeficiencies might be instructive to immunotoxicologists in that much has also been learned concerning reconstitution of immune function in immunodeficiency patients (Buckley 1988; Waldman 1988).

C. VULNERABLE POINTS IN THE IMMUNE SYSTEM

The immune system possesses so many components and functions through different pathways that result in the elaboration of so many mediators that numerous opportunities exist for potential immunotoxicants to exert effect. Toxic effects are possible in any of the cell types involved in either the afferent or efferent limb of the immune response, including hematopoietic stem cells. Modifications of special concern are those that alter functions, especially those concerned with production of secretory products or expression of key receptors, for it is these substances that play such a critical role in regulation and cell-to-cell cooperation. Although cell lysis of immunocompetent cells is always possible, such extreme effects would most likely result in profound alteration in immune function, which in the main is not seen in immunotoxicity. Rather, most alterations of immune system parameters are more subtle, which implies that it is the regulatory functions that are those usually affected.

Two of the most critical areas of vulnerability are the stem cells and any of the antigen-processing cells. Damage to the former would be expected to result in the most profound defects. It is defects in specific stem cell lines that characterize many of the genetic or developmental immunodeficiencies, and these same stem cells are the targets of some forms of chemotherapeutic immunosuppression. Macrophages and other antigen-presenting cells are especially vulnerable because of their xenobiotic uptake functions and anatomic location. Since the cells are among the first lines of defense and most likely to encounter a toxin first, they are more prone to damage. Their functions of antigen presentation and lymphocyte regulation are critical to induction of primary immune responses, so that any damage to antigen-presenting cells will reduce the effectiveness of immune responses. Moreover, damage to phagocytic cells will become immediately manifest by the presence of opportunistic microbes that will fail to be contained or killed.

Toxicants that affect protein synthesis, gene expression, and receptor expression will also have profound effects. Such alterations are unlikely to be detectable morphologically, but only through more complicated assays. Molecular biology has provided much additional insight into not only how critical such products are themselves but also how important expression of the product is at the exact critical time required for optimum effect on receptive targets. Failure to produce the required mediator or receptor in a timely fashion could affect coordination of a given immune response but would not be detectable in currently popular routine assays.

Finally, efferent expression of immune responses can be altered by toxicants that affect target tissue functions. Increased release of histamine, alteration in cAMP or substance P production, stimulation of adhesion molecules, etc. are all examples that would give the appearance of altering the immune system.

A summary of some of the most important points of vulnerability to immunotoxicants is depicted in Fig. 7–1. Selected vulnerable components or steps are discussed below using well-studied examples pertaining to each. The examples selected involve those with the greatest human application but do not include those brought about by intentional immunosuppression (for these, see Chapter 8). The reader is referred to the excellent reviews of Dean, Luster, and their colleagues described in Chapter 1 for further details concerning immunotoxicologic studies performed in animals.

1. Stem Cells

Great advances have been made in the last decade toward understanding the molecular and cellular biology of hemato- and myelopoiesis. Formerly, any thought of such damage was confined to lysis or ablation of an entire stem cell lineage, but except for such extreme situations as irradiation, such absolute toxicity is

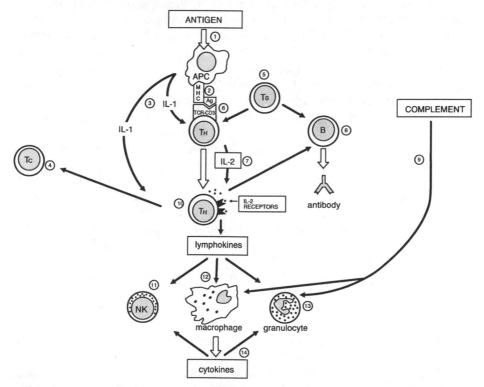

FIGURE 7–1.   Overview of the the immune response indicating some of the major points of vulnerability to xenobiotic toxicity. (1) Antigen uptake; (2) antigen presentation; (3) macrophage regulatory functions; (4) generation of T-cytotoxic cells; (5) T-suppressor-cell modulation; (6) interference with T-helper-cell induction; (7) T-helper-cell function; (8) immunoglobulin synthesis; (9) complement regulation and activation; (10) lymphokine production; (11) NK-cell function; (12) macrophage chemotaxis and cytotoxic functions; (13) neutrophil functions; and (14) inflammatory cell cytokine production.

rare. Rather, it is more likely that a particular lineage would be depressed, that production of a critical cytokine such as a colony-stimulating factor (CSF) or IL-3 might be depressed or that damage might occur to *another* cell type critical to immune cell development. When one considers that macrophage or stromal cell production of IL-1 and IL-6 in the bone marrow influences colony formation by hematopoietic precursor cells in the presence of CSF, it is apparent that a potential immunotoxicant can profoundly affect the immune system in ways far more subtle than stem cell lysis. Moreover, some cytokines (e.g., TNF, IFN-γ, transforming growth factor β) capable of being stimulated by an immunotoxicant, can depress CSF responses. Unfortunately, few contemporary immunoassay systems screen for alterations as complicated as this.

One of the xenobiotics that has been studied extensively with regard to stem cell immunotoxicity has been benzene. It has long been recognized that acute toxicity to benzene may lead to pancytopenia (decreased numbers of all circulating cells), aplastic anemia, and occasionally leukemia, the clinical condition and severity being dependent on length and concentration of the dose (Snyder et al. 1981). Although much of the bone marrow toxicity of benzene is predictable knowing exposure parameters, that related to leukemia is not. Some of these effects (excluding leukemia) can be reproduced experimentally in rodents.

Benzene is an example of an individual molecule that is not toxic in its native state but becomes so only after being oxidatively metabolized to toxic materials (Snyder et al. 1981). Oxidation to phenol is effected via the cytochrome P-450 oxidase system, most probably in the liver and to a much lesser extent in the bone marrow, and can be partially inhibited with antioxidants. Various other types of benzene metabolism include hydroxylation to substances like hydroquinone or dehydrogenation to catechols. The major effects are on red blood cell precursors, but in high enough concentration lymphoid and myeloid stem cells may also be affected. In high doses, benzene has profound effects on other types of bone marrow cells of immune interest, resulting in decreased function and increased lethality to infections. Although not clearly defined, the toxicity induced by benzene metabolites may occur through mutagenesis of stem cells, alteration of accessory cells, or a decrease in cytokine production. Because the metabolites of this substance remain in the marrow even after exposure ceases, there is a concern for the appearance of long-term immunotoxic effects, even though new occupational exposure standards have been set much lower than previously. Workers chronically exposed to benzene in doses in excess of 100 ppm have increased rates of such diseases as acute myelogenous leukemia and possibly lymphoma (Decoufle, Blattner, and Blair 1983), both of which may be accompanied by an increased risk to infection. However, claims of depressed immunity (in the absence of malignancy) resulting from benzene exposure need to be examined more carefully.

There is a great disparity in quality between experimental animal data and those obtained from human studies. Initial studies from acute inhalation exposure (6 hr/day for 6 days, 10 ppm) studies in rats indicated limited suppression of B-lymphocyte mitogenesis without a significant decrease in circulating B cells (Rozen, Snyder, and Albert 1984). Conversely, benzene metabolite injection in rabbits or mice led to a selective decline of immunoglobulin-bearing B cells and concomitant decreases in mitogen responses of bone marrow B lymphocytes as well as attenuation in antibody responses (Irons and Moore 1980; Wierda and Irons 1982). The nature of the depressed mitogenic response was explained further by the studies of King, Landreth, and Wierda (1989), who showed that the primary effect of the hydroquinone metabolite was in depressing IL-1 production by macrophages. This cytokine influences the subsequent production of IL-4 by bone marrow stromal cells, an essential ingredient in the transformation of pre-B cells to induce immunoglobulin production. Thus, although the distal effect of the immunotoxicity involves precursors of macrophages, the most proximal effect appears to be on lymphocytes.

That such findings could have meaning to the systemic well-being of the animals was demonstrated by the findings of depressed resistance to *Listeria* infection in mice exposed to 5-day (6 hr/day) benzene inhalation at concentrations of 30 ppm but not 10 ppm (Rosenthal and Snyder, 1985). At the time of the study, 10 ppm was the permissible standard for exposure to benzene.

In vitro data with human lymphocytes exposed to these materials indicate similar depressions in mitogenic responses; however, the metabolite catechol (and, to a lesser extent, hydroquinone) rather than benzene has been identified as the major incitant of the alteration (Morimoto and Wolff 1980). Depressed serum IgG, IgA, and hemolytic complement activity levels with increased IgM have been reported in workers chronically exposed to benzene (Lange et al. 1973; Smolik et al. 1973). Unfortunately, no quantitative data regarding benzene exposure were available from these studies. Although these workers were also exposed to toluene and xylene, experimental data suggest that the presence of these additional solvents attenuates the metabolism of benzene (reviewed in Snyder et al. 1981). Had exposure been restricted to benzene alone the observed depressions might have been even lower. Yardley-Jones, Anderson, and Jenkinson (1988) could not find depressed lymphocyte mitogen responsiveness to phytohemagglutinin (PHA) in workers with long-term exposure to 1–5 ppm with occasional exposures up to 100 ppm. Unfortunately, PHA is a T-cell mitogen in humans, and animal studies suggest that it would have been more appropriate to have examined B-cell function in these workers.

Those interested in the human relevance of immunotoxicology need to approach a greater degree of sophistication, as best exemplified by the experimental studies of King, Landreth, and Wierda (1989), instead of the single-parameter surveys of exposed populations of the past. More effort needs to be placed on mechanisms rather than effects, a warning sounded by Sharma and Zeeman over a decade ago (1980). At the same time, the experimentalists need to recognize the vast differences between short-term, high-dose exposure (not even given by inhalation) that they have used and long-term, low-dose inhalation exposure to which humans are subjected.

2. Macrophages/Monocytes

As was seen in the assessment of benzene immunotoxicity, what began as a study of effects on lymphocyte maturation ended up incriminating altered macrophage function as ultimately responsible for the chain of events leading to the impairment. In addition to their defensive, phagocytic role, cells of the macrophage/monocyte lineage, as well as other cells involved in antigen presentation (see Table 2-2, Chapter 2), are critical in induction of antigen-specific immune responses. Their role lies in producing cytokines that regulate immune responses, and, in themselves, they are also important in responding to mediators produced by various types of inflammation including interaction with effector cells and molecules of immune recognition. Thus, monocytes/macrophages are equally important in both afferent and efferent pathways and of both antigen-specific and nonspecific reactions. Damage to these cells could result in several types of immune impairment. Two key steps of antigen presentation are especially critical and subject to environmental variation: (1) antigen processing and expression of peptide fragments on the cell membrane (see Fig. 2–9, Chapter 2); and (2) presentation of these peptides in MHC class II context (see Fig. 2–10, Chapter 2). If metabolic processing of the native antigen is blocked, or if conditions of the microenvironment are altered, the result could well have a profound effect on the quality of antigen processing. If MHC class II expression is inhibited, there will be no afferent pathway induction. Such inhibition can occur through very indirect and subtle pathways. For example, many toxicants can induce PGE_2 production in a number of cells including macrophages. This cyclooxygenase pathway product inhibits macrophage expression of MHC molecules and also inhibits proliferation of human myeloid stem cells in the bone marrow (Pelus 1982).

The phagocytic process can be enhanced or depressed by a number of environmental substances depending on concentration (Table 7–3). For simplification, both chemotaxis and engulfment are included under phagocytic functions. One of the best-studied macrophage toxins is certain crystalline forms of silicon dioxide or silica (Allison, Harington, and Birbeck 1966; Kessel, Monaco, and Marchisio 1963); however, the effects are much more pronounced in vitro than in vivo (Davis 1986). When silica is added to macrophage cultures, cytopathic effects are soon noticed, followed by lysis. There is no question that high doses of silica given intraperitoneally or intravenously abrogate the immune response, making recipient animals more susceptible to tumors and infectious agents and prolonging allograft acceptance (reviewed by Burrell 1981). Yet pulmonary macrophages obtained from Vermont granite workers naturally exposed to silicaceous dusts possessed normal viability and function even though up to 90% of the cells contained refractile silica particles (Christman et al. 1985). It is likely that two reasons account for the great differences between experimental studies and those from normally exposed subjects. Doses used by experimentalists (e.g., > 100 μg/ml in culture; 3–5 mg/IV dose) are very likely to be much in excess of those that alveolar macrophages encounter under natural conditions. More importantly, the

TABLE 7–3.   Selected Environmental Agents That Affect Macrophage Function

Agent	Effect
Silica	Cytotoxic; in small quantities, depression
Crocidolite asbestos	Enhancement
Fly ash	As particle size decreases, enhancement; also cytotoxic
Coal mine dust	Depression
Manganese dioxide	Depression and cytotoxicity
Cigarette smoke	Depression
Carbon monoxide	Enhancement
SO_2	5–20 ppm, enhancement
NO_2	25 ppm, depression
Formaldehyde	10 ppm, enhancement; 20 ppm, depression
Aflatoxin, mycotoxins	Depression and cytotoxicity

Source: Modified from Burrell (1985).

toxicity of silica particles in inhalation studies may possibly be blunted by being coated with endogenous surfactant lipids (Davis 1986).

Prolonged exposure to silica dusts at 50 mg/m^3 recruits low levels of alveolar macrophages and eventually neutrophils into the terminal air spaces (Donaldson et al. 1990), although the almost certain presence of infections may confound this as well. Bronchoalveolar lavages from silica-exposed animals and humans show an increase in number of macrophages with increased functions, e.g., enhanced chemiluminesence and changes in membrane properties. Furthermore, activated macrophages or their products influence other types of cells by such mediators as toxic oxygen radicals, tumor necrosis factor, prostaglandins, and IL-1 (Burns and Zarkower 1982; Driscoll et al. 1990). Some of these cytokines would not have an immediate effect on inflammation, but others would have an effect on subsequent lymphocyte functions (Miller and Zarkower 1974, 1976). Finally, silica-dust-stimulated macrophages produce fibroblast-stimulating and collagen-generating factors, e.g., IL-1, macrophage-derived growth factor, and fibronectin, which are important in fibrosis development in pulmonary silicosis (Davis 1986).

One of the most interesting new ideas in the study of silica toxicity concerns the production of reactive oxygen radicals on the surface of the freshly fractured quartz particles. Freshly ground quartz yields a much higher amount of silica-based radicals per gram of dust capable of reacting with aqueous media to produce hydroxyl ions than do older dusts, which have been stored (Vallyathan et al. 1988). These radicals, as well as their ability to generate hydroxyl radicals, decrease quickly after grinding with a half-life of about 30 hr and even faster if stored in aqueous media, within minutes. Freshly ground quartz produced a greater respiratory burst in alveolar macrophage cultures as measured by superoxide anion production, hydrogen peroxide release, and dye reduction. It is hypothesized that the free radicals initiate an oxidative chain reaction leading to macrophage membrane damage through peroxidation (Dalal, Shi, and Vallyathan 1990). Thus, although the toxicity of oxygen radicals is well known, the idea that the particle itself can generate them without biological interaction is novel and provides an additional toxicologic parameter to consider.

3. B Lymphocytes

Phenytoin, a drug widely used to treat generalized and focal seizure disorders, has been linked to many immunologic side effects. Outward signs and symptoms include a variety of cutaneous reactions with rashes (some of which may be caused by hypersensitivity mechanisms), serum sickness, collagen vascular diseases, declining but reversible levels of IgA, transient hypogammaglobulinemia of all classes with lymphocytosis possibly linked to abnormal T_s activity, and, in at least one severe instance, permanent B-cell impairment. In addition to phenytoin, several drugs with related chemical structures, e.g., phenobarbital and carbamazepine, have also been reported to provoke similar reactions, suggesting that some unique chemical prosthetic group is required to induce the reaction in susceptible individuals (Knutsen et al. 1984). These observations as well as those reports of in vitro proliferative responses to the drug in lymphocytes from treated patients (Josephs, Rothman, and Buckley 1980; Lillie et al. 1983) suggest that at least some of the untoward reactions to phenytoin also consist of a cell-mediated hypersensitivity reaction in addition to the toxicity. However, the immune defects of decreased B lymphocytes and immunoglobulin production are not the kind of impairments seen in hypersensitivity reactions (see Chapter 6). Usually, physical symptoms improve and immune parameters return to normal following cessation of the phenytoin therapy. The use of corticosteroids has brought about great improvement in some, but in others it appears to contribute further to the immunosuppression (Josephs, Rothman, and Buckley 1980).

Bardana et al. (1983) carried out a prospective longitudinal study of 118 patients treated with phenytoin, allowing comparisons to be made before commencing therapy and at 6-month intervals thereafter. Phenytoin administration was associated with an increased incidence of significantly low IgA and IgE values at the first 6-month interval. The IgA decrease tended to occur in certain types of patients, i.e., those with idiopathic epilepsy. This group had an unexpected incidence of low IgA before initiation of treatment. The decrease in IgE was distributed evenly in all groups. Further decline in immunoglobulin levels occurred in only a few patients after that time. The IgG and IgM values also fell, but the decline per group was not statistically significant; IgD, C3, and C4 were unaffected.

In one somewhat typical case study, a patient was described as having erythroderma and exfoliative dermatitis with panhypogammaglobulinemia as well as a marked increase in T lymphocytes that responded poorly to T-cell mitogens in vitro (Lillie et al. 1983). These authors concluded that the T-cell lymphocytosis was caused by an increase in T_s cells, but no examination for suppressor subset markers or function was attempted. In another study, functional suppressor activity was indeed demonstrated in lymphocytes from a patient with hypogammaglobulinemia and a virtual absence in B cells (Dosch, Jason, and Gelfand 1982). This suppressive effect was not seen in any of 100 lymphocyte suspensions from normal subjects or from patients with normal immunologic values undergoing phenytoin therapy.

A most remarkable case of severe permanent B-cell deficiency induced by phenytoin was described in one patient who developed a rash, lymphadenopathy, and subsequent severe depressions in all immunoglobulin isotypes within 3 weeks after receiving the drug (Guerra et al. 1986). In vitro cellular immunology studies failed to find any abnormalities in T-cell subset distribution or function, but very few, if any, circulating B cells could be found (see Table 7-4). Other B-cell function tests, e.g., PWM stimulation studies, were exceedingly low. No evidence of suppression or increased number of CD8$^+$ cells could be documented. Panhypogammaglobulinemia was present, and the patient failed to demonstrate isohemagglutinins or antibody responses to diphtheria or tetanus toxins, although this is not the usual finding in most patients. The depression in immune function remained for at least 3 years after exposure to the drug. The patient continued to experience increased bouts of mild gastrointestinal and respiratory infections and required maintainance on intravenous γ-globulin therapy. Although most evidence seems to point circumstantially to phenytoin's immunotoxic effect as an indirect one resulting from an imbalanced T-cell regulation of B cells, this latter case seems to have a more direct effect on B-cell precursors. This episode might in some ways be considered the worst-case scenario in immunotoxicology, i.e., exposure to a single compound resulting in a near absolute disappearance of a definable immune function. This is the kind of reaction immunotoxicologists have feared and have searched for, but fortunately it is extremely rare. If any

TABLE 7-4.   Laboratory Data from Patient with Phenytoin Immunotoxicity

	Months after Initiating Rx					
	1	8	10	21	33	Control Range
Globulin	0.7	0.3	0.1	ND	ND	0.7 to 1.7 g/dl
IgG	ND	180	209	291	259	639–1,349 mg/dl
IgA	ND	15	29	31	28	70–312 mg/dl
IgM	ND	0	11	12	13	56–352 mg/dl
IgE	105	ND	ND	6	1	3–382 IU/ml
B cells						
sIg				0[a]	0	5.1–17.5
CD20				0.9	0.3	1.8–13.6
T cells						
E rosettes				77.9	67.7	42.5–73.7
CD3				71.5	77.3	38–86.4
CD4				49.9	56.8	23–57.8
CD8				19.9	24.4	12.5–32.5
In vitro Ig production						
Unstimulated PFU MNC[b]				247	50	1,753 IgSC/10^6
PWM-stimulated CFU MNC				435	280	8,946 IgSC/10^6

[a]Percentage positive.

[b]Number of Ig-secreting cells/10^6 mononuclear cells.

Source: Data from Guerra et al. (1986).

drug or chemical were often responsible for such a profound type of immunodeficiency happening, it would most likely be unusable.

No molecular or cytokine studies are available, so it is not possible to construct the sequence of events leading to this impairment or to determine whether the B cell is directly affected by the drug or if the B-cell defect is caused by an imbalance in T-cell regulation. The superimposition of definite hypersensitivity on this defect complicates the understanding, but possibly this is an example of how one agent can lead to an immunotoxicity and hypersensitivity occurring in the same patient.

4. T Lymphocytes

Certainly the worst-case scenario for a T-cell immunotoxin would be the human immunodeficiency virus (HIV), the putative cause of the acquired immunodeficiency syndrome (AIDS). Although immunotoxicologists usually think strictly in terms of chemicals as agents of immunotoxicity, there are a number of cogent reasons for discussing the mechanism of HIV immunotoxicity in some detail. One of the purposes of this treatise has been to present evidence that factors other than a given etiologic agent in the environment are important in the development of immunotoxic effects and that very often those other factors involve infectious or microbial agents. In the case of AIDS, the infective agent and the immunotoxic agent happen to be one and the same. Great research effort has been directed toward understanding HIV pathogenicity, and there has been enormous spinoff in that the findings are directly applicable to immunotoxicity studies.

↝ AIDS could be considered the worst possible type of immunotoxicity, the type that fortunately is not produced by any known chemical. This fact has not daunted "yellow journalists" and others bent on persuading the public that our environment is simply awash in too many chemicals, that we are poisoning ourselves to extinction, and that the only solution is to prohibit their production and usage. The term "chemical AIDS" is frequently used by such groups but is utterly without scientific foundation. Nevertheless, a serious discussion of just what comprises the immunologic lesions of AIDS should be worth any immunotoxicologist's consideration. The following discussion only considers those matters pertaining to how HIV interacts with cells of immune importance and is not concerned with such equally important matters as clinical signs and symptoms, epidemiology, and social consequences. The discussion presumes that HIV is the causative agent, and although persuasive evidence exists that it does not act alone in its pathogenesis, and there is also serious argument that HIV is not even the causative agent (Duesberg, 1991), no attempt is made to examine these claims.

Although a brief synopsis of the most important details in immunopathogenesis is presented, the reader is referred to Rosenberg and Fauci (1990) for a further description of HIV pathogenesis. The basic effect begins with interaction between glycoprotein molecules present on the virus and cells bearing the transmembrane CD4 receptor, i.e., T-helper cells and macrophages. HIV is a retrovirus capable of long-term latent infections by inserting its own genes into the host genome. This retroviral genome can be replicated for many generations along with the host genome, or it can be transcribed into complete viral particles capable of killing or lysing the host cell and/or infecting new cells. These factors account for the often long incubation periods of AIDS and the general loss of some of the T-helper cells. Specific nucleotide sequences in the HIV genome are responsible for encoding envelope glycoproteins (*env* genes), one of which, *gp120*, is critical in the infectious process. The *gp120* is the high-affinity binding protein that intially binds the viral particles to primate CD4. Either free viral particles can bind to uninfected cells or infected cells expressing *gp120* before particle release can bind to uninfected CD4$^+$ cells, causing a fusion of the membranes of the two cells that permits direct transfer of viral genome.

The transcribed viral DNA may not necessarily undergo further replication in the host cell for many years. At this point, certain HIV sequences (long terminal repeats [LTRs]) that regulate DNA transcription are influenced by activation of the T-cell receptors or cytokine production (e.g., TNF) by the host cells. A common way that these cells become activated is by the presence of other coinfective agents (Gowda et al. 1989), e.g., herpes, hepatitis, gonococci, or infective agents already present at the time of HIV exposure (e.g., parasites in much of the Third World). These infections can activate the cells in a variety of ways, but one of the most important is by inciting TNF production (Clouse et al. 1989). It is unfortunate that the same stimuli responsible for T-cell growth are also responsible for enhancement of HIV replication.

Normally the CD4$^+$/CD8$^+$ ratio of healthy humans is 2:1, but in advanced AIDS this ratio is often reduced to as low as 0.5. Although it is generally known that this latter value represents serious compromise, what is unknown is at what point in declining ratio does clinical immunosuppression begin, because signs and symptoms appear before much loss in CD4$^+$ cells. Paradoxically, this loss of cells occurs in spite of evidence that perhaps only 1% of CD4$^+$ cells present are infected with viral particles, and in most of these there is no evidence of viral transcription. Among the possible reasons to account for this are these: accumulations of viral RNA may be functionally toxic to host cells; *gp120* may be binding recycled CD4 molecules within the cytoplasm; and those cells that had produced complete particles have already lysed from permeabilty malfunctioning caused by the excessive *gp120* production on the cell membrane. Other CD4$^+$ cells may be affected indirectly in that critical supplies of cytokines necessary for developing T cells are limited because of infection in cells producing them. Some investigators feel that destruction is an autoimmune event mediated by host anti-*gp120* antibodies and brought about by ADCC (Lyerly et al. 1987) or cytotoxic lymphocytes (Siliciano et al. 1988) reacting with soluble glycoproteins that have adsorbed to CD4 receptors of normal cells. Moreover, IL-2 and *gp120* share regions of homology (Reiher et al. 1986), and it is possible that *gp120* antibodies may cross-react and interfere with IL-2 function. Even without physical destruction, infected T_h cells could suffer loss in such critical functions as IL-2 binding or MHC class II interaction with antigen-presenting cells.

Other cells are also affected in HIV infection. Macrophages/monocytes bear CD4 molecules but do not seem to be lysed or killed by the infection and are considered to be the major reservoir of viral particles in infected hosts. Moreover, essential macrophage functions such as phagocytosis, antigen presentation, and IL-1 production are impaired in part because infected lymphocytes have defective release of IFN-γ, a potent stimulator of macrophage function (Murray et al. 1985). B cells undergo a profound hyperreactivity, most likely because of the impairment in T-cell regulation, and results in heightened polyclonal immunoglobulin levels. Unfortunately, this production is not directed to new antigens, and most of it is of little help to the infected individual.

Immunotoxicologists may well profit from the sophisticated studies that have been made regarding HIV pathogenesis in that numerous pathways are suggested for studying immunotoxic reactions to other materials. HIV is unique in that it interferes with a molecule, i.e., CD4, in such a way that numerous other immune functions are compromised. Should some chemical compound analogous to *gp120* exist in the workplace or the environment, the results could be equally serious. HIV has two other unique properties with which immunotoxicologists usually do not have to contend, and both are related to the fact that HIV is a self-replicating immunotoxin; i.e., not only does the amount of immunotoxic principle increase within a single infected individual, but the reproductive property enables the agent to be communicable from person to person.

5. NK Cells

Understanding of the role of NK cells is rather new in toxicology and even in immunology. Indeed, their stem cell origin and precise relationship to lymphocytes have not yet been defined. For these reasons, little is known about what sort of xenobiotics can alter NK cells and function.

A disquieting concept has recently appeared regarding the possibility of immunotoxicity by micronutrients. Although in vitro evidence indicates that selenium (Nair and Schwartz 1990) can suppress NK, LAK, and lymphocyte functions in concentrations about 1.0 μg/ml, in vivo evidence from humans is lacking. Such minerals currently have a good reputation among nutritionists, and possible trouble might be encountered by food faddists who tend to overdo things when new information becomes available concerning the salutary effects of nutrients. Although it is doubtful that tissue levels could reach 0.2–1.0 μg/ml through ingestion of natural food sources, possible toxic levels might be reached if it is taken in concentrated supplement form. Selenium has been shown to depress target cell cytotoxicity when added to NK-cell assays, to inhibit generation of LAK cells (i.e., when NK cells are activated by IL-2), and to inhibit T-cell proliferation responses to standard mitogens (Nair and Schwartz 1990). Selenium did not affect cell viability or NK target cells.

Of greater concern perhaps is the possible NK-cell suppressive activity of agents like theophylline, taken by asthmatics at therapeutic concentrations. This drug is widely and successfully used to alleviate bronchoconstriction by inhibiting the phosphodiesterase breakdown of cAMP in chronic asthmatics and in this use has literally made living possible for an enormous number of people. When aminophylline was added to in vitro NK-cell assays, concentrations in excess of 5×10^{-5} M significantly inhibited cytotoxicity of target cells (Yokoyama et al. 1990). In one of the few studies to extend such findings to use in vivo in patients, these same authors administered sustained-release tablets (400–500 mg/day for 7 days) to five normal volunteers and again found significant inhibition of NK cytotoxicity. Of even greater relevance was their finding that the serum concentration reached by this treatment was only 2×10^{-5} M, i.e., less than that minimum concentration giving similar results in vitro. The long-term immunologic effects of theophylline administration to asthmatics is unclear in that, on the one hand, a lower than normal incidence of malignancies has been recorded for all asthmatics regardless of therapy (Alderson 1974), but on the other, asthmatics appear to have more viral respiratory infections than normal people (Mills 1986).

The local anesthetic lidocaine has been shown to inhibit human NK cell activity when added to in vitro cultures (Renzi and Ginns 1990b). Although this agent receives some human use in patients undergoing bronchoscopy, it is unlikely that this limited contact would bring about relevant in vivo immunosuppression. However, the findings are especially germane to experimental pulmonary immunologists who frequently use lidocaine to increase cell yields obtained by bronchoalveolar lavages. If lidocaine is used in such procedures, NK-cell activity is significantly inhibited at doses normally employed for this purpose (Renzi and Ginns 1990a).

It is possible that xenobiotics may have an up-regulating effect on human NK cells as well. One of the most intriguing findings of the immunologic studies performed on those exposed to polybrominated biphenyls in a Michigan incident involving widespread exposure to a feed supplement accidentally contaminated with a fire retardant containing the PBB (see Chapter 11 for details) was that there was a marked and apparently permanent increase in the number of what we now regard as circulating NK cells (Bekesi et al. 1985). This exposure occurred during the mid-1970s, and to date no unusual incidence of infectious disease or malignancies has been reported in these people. Ironically, it is possible that the PBB actually may have enhanced tumor resistance by inducing this NK-cell effect, although no NK-cell function studies have been performed.

6. Neutrophils

Perhaps some of the earliest incidents of immunotoxicity involving drug toxicity to neutrophils were reported during the 1920s and 1930s and were summarized by Kracke in 1938. As a result of the tremendous advances being made in organic synthesis at that time, drugs like arsphenamines and aminopyrine first became available and widely used with the subsequent observations of neutropenia. These first-line defense cells seem particularly vulnerable to a wide array of drugs (see Table 7-5 for examples), and although no individual drug-related complication of therapy is very common, the specter of the possibility of such an event with any drug use certainly is a serious consideration. Although many of these drugs induce side effects more common than neutrophil toxicity, this discussion is limited to those of immune consequence. Similarly, the discussion is limited to those causing changes only in neutrophils, although it is known that several hematopoietic lineages including erythrocytes and platelets are capable of being affected. Neutropenia simply refers to an abnormally low number of circulating neutrophils, regardless of cause (>2 S.D. below normal). Agranulocytosis refers to a more profound absence (or $<0.5 \times 10^6$/ml) of these cells as a result of an effect on the CFU-GM stem cells responsible for neutrophil development and proliferation. Aplastic anemia is an even more serious effect of drug toxicity in that the effect is on pluripotential stem cells that give rise not only to CFU-GM stem cells but also those of platelet and erythrocyte lineages. Aplastic anemia is rarer than agranulocytosis but has a higher mortality.

There are two main types of mechanisms to account for the development of agranulocytosis. The first is dose related, affects DNA and protein synthesis, and involves either committed neutrophil stem cells or the proliferating pool of granulocyte precursors (Vincent 1986). There is likely to be a delay seen between

TABLE 7-5.   Selected Drugs Associated with Neutrophil Immunotoxicity[a]

Anti-inflammatory agents	Antimalarials
Indomethacin	Chloroquine
Phenacetin	Dapsone
Aminopyrine	Pyrimethamine
Phenylbutazone	Quinine
Antibiotics	Antithyroid drugs
Chloramphenicol	Carbimazole
Gentamycin	Methimazole
Isoniazid	Propylthiouracil
Semisynthetic penicillins	Cardiovascular drugs
Sulfonamides	Captopril
Tetracyclines	Methyldopa
Trimethoprim–sulfamethoxazole	Procainimide
Anticonvulsants	Propanolol
Carbamazephine	Quinidine
Phenytoin	Diuretics
Antidepressants	Chlorthalidone
Amitriptyline	Ethacrynic acid
Desipramine	Hypoglycemic agents
Doxepin	Chlorpropamide
Histamine receptor blockers	Tobutamide
Metiamide	Miscellaneous
Hypnotics and sedatives	Phenothiazines
Benzodiazepines	Levamisole
Meprobamate	Penicillamine

[a]This is not a complete list. For more complete coverage, the reader is referred to the annual series, *Meyler's Side Effects of Drugs*, New York: Elsevier.

Source: Adapted from Dale (1990).

drug exposure and onset of damage, as it will take a while for developing cells to move through the full maturation sequences and enter the blood. Examples of drugs inciting this kind of effect are pyrazolone derivatives, chlorpromazine, antithyroid drugs, and chloramphenicol, although the latter is more often associated with aplastic anemia. Patients with high plasma levels of drugs as a result of such complicating factors as receiving multiple drugs, slow metabolism, or impaired renal function exhibit a greater incidence of this type of toxicity (Dale 1990). It has been argued that induction of these disorders may not be so often from single, specific drugs but rather from combinations of drugs (Heit et al. 1985), a very difficult proposition to assess.

The second major mechanism of drug injury appears to be immune mediated (as discussed in Chapter 6). In this instance, injury *by* the immune system would precede injury *to* the immune system. Antibodies reactive with either granulocytes (or stem cells) or more likely with drugs adsorbed to granulocyte membranes account for their subsequent inhibition or destruction. Sulfonamides, quinidine, propylthiouracils, and semisynthetic penicillins are examples of drugs associated with the development of such antibodies. An interesting example of how slight differences in drug structure may account for this kind of toxicity is illustrated by analogs of the histamine H_2-receptor blockers metiamide and cimetidine. The former was the first H_2 antagonist in clinical use but soon was withdrawn because of its unacceptably high rate of agranulocytosis induction. It was succeeded by cimetidine, which differs only by the replacement of a thiourea side chain with cyanoguanidine. Cimetidine has been extensively used with very little incidence of agranulocytosis and, unlike metiamide, is not taken up by bone marrow cells in experimental animals (Brimblecombe et al. 1978).

This is one type of immunocytotoxicity where there is a clear, inverse relationship between the laboratory parameter observed and the clinical risk as well as severity of disease. Those with neutrophil counts of $1.0–1.8 \times 10^6$/ml are at little risk, those with $0.5–1.0 \times 10^6$/ml are at moderate risk, and those below this level are at substantial risk (Dale 1990). Many other factors modify the severity of the clinical expression, including the cause and duration of the disease, integrity of the skin and mucous membranes, vascular supply, and nutritional status. Initial symptoms that include fever, chills, headache, sore throat, and infections beneath the skin and mucous membranes represent a serious situation calling for prompt therapy. In its most serious forms, fatality often follows overwhelming infections.

D. ADDITIONAL CONSIDERATIONS

Other types of cells concerned with the efferent phases of the immune response, e.g., mast cells, basophils, and platelets, are also capable of being affected by a variety of drugs and external agents. However, when such cells are adversely affected, rather than inducing depressed resistance to infective agents or oncogenic processes, inflammatory conditions are brought about through enhanced mediator release. Platelets can be destroyed by immune complexes (in which drugs are haptens) that become attached to Fc receptors. Mechanisms for these types of injury were discussed in the previous chapter. Similarly, any type of external agent that would specifically react with a complement component would most likely initiate the cascade sequence resulting in secondary inflammation. One additional question that has not been studied is the possibility that a xenobiotic might interfere with immunoglobulins after transcription. Staphylococcal protein A and certain plant tannins can certainly combine with the Fc end of immunoglobulins. In these instances, the substance reacts with immunoglobulins, sometimes particular isotypes, but without regard to their antigen-binding specificity. The binding is usually directed to heavy-chain constant regions. Staphylococcal protein A is a 42,000–Da cell wall polypeptide of a very common microorganism found growing opportunistically in a variety of human habitats. Such interaction with immunoglobulins leads to complement activation, which in turn mediates consequences such as blood coagulation and platelet injury that in vivo could participate in the inflammation and capillary thromboembolus formation common to staphylococcal infections (Forsgren et al. 1983). It is possible that the protein A released from the bacterial cells provides a phagocytic escape mechanism because the substance, when added to neutrophil suspensions, inhibits their subsequent ability to ingest whole cells without inhibiting the phagocytic cells per se. It most likely does this by inhibiting Fc attachment of opsonizing immunoglobulins.

Doubtless, protein A is important in the pathogenesis of staphylococcal infections, but the point for immunotoxicologists to consider is whether there is a possibility of xenobiotics being able to initiate similar effects. Another likely way for xenobiotics to react nonspecifically with immunoglobulins would be as lectins with a specificity for the carbohydrate residues of the glycoprotein immunoglobulins. If a substance were large enough to sterically hinder the Fab function of an immunoglobulin, there would in effect be neutralization, but unless there were a constant supply of the neutralizing substance, the effect would be short-lived because of immunoglobulin turnover. For such a material to be more effective, it would have to interfere with globulin production, i.e., by affecting B cells or their receptors. A more likely way for lectin-binding substances to affect immunoglobulins adversely would be by cross-linking two or more antibody molecules bound to cell membrane receptors, in effect inciting membrane perturbation. Were such a substance to cross-link IgE molecules, the effect would be indistinguishable from an allergen reacting with antigen-specific IgE.

In assessing the sites of immuntoxic effects, it is important to realize that these may be indirect and that the primary toxicity may occur elsewhere. Endocrinological disturbances are well known, and many corticosteroid hormones have profound immunomodulation effects (Besedovsky, del Ray, and Sorkin 1983). Some of these effects, including physical and psychological stress, can result in thymic and lymphoid tissue alteration. A variety of extraneous materials can induce release of neuropeptides that have effects on immunoregulation and modulation of hypersensitivity (McGillis, Organist, and Payan 1987; Payan, Levine, and Goetzl 1984). It is also important to realize that immunotoxicology should not be concerned only with chemical substances. Although it is not the intent of immunotoxicology to explain microbial pathogenesis, there are a number of microbial components that become manifest either through infection or exposure in other forms (e.g., inhalation) that in effect exert immunotoxic effects or enhance the immunotoxic effects of other agents present in the environment (see Chapter 9). Immunotoxicologists can profit from this information in that it might point the way to understanding how organic chemicals from other origins might affect the immune system.

It must also be pointed out that laboratory-based research is necessarily focused on investigating single, isolated xenobiotics, but in nature exposure to complex mixtures is much more likely. Workers who deal in agricultural products or who process these materials are subject to concentrated aerosols of complex mixtures of organic dusts (Rylander 1986; Von Essen et al. 1990), and determining which of the many components, alone or in concert, is responsible for the toxicity has been very difficult. In cotton dust alone, one may find bacterial endotoxin, histamine, a histamine-releasing agent, tannins, the nonspecific immunoglobulin-precipitating polymer, and a bronchoconstrictive agent, among others that are capable of individually causing immunotoxic responses (Nichols 1991). Exposure to these or even simpler materials is invariably confounded by exposure to other agents present in the same environment, e.g., infectious agents, cigarette smoke, or heavy air pollution, which may make determination of specific pathogenesis even more difficult. This is not to say that making an attempt to study the pathogenesis of complicated mixtures is futile—only that one needs to be cognizant of the pitfalls likely to be encountered.

E. CONCLUSIONS

Most efforts in the past have been directed at looking for effects rather than mechanisms; however, greater insight is currently being provided by looking at the mechanisms by which immunotoxic reactions are brought about. Although there is still value in determining which cell type is affected, e.g., macrophages, lymphocytes, more relevant information is to be obtained by examining such important aspects of the immune response as interferon production, interaction with cell membrane receptors, MHC molecule production, and expression of the various genes concerned with these processes. With respect to studying effects, more attention should be made with respect to long-term follow-up studies of those exposed to agents under study. The experimentalists will also need to adopt similar approaches in the animals they study and not rely entirely on acute effects.

References

Alderson, M. 1974. Mortality from malignant disease in patients with asthma. *Lancet* 2:1475–77.

Allison, A. C., J. S. Harington, and M. Birbeck. 1966. An examination of the cytotoxic effects of silica on macrophages. *J. Exp. Med.* 124:141–54.

Bardana, E. J., Jr., J. D. Gabourel, G. H. Davies, and S. Craig. 1983. Effects of phenytoin on man's immunity. Evaluation of changes in serum immunoglobulins, complement, and antinuclear antibody. *Am. J. Med.* 74:289–96.

Bekesi, J. G., J. Roboz, A. Fischbein, et al. 1985. Immunological, biochemical, and clinical consequences of exposure to polybrominated biphenyls. In *Immunotoxicology and Immunopharmacology*, ed. J. H. Dean, M. I. Luster, A. E. Munson, and H. Amos, pp. 393–406. New York: Raven Press.

Besedovsky, H. O., A. E. del Ray, and E. Sorkin. 1983. What do the immune response and the brain know about each other? *Immunol. Today* 4:342–46.

Brimblecombe, R. W., W. A. M. Duncan, G. J. Durant, et al. 1978. Characterization and development of cimetidine and metiamide as a histamine H_2 receptor antagonist. *Gastroenterology* 74:339–47.

Buckley, R. H. 1988. Normal and abnormal development of the immune system. In *Zinsser Microbiology,* 19th ed., ed. W. K. Joklik, H. P. Willett, and D. B. Amos, pp. 226–42. Norwalk: Appleton-Century-Crofts.

Burns, C. A., and A. Zarkower. 1982. The effects of silica and fly ash dust inhalation on alveolar macrophage effector cell function. *J. Reticuloendothel. Soc.* 32:449–59.

Burrell, R. 1981. Immunological aspects of silica. In *Health Effects of Synthetic Silica Particulates*, ed. D. D. Dunnom, pp. 82–93. Philadelphia: American Society for Testing and Materials.

Burrell, R. 1985. Immune system. In *Environmental Pathology*, ed. N. K. Mottet, pp. 320–43. New York: Oxford UniversityPress.

Christman, J. W., R. J. Emerson, G. B. Graham, and G. S. Davis. 1985. Mineral dust and cell recovery from the bronchoalveolar lavage of healthy Vermont granite workers. *Am. Rev. Respir. Dis.* 132:393–99.

Clouse, K. A., D. Powell, I. Washington, et al. 1989. Monokine regulation of human immunodeficiency virus-1 expression in a chronically infected human T cell clone. *J. Immunol.* 142:431–38.

Dalal, N. S., X. Shi., and V. Vallyathan. 1990. Role of free radicals in the mechanisms of hemolysis and lipid peroxidation by silica: Comparative ESR and cytotoxicity studies. *J. Toxicol. Environ. Health.* 29:307–16.

Dale, D. C. 1990. Neutropenia. In *Hematology*, 4th ed., ed. W. J. Williams, E. Beutler, A. J. Erslev, and M. A. Lichtman, pp. 807–16. New York: McGraw-Hill.

Davis, G. S. 1986. Pathogenesis of silicosis: Current concepts and hypotheses. *Lung* 164:139–54.

Decoufle, P., W. Blattner, and A. Blair. 1983. Mortality among chemical workers exposed to benzene and other agents. *Environ. Res.* 30:16–25.

Donaldson, K., G. M. Brown, D. M. Brown, et al. 1990. Contrasting bronchoalveolar leukocyte responses in rats inhaling coal mine dust, quartz, or titanium dioxide—effects of coal rank, airborne mass concentration, and cessation of exposure. *Environ. Res.* 52:62–76.

Dosch, H.-M., J. Jason., and E. W. Gelfand. 1982. Transient antibody deficiency and abnormal T suppressor cells induced by phenytoin. *N. Engl. J. Med.* 306:406–8.

Driscoll, K. E., R. C. Lindenschmidt, J. K. Maurer, et al. 1990. Pulmonary response to silica or titanium dioxide: Inflammatory cells, alveolar macrophage-derived cytokines, and histopathology. *Am. J. Respir. Cell. Mol. Biol.* 2:381–90.

Duesberg, P. 1991. AIDS epidemiology: Inconsistencies with human immunodeficiency virus and with infectious disease. *Proc. Natl. Acad. Sci. U.S.A.* 88:1575–79.

Dukes, M. N. G., and L. Beeley. *Side Effects of Drugs Annual.* Amsterdam: Elsevier.

Forsgren, A., V. Ghetie, R. Lindmark, and J. Sjöquist. 1983. Protein A and its exploitation. In *Staphylococci and Staphylococcal Infections*, ed. C. S. F. Easmon and C. Adlam, pp. 429–80. New York: Academic Press.

Frank, M. M. 1988. The complement system. In *Immunological Diseases*, 4th ed., ed. M. Samter, D. W. Talmage, M. M. Frank, K. F. Austen, and H. N. Claman, pp. 963–78. Boston: Little, Brown.

Gallin, J. I., and E. S. Buescher. 1983. Abnormal regulation of inflammatory skin responses in male patients with chronic granulomatosis disease. *Inflammation.* 7:227–32.

Gowda, S. D., B. S. Stein, N. Mohagheghpour, et al. 1989. Evidence that T cell activation is required for HIV-1 entry in CD4$^+$ lymphocytes. *J. Immunol.* 142:773–80.

Guerra, I. C., W. A. Fawcett IV, A. H. Redmon, et al. 1986. Permanent intrinsic B cell immunodeficiency caused by phenytoin hypersensitivity. *J. Allergy Clin. Immunol.* 77:603–8.

Heit, W., H. Heimpel, A. Fischer, and N. Frickhofen. 1985. Drug-induced agranulocytosis: Evidence for the commitment of bone marrow hematopoiesis. *Scand. J. Haematol.* 35:459–68.

Irons, R. D., and B. J. Moore. 1980. Effect of short-term benzene administration on circulating lymphocyte subpopulations in the rabbit: Evidence of a selective B-lymphocyte sensitivity. *Res. Commun. Chem. Pathol. Pharmacol.* 27:147.

Josephs, S. H., S. J. Rothman, and R. H. Buckley. 1980. Phenytoin hypersensitivity. *J. Allergy Clin. Immunol.* 66:166–72.

Kessel, R. W. I., L. Monaco, and M. A. Marchisio. 1963. The specificity of the cytotoxic action of silica—a study in vitro. *Br. J. Exp. Pathol.* 44:351–64.

King, A. G., K. S. Landreth, and D. Wierda. 1989. Bone marrow stromal cell regulation of B-lymphopoiesis. II. Mechanisms of hydroquinone inhibition of pre-B cell maturation. *J. Pharmacol. Exp. Ther.* 250:582–90.

Knutsen, A. P., J. Anderson, S. Satayaviboon, and R. G. Slavin. 1984. Immunological aspects of phenobarbital hypersensitivity. *J. Pediatr.* 105:558–63.

Kracke, R. R. 1938. Relation of drug therapy to neutropenic states. *J.A.M.A.* 111:1255–59.

Lange, A., R. Smolik, W. Zatonski, and J. Szymanska. 1973. Serum immunoglobulin levels in workers exposed to benzene, toluene, and xylene. *Int. Arch. Arbeitsmed.* 31:37–44.

Lillie, M. A., L. C. Yang, P. J. Honig, and C. S. August. 1983. Erythroderma, hypogammaglobulinemia, and T-cell lymphocytosis. *Arch. Dermatol.* 119:415–18.

Lyerly, H. K., D. L. Reed, T. J. Matthews, et al. 1987. Anti-GP 120 antibodies from HIV seropositive individuals mediate broadly reactive anti-HIV ADCC. *AIDS Res. Hum. Retoviruses* 3:409–22.

Malech, H. L., and J. I. Gallin. 1987. Neutrophils in human disease. *N. Engl. J. Med.* 317:687–94.

McGillis, J. P., M. L. Organist, and D. G. Payan. 1987. Substance P and immunoregulation. *Fed. Proc.* 45:196–99.

Miller, S. D., and A. Zarkower. 1974. Alterations of murine immunologic responses after silica dust inhalation. *J. Immunol.* 113:1533–43.

Miller, S. D., and A. Zarkower. 1976. Silica-induced alterations of murine lymphocyte immunocompetence and suppression of B lymphocyte immunocompetence: A possible mechanism. *J. Reticuloendothel. Soc.* 19:47–61.

Mills, E. L., and P. G. Quie. 1983. Inheritance in chronic granulomatous disease. In *Advances in Host Defense Mechanisms*, Vol. 3, ed. J. I. Gallin and A. S. Fauci, pp. 25–54. New York: Raven Press.

Mills, J. 1986. Respiratory tract infections and asthma. In *Bronchial Asthma*, 2nd ed., ed., M. E. Gershwin, pp. 191–212. New York: Grune & Stratton.

Morimoto, K., and S. Wolff. 1980. Increase of sister chromatid exchanges and perturbations of cell division kinetics in human lymphocytes by benzene metabolites. *Cancer Res.* 40:1189–93.

Murray, M. J., N. I. Kerkvleit, E. C. Ward, and J. H. Dean. 1985. Models for evaluation of tumor resistance following chemical or drug exposure. In *Immunotoxicology and Pharmacology,* eds. J. H. Dean, M. I. Luster, A. E. Munson, and H. Amos, pp. 113–122. New York: Raven Press.

Nair, M. P. N., and S. A. Schwartz. 1990. Immunoregulation of natural and lymphokine-activated killer cells by selenium. *Immunopharmacology* 19:177–83.

Nichols, P. J. 1991. The search for the etiologic agents and pathogenic mechanisms of byssinosis: In vivo studies. *Proc. Cotton Dust Res. Conf.* 15:307–20.

Payan, D. G., J. D. Levine, and E. J. Goetzl. 1984. Modulation of immunity and hypersensitivity by sensory neuropeptides. *J. Immunol.* 132:1601–4.

Pelus, L. M. 1982. Association between colony forming units-granulocyte macrophage expression of Ia-like (HLA-DR) antigen and control of granulocyte and macrophage production. *J. Clin. Invest.* 70:568–78.

Quie, P. G. 1982. Neutrophil dysfunction and recurrent infection. In *Advances in Host Defense Mechanisms*, Vol. 1, ed. J. I. Gallin and A. S. Fauci, pp. 163–85. New York: Raven Press.

Reiher, W. E., J. E. Blalock, and T. K. Brunck, et al. 1986. Sequence homology between acquired immunodeficiency syndrome virus envelope protein and interleukin-2. *Proc. Nat. Acad. Sci. U.S.A.* 83:9188–92.

Renzi, P. M., and L. C. Ginns. 1990a. Effect of lidocaine on natural killer activity—rapid inhibition of lysis. *Immunopharmacol. Immunotoxicol.* 12:417–37.

Renzi, P. M., and L. C. Ginns. 1990b. Natural killer activity is present in rat lung lavage and inhibited by lidocaine. *Immunopharmacol. Immunotoxicol.* 12:389–415.

Rosenberg, Z. F., and A. S. Fauci. 1990. Immunopathogenic mechanisms of HIV infection: Cytokine induction of HIV expression. *Immunol. Today* 11:176–80.

Rosenthal, G. J., and C. A. Snyder. 1985. Modulation of the immune response to *Listeria monocytogenes* by benzene inhalation. *Toxicol. Appl. Pharmacol.* 80:502–10.

Rozen, M. G., C. A. Snyder, R. E. Albert. 1984. Depressions in B- and T-lymphocyte mitogen-induced blastogenesis in mice exposed to low concentrations of benzene. *Toxicol. Lett.* 20:343–49.

Rylander, R. 1986. Lung diseases caused by organic dusts in the farm environment. *Am. J. Ind. Med.* 10:221–28.

Sharma, R. P., and M. G. Zeeman. 1980. Immunologic alterations by environmental chemicals: Relevance of studying mechanisms versus effects. *J. Immunopharmacol.* 2:285–307.

Siliciano, R. F., T. Lawton, C. Knall, et al. 1988. Analysis of host-virus interactions in AIDS with anti-*gp120* T cell clones: Effect of sequence variation and a mechanism for CD4+ cell depletion. *Cell* 54:561–75.

Smolik, R., K. Grzybek-Hryncewicz, A. Lange, and W. Zatonski. 1973. Serum complement level in workers exposed to benzene, toluene, and xylene. *Int. Arch. Arbeitsmed.* 31:243–47.

Snyder, R., S. L. Longacre, C. M. Witmer, and J. J. Kocsis. 1981. Biochemical toxicology of benzene. *Rev. Biochem. Toxicol.* 3:123–53.

Vallyathan, V., X. Shi., N. S. Dalal, et al. 1988. Generation of free radicals from freshly fractured silica dust. *Am. Rev. Respir. Dis.* 138:1213–19.

Vincent, P. C. 1986. Drug-induced aplastic anemia and agranulocytosis. Incidence and mechanisms. *Drugs* 31:52–63.

Von Essen, S., R. A. Robbins, A. B. Thompson, and S. I. Rennard. 1990. Organic dust toxic syndrome—an acute febrile reaction to organic dust exposure distinct from hypersensitivity pneumonitis. *J. Toxicol. Clin. Toxicol.* 28:389–420.

Waldman, T. A. 1988. Immunodeficiency diseases: Primary and acquired. In *Immunological Diseases*, 4th ed., ed. in M. Samter, D. W. Talmage, M. M. Frank, et al. pp. 411–66. Boston: Little, Brown.

Wierda, D., and R. D. Irons. 1982. Hydroquinone and catechol reduce the frequency of progenior B lymphocytes in mouse spleen and bone marrow. *Immunopharmacology* 4:41–54.

Yardley-Jones, A., D. Anderson, and P. Jenkinson. 1988. Effect of occupational exposure to benzene on phytohaemagglutinin (PHA) stimulated lymphocytes in man. *Br. J. Ind. Med.* 45:516–22.

Yokoyama, A., N. Yamashita, Y. Mizushima, and S. Yano. 1990. Inhibition of natural killer cell activity by oral administration of theophylline. *Chest* 98:924–27.

8

Intentional Modulation of the Immune Response: Immunopotentiation and Immunosuppression

A. INTRODUCTION

Immunomodulation is literally the regulation or modulation of the immune response. It refers to naturally occurring events influenced by a variety of endogenous controls in vivo but also refers to the purposeful modulation of the immune response by external agents or therapeutics. Since this latter situation is essentially immunotoxicology, i.e., modification of the immune response by xenobiotics, albeit for useful purposes, it is worth our attention to examine by what mechanisms such agents exert their effects. Much has been learned from the study of immune modulators that has led to an increased understanding of the basic immune response, and knowing how these agents work helps in the understanding of how immunotoxicants might function. Modulation could be in the form of enhancement of immune responses, immunosuppression, or even those mechanisms that lead to immunopathology or host tissue injury. This chapter focuses on the purposeful induction of the first two of these forms.

Purposeful enhancement of the immune response is accomplished either specifically (by giving antigen together with an adjuvant) or nonspecifically by therapeutic pharmacology (through the use of natural immunomodulators, e.g., cytokines or immunologic hormones: Hadden 1989). An immunologic adjuvant is any material that enhances any part of antigen-driven immune responses although it is not necessarily antigenic in itself. Adjuvants are used to enhance vaccine effectiveness, especially if the antigen concentration or potency is low. They also often sustain an immune response over a longer period of time and achieve higher levels of effector production. In addition to their uses to enhance vaccine or immunogen response in animals and humans, many of these substances have been used as adjunctive aids in reconstituting immunodeficiency diseases and in the immunotherapeutic treatment of a number of tumors. Experimentally, they are often used to induce immune responses to relatively inactive materials when only minute quantities of antigen are available.

Therapeutic immunosuppression has been used for prevention of rejection in transplantation surgery. Consequently, most of what is known refers to suppression of primary responses to antigens present in transplanted tissues. Although very effective in suppressing immune responses to foreign tissue antigens at the time of transplantation, such measures are not antigen specific, and, unfortunately, immune responses to potential pathogens harboring in the transplanted tissue, e.g., cytomegalovirus, are also inhibited. Even though most chemotherapeutic immunosuppressants are aimed at suppressing primary immune responses, some effort is also made to suppress existing immune responses in various types of autoimmune diseases (Herrmann and Bicker 1990). Even in these cases, it is difficult to suppress existing antigen-specific immune responses safely, and much of the ameliorative effects of treating such diseases is aimed at controlling mediator production or inflammatory cell elicitation. This latter form of immunosuppression is beyond the purposes of this chapter, which deals only with suppression of afferent responses.

B. IMMUNOLOGIC ENHANCEMENT

Adjuvants promote immunologic responses in at least three ways (Lise and Audibert 1989). One way is by affecting antigen localization. This can be accomplished by precipitating the antigen (e.g., with aluminum potassium sulfate) or by incorporating it in lipid emulsions or in liposomes. Antigen degradation is slowed down, sustained release is afforded, and phagocytosis is promoted. Adjuvants also promote antigen presentation by enhancing IFN-γ release, which increases the density of MHC class II molecule expression. And finally, macrophages and lymphocytes are nonspecifically activated to produce IL-1 and IL-2, respectively.

1. Prototypes

Experimental immunologists have long used two particular adjuvants for laboratory work, and one of them, alum, is the only one currently licensed for use in humans. It has long been known that various species of mycobacteria, including the BCG vaccine strain, have the ability to enhance both antibody and cell-mediated responses to antigens administered simultaneously with the mycobacteria. Indeed, this has long been the basis for incorporating mycobacteria in the classical Freund's complete adjuvant (FCA) before mixing with the desired antigen. Freund's adjuvant consists of an aqueous antigen phase emulsified into mineral oil with an emulsifying agent such as a lanolin derivative or Arlacel-A (mannide monooleate). In the complete adjuvant form, killed mycobacteria (either *M. butyricum* or the bovine Ravenel strain of *M. tuberculosis*) are added (0.5 mg/ml). Not only do these materials activate macrophages and mononuclear cells, but they also result in secondary activation of T lymphocytes and may even stimulate NK cells. Moreover, phagocytized, living BCG are stimulated to synthesize heat shock or stress proteins, and these molecules are highly conserved targets of vertebrate humoral and cellular immune effectors (Young 1991). But Freund's adjuvant has a number of undesirable properties. Not only does the presence of killed mycobacteria induce tuberculin hypersensitivity and DTH-dependent granuloma formation, but mineral oil is undegradable and, together with the mycobacteria, leads to sterile abscess formation. It is highly inflammatory at the site of deposition as well as in organs such as the lung, where small droplets are carried by the circulation. In some species, e.g., the rat, its use leads to an arthritic disease. For these reasons, it has never been approved for human use. In addition, the complete form is antigenic in itself, which may confuse responses and may even compete strongly with weak antigens present to which the responses are desired. Many of these problems can be circumvented by using mycobacterial derivatives or synthetic analogs of the active components together with metabolizable vegetable oils or other noninflammatory lipids.

The other prototype in experimental immunology as well as in vaccines for human use is alum. Originally, alum was defined as aluminum potassium sulfate, but contemporary use has extended the term to include aluminum hydroxide. Protein solutions are precipitated with equal volumes of 10% alum at pH 6.5. In this particulate form in tissue, mild inflammation attracts inflammatory cells, phagocytosis is enhanced, and slow, sustained antigen release is promoted. Mild granulomata are produced, which may persist for weeks.

Alum is used primarily to enhance antibody production, and there is some concern that IgE responses may be enhanced as well. Although FCA enhances antibody production, it also promotes cell-mediated immune responses. Possibly these preferences may be related to the induction of different subsets of CD4$^+$ T_h-cell populations, which are known to produce distinctly different cytokines and thereby augment different immune response types (Grun and Maurer 1989). T_h2 cells seem predominantly induced by alum, and these cells preferentially mediate IL-4, IL-5, and IL-6 production, hapten-carrier helper activity, and IgG_1 and IgE augmentation. Conversely, T_h1 cells, preferentially induced by FCA, induce more IL-2 and IFN-γ, augment IgG_{2a} production, and mediate DTH reactions through macrophage activation (Bottomly 1989).

2. Mineral Compounds

Mineral oil and alum are both in this class, and, except for the toxicity of the former limiting its human use, both have acceptable uses in immunology. Aluminum hydroxide, which forms more of a gel than a precipitate, and calcium phosphate have also received a fair amount of use in experimental studies. Other minerals known to influence immune responses are coal mine dust, certain mineral crystalline forms of asbestos fibers, and beryllium salts, and although these minerals under certain circumstances can up-regulate immune effectors, and the latter have been used as an adjuvant, these materials are usually thought of as immunotoxicants and are discussed in Chapter 11.

3. Bacterial Stimulants

Microbial products have long been known to possess immunomodulating activities (Burrell 1988). For Gram-positive bacteria, cell walls are largely composed of peptidoglycans, and these are responsible for much of their immunostimulating activity. Peptidoglycans consist of multiple layers of linear polymers of N-acetylglucosamine and N-acetylmuramic acid held together by peptide bridges cross-linked with muramic acid. Another important structural component of Gram-positive bacteria is the teichoic acids, polymers of either ribitol phosphate or glycerol phosphate held together through diester linkages. Some of these polymers are linked to the peptidoglycan muramic acid, whereas others, known as lipoteichoic acid, are linked to the glycolipid portion of the cytoplasmic membranes.

Gram-negative bacteria possess only a limited amount of peptidoglycan and no teichoic acids. Instead, their outer cell membranes are lipid bilayers, the outermost of which are rich in lipopolysaccharides. This structural component consists of outer oligosaccharide chains responsible for antigenic specificity of individual species, an inner, unique core polysaccharide that is common to almost all Gram-negative bacteria, and a terminal lipid A structure, which contains most of the toxic and immunomodulating properties of Gram-negative bacteria. Lipid A is essentially a phosphorylated D-glucosamine disaccharide to which are attached various ester- and amine-linked fatty acids.

$$
\begin{array}{c}
\text{FA} \\
| \\
\text{FA - Gl c N -}\textcircled{P}\!:\!\textcircled{P}\text{-O - NH}_2\text{Eth} \\
| \\
\textcircled{P}\text{- O --- Gl c N - FA} \\
| \\
\text{FA}
\end{array}
$$

LIPID A

These products together with other immunomodulatory microbial substances are presented in Table 8–1. Although many of these substances are too toxic for human administration, knowledge of their structures and mode of actions has facilitated the identification of the active fragments and the separation of these from the toxic principles.

4. Muramyl Dipeptides

The search for a nontoxic immunostimulating subcellular component from myco-bacteria led to the identification of a tripeptide-monosaccharide from the peptido-glycan cell walls. The smallest remnant of mycobacterial cell walls retaining

TABLE 8–1.   **Microbial Products with Immunostimulating Activity**

Substance	Source	Activity
Lipopolysaccharide	All Gram-negative bacteria	Extremely varied; affects all systems
Peptidoglycans	All Gram-positive bacteria; present in lesser amounts in Gram-negative	Various
Lipoteichoic acid	Gram-positive bacteria	Various
Protein exotoxin	*Bordetella pertussis* (whooping cough bacillus)	Alters balance of T_h cells
Heat-stable enterotoxin	*Escherichia coli*	Modulates IgM–IgG
Toxic shock syndrome toxin (TSST-1)	Staphylococci	T-cell mitogen
		Suppresses induced Ig secretion of B cells
		Stimulates macrophages
Pyrogenic exotoxins	Streptococci	Similar to TSST-1

adjuvant activity is N-acetylmuramyl-L-alanyl-D-isoglutamine, better known as muramyl dipeptide (MDP).

MURAMYL DIPEPTIDE

Using knowledge of the structure of these peptidoglycans, various synthetic glyco-peptides have been prepared and studied for adjuvant effects. Some of the most active synthetic analogs have a molecular weight of only 500 but are powerful adjuvants, even when administered by the oral route. Although most effects are on the macrophages, MDPs are mitogenic for murine but not human B lymphocytes. They induce release of immunoglobulins from murine cells and induce carrier-specific T_h cells (Bahr and Chedid 1986). Another interesting property of MDPs is their ability to modify the specificity of an antigen with which it may be conjugated. The response to that antigen may be modified depending on what forms the MDP and antigen are in (i.e., whether separate or conjugated) for initial priming (Bahr and Chedid 1986). Hydrophilic MDP, when mixed with antigen, induces excellent immunoglobulin responses, whereas incorporation into oil or liposomes promotes DTH induction. When given in high doses prior to antigen, MDP may even exert suppressive effects (LeClerc et al. 1979). Aqueous solutions of MDP may be cleared too rapidly from the circulation for sustained effect, but its activity may be substantially enhanced by administration with synergistic partners, e.g., trehalose dimycolate or IFN-γ, incorporation into liposomes, or modification of the peptide side chain in such a way as to retard degradation.

5. Nontoxic Analogs of Bacterial Lipopolysaccharide

Purified lipopolysaccharide (LPS) prepared from bacterial endotoxin is an extremely versatile immunomodulatory substance but in its native form is also highly
toxic (Burrell 1990). Lipopolysaccharide is the prototypical macrophage activator
and IL-1 stimulator. Indeed, fever caused by the pyrogenic effects of IL-1 is regarded as the hallmark of the presence of LPS. Extremely small doses of LPS also
affect circulating leukocytes and platelets in a variety of ways, activates both complement pathways in the absence of antibodies, interacts with a variety of acute-
phase proteins, enhances histamine sensitivity, induces hypotensive changes,
increases capillary permeability, and affects the coagulation systems. Macrophages/
monocytes, endothelial cells, and granulocytes are especially sensitive to LPS.
Inflammatory effects include attachment of inflammatory cells to endothelium,
increased production of lysosomal proteolytic enzymes, increased prostaglandin
and leukotriene production, and stimulation of toxic hydroxyl radicals. Immunomodulation is accomplished through its actions as a nonspecific B-cell mitogen,
as a specific lymphocyte activator by being a carrier for other antigens, as a
regulator of the expression of class II MHC antigen expression on the surfaces
of antigen-presenting cells, and possibly as a specific T_s activator.

Since much (but not all) of the inflammatory and immunomodulating activities of LPS resides in the lipid A portion of the molecule, great effort has been
directed toward either modifying native lipid A or constructing synthetic analogs.
Hydrolyzing native LPS to a monophosphoryl derivative has proven effective in
eliminating much of the toxicity, yet retaining the immunostimulating properties
(Ribi 1984). Toxicity is largely determined by the presence of the disaccharide
and the two phosphates at the 1' and 4' positions. Combining this fact with
knowledge concerning the nature of additional determinants of toxicity on the
lipid A moiety, e.g., the number of fatty acid acyl groups, the number of carbons
in the fatty acid chains, and the nature of the sugar in the backbone, has allowed
other modifications to be made in the native molecule (Takayama et al. 1984).

Great progress has been made in preparing synthetic analogs of lipid A (Kotani
et al. 1984, 1985; Takada et al. 1985). Analogs that have two amide and two ester
groups bound to glucosamine disaccharide mono- or diphosphates possess most
of the activities, with one diphosphate derivative being almost as lethal as unmodified lipid A. Certain analogs in particular (compound 506, for example)
were found to be almost as bioactive or even more so than a wild-type reference
lipid A (Kotani et al. 1985). Much current screening of these kinds of analogs is
being carried out in many laboratories to find ones that possess the least toxicity
yet retain desirable immunomodulating properties.

6. Other Synthetic and Natural Peptides

A variety of peptides newly synthesized or derived from natural products have
been examined for immunostimulating properties (St. Georgiev 1990). Immunostimulating and immunosuppressive peptides have been derived from diverse
sources: bacterial cell wall peptidoglycans, microbial metabolites, serum proteins, and milk proteins as well as synthetic analogs.

Bestatin is an orally effective peptide originally extracted from *Streptomyces*.
It stimulates IL-1 production by macrophages and IL-2 production from mitogen-

stimulated lymphocytes by suppressing the activity of membrane-associated peptidases (Umezewa and Ishizuka 1985). It has also been used to increase the reduced T-cell levels in tumor patients.

Lipopeptides are molecules consisting of a fatty acid covalently bound to a peptide (St. Georgiev 1990). Such molecules combine features found in immuno-stimulating peptides and liposomes, the lipid tail being considered by many contemporary vaccine biologists as being very important in antigen delivery. A synthetic analog of a bacterial lipoprotein, tripalmitoyl pentapeptide, was mitogenic and capable of stimulating polyclonal antibody production if given at the time of antigen administration (Lex et al. 1986).

A number of naturally occurring hormones have also been investigated, and their mechanisms of action are of interest since they shed light on the very nature of the normal immune response. A number of thymic peptides (e.g., thymopoietin, thymulin, and thymosin) have been isolated, and some synthetic derivatives (e.g., thymopentine) have been produced from their study. Thymosin is the best studied and is actually a mixture of several similar peptides important in T-cell maturation and differentiation. Splenin (splenopentin, the synthetic analog) is a peptide isolated from normal spleens that is important in generating and restoring B-cell function. It is chemically and functionally very similar to thymopoietin, although the immunomodulatory roles of the two are quite different. Bursin is a B-cell-differentiating hormone isolated from avian bursa of Fabricius, the site of origin of B stem cells in avian species.

Tuftsin represents a unique approach to immunostimulating peptides in that it is a four-amino-acid sequence derived from the constant region of human IgG chains. It stimulates various macrophage and neutrophil functions, including phagocytosis, antigen processing, and tumoricidal activity (Najjar 1978). In addition to being present within the IgG heavy chain, it is also produced separately in the spleen, where it is released from cytophilic γ-globulins by an endocarboxypeptidase. This may explain why people who have been splenectomized are prone to developing certain types of overwhelming infections. It is also lacking in a rare phagocyte dysfunction syndrome and is depressed in AIDS (Corazza et al. 1991).

7. Liposomes

Liposomes are artificially prepared lipid mixtures that form small concentric spheres consisting of phospholipid bilayers separated by aqueous compartments (Fig. 8–1). These spheres are biodegradable and in themselves nonimmunogenic; however, they are good adjuvants when antigen is trapped in the aqueous phase and have been used with a wide variety of antigens (Gregoriadis 1990). Although there are many formulations for lipid composition and lipid : antigen ratios, as well as many methods of preparation, a mixture of lecithin, cholesterol, and stearylamine in a 7 : 2 : 1 ratio may serve as an example and one that has been used to obtain better antibody responses to diphtheria toxoid (Allison and Gregoriadis 1974). Certainly, antigen incorporated into liposomes has an extended survival time (although the stability of some liposome mixtures is a problem), but the nature of the lipid surface is undoubtedly an important factor in antigen acquisition by lipid bilayer membranes of immunologic cells. This would facilitate antigen uptake and presentation by macrophages. No adjuvant activity is seen if empty lipid particles and antigen untrapped in the liposomes are injected separately, thus stressing the importance of the physical association. Both cellular and humoral forms of immunity are stimulated. Liposome adjuvants can be given orally

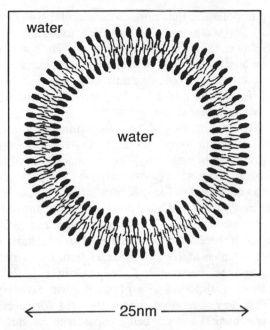

water

water

← —————— 25nm —————— →

FIGURE 8-1.   Diagrammatic cross-sectional view of a liposome. Note the concentric orientation of the phospholipid bilayer surrounding the aqueous phase of solute.

to stimulate mucosal immunity (Michalek et al. 1989). Current investigations combine other adjuvants, e.g., MDP or lipid A into the liposome–antigen combinations.

8. Synthetic Polymers

Nonionic, hydrophobic polymer surfactants have been developed to incorporate antigen into an emulsion, thereby concentrating it in such a fashion that the antigen not only binds to the polymer particle surfaces but also adheres to cell membranes (Hunter, Strickland, and Kezdy 1981). Synthesis of these polymers must carefully take into consideration the relative balance of hydrophilic polyoxyethylene and lipophilic polyoxypropylene, since certain formulations lead to adjuvanticity and others induce granulomatous inflammation (Hunter and Bennett 1984). Exploration of these polymers administered with MDP or nontoxic lipid A appears to be an area of productive investigation.

Synthetic ionic polymers have also been investigated, particularly double-stranded polynucleotides consisting of one strand each of polyadenylate and polyuridylate, for example. Such a material stimulates helper T cells, DTH, and cell-mediated cytotoxicity. It may also affect B cells, most likely by IL-6 induction by fibroblasts (Pignol et al. 1991), and enhance antibody production. Other polynucleotides are especially effective in promoting IFN-γ production.

A somewhat different use of polymers is being made by allergists in an attempt to induce antigen-specific desensitization in patients suffering allergic rhinitis to particular inhalants. The rationale of such therapy is to induce antigen-specific IgG to competitively inhibit IgE reactions with antigen and at the same time to induce IgE suppressor cells. Currently, patients undergoing conventional desensitization must take weekly injections for several months prior to the allergen season before benefits are realized. Precipitation of the allergen extracts with polyethylene glycol results in a preparation called *allergoids* (Lee and Sehon

1978). These result in polymers that raise the molecular weight of a typical antigen from 30,000 to 1,000,000 or more. Use of these materials reduces the number of outpatient visits and enhances IgG responsiveness. For some reason, this modification reduces the allergenicity of the products many hundredfold while maintaining the ability to induce IgG blocking antibody. Immunotoxicologists should note how chemical processing might similarly alter immunologic properties of other industrial or environmental chemicals.

Somewhere between polymers and true liposomes is a different approach known as immunostimulating complexes or ISCOMs. In this system, many copies of antigen are presented in a polymer-like manner attached as multimers to a matrix composed of a triterpenoid (short polymers of an isoprene-based molecule) combined with cholesterol to form 40–nm cage-like particles (Morein 1990). These act as a built-in adjuvant and have no components antigenic in themselves, unlike Freund's complete adjuvant. The antigens placed in ISCOMs are rapidly transported from the injection site to the draining lymphatic organ. ISCOM-borne antigens induce higher antibody responses than the same amount of antigen in micelle form and are able to elicit T_c-cell responses. In this transport form, aqueous-phase antigen is dispersed in a physical form favoring absorption by cell membranes. They have been experimentally used for several viral antigens (particles as well as subunits) and are being considered for human use.

9. Miscellaneous Synthetic Immunostimulating Drugs

Levamisole (phenylimidazolethiazole)

LEVAMISOLE

has been used extensively as an antiparasitic drug in veterinary medicine but incidentally has been found to possess peculiar immunopotentiating activities. It acts on a wide variety of cells, but its main effect is on monocyte chemotaxis and other activation functions. Dose and timing with respect to antigen administration appear to be critical because immunosuppressive effects may occur as well. In humans, there is little effect on humoral antibody production, but cellular functions are enhanced in those with impaired immune functions, not in those with intact systems. Thus, it was of most value for restorative purposes, but the inconsistency of its results and the number of undesirable side effects have limited its clinical usefulness (Bardana 1985; Fudenberg and Whitten 1984).

Methisoprinol or ISO (Inosiplex or Isoprinosine) is the *p*-acetamidobenzoic acid salt of N,N-dimethylamino-2–propanol:inosine complex in a 3:3: molar ratio.

METHISOPRINOL (ISO)

It is mainly used in viral diseases because it inhibits replication of a variety of DNA and RNA viruses, and it also stimulates T- and NK-cell functions, particularly in patients with low levels before treatment. The major effect of this compound may be related to its ability to stimulate T-cell proliferation in response to viral antigens (perhaps by enhancing IL-2 production). It also prevents depression of cellular immunity that often accompanies certain viral infections.

10. Host Mediators

As knowledge concerning the regulatory and enhancement roles of immunologic cytokines grows, more attention has been given to using these agents as immunostimulants, particularly in situations of restoring immune competence in genetic or acquired immunodeficiency syndromes (Hadden 1989). Now that many of these cytokines are available as recombinant products, interest in therapeutic use will certainly increase. Interferon, of course, has received the most use, and IFN-α has been and is being used in clinical trials for cancer immunotherapy (Goldstein and Laszlo 1989). Certain tumors, e.g., hairy cell and chronic myeloid leukemias, mycosis fungoides, venereal papillomas, and certain types of lymphoma, respond well; however, other types respond only moderately (melanoma and renal cancer) or not at all (breast, lung, and colon cancers). Attention is being turned to its use as a possible synergistic partner to other modalities.

Interleukin 1 and IL-2 may function as enhancing agents if given with antigen. Indeed, certain adjuvants owe part of their effectiveness to induction of these same mediators. Interleukin 1 augments proliferating T lymphocytes when in the presence of mitogen and enhances secondary antibody production in primed animals. Interleukin 2 has received particular interest because of its known ability to support the growth and proliferation of antigen-activated T_h cells, which, together with other cytokines, influence B-cell function. Not only has IL-2 been used to enhance animal immunizations, it also has been considered in AIDS therapy and in the production of LAK cells (lymphokine-activated killer cells) from NK cells. One of the drawbacks of IL-2 administration is the serious amount of pulmonary edema that may be induced (Rosenberg et al. 1985).

One of the most intriguing natural product immunostimulants is transfer factor. Originally prepared as aqueous dialyzable extracts from lysed human leukocytes, this material was shown to be able to passively transfer antigen-specific delayed-type skin sensitivity and lymphokine production to the same antigen to which the donor was sensitive (Fudenberg et al. 1980). The material has been characterized as at least two nucleopeptides with a molecular weight of only 2,000–2,500 containing RNA but not DNA. Mechanistically, transfer factor may recruit antigen-specific lymphocytes or derepress specific stem cells. Preparations of the substance have received extensive clinical application in a wide variety of disorders. Some examples have been seen in restoring immune competence in individuals with Wiskott–Aldrich immunodeficiency, certain progressive forms of infectious disease, e.g., recurrent shingles, or systemic candidiasis, and used together with other therapies in tuberculosis and certain of the systemic mycoses among many other types of disease (Fudenberg 1985).

C. IMMUNOSUPPRESSION

The immune response is under several forms of regulation or natural suppression: antigen-specific tolerance, antibody-dependent regulation, suppressor–contrasuppressor circuits, and regulation by the endocrine and nervous systems.

1. Immunologic Tolerance

The magnitude of an immune response is controlled by characteristics associated with the antigen, i.e., the dose, physical state, frequency and timing of contact, etc. In most cases, optimal presentation of antigen leads to an immune response, but there are a number of situations in which presentation in certain manners leads to specific tolerance, i.e., failure of an immune response to be generated to that particular antigen. There are several possibilities for tolerance induction. Presentation of antigen to prenatal or neonatal animals may lead to abortion of an antigen-specific clone because of presentation of antigen to immature B- or T-cell clones. Repeated antigenic challenge (particularly with T-independent antigens) may lead to exhaustion of specific B-cell clones. If the antigen-presentation step is bypassed and antigen binds directly to B cells without either processing or T-cell help, tolerance may occur. Similarly, if high concentrations of T-independent antigens are administered or given in such a physical form that B-cell receptors cannot be cross-linked, high-dose tolerance may occur. Very high doses of antigen may block surface receptors of B cells to such an extent that antibody secretion may be inhibited. It is also possible that individual T-cell subsets may be deleted, causing the loss of that particular function (e.g., cytotoxicity or helper activity). Finally, selective loss of T_h cells or selective enrichment of T_s cells may lead to functional tolerance in either B cells or other T-cell subsets. Although the existence of a definable T_s-cell population with antigen-specific suppressor determinants has been questioned, the accumulation of data leans toward establishing their bona fide existence (Sercarz and Krzych 1991).

2. Natural Means of Immunosuppression

Aside from matters of antigen-specific tolerance induction, the body also has a number of ways of down-regulating the immune response once suitable effectors have been produced. For example, the mere presence of circulating antibody functions as a feedback inhibitor, possibly because antibody being produced competes with lymphocyte antigen receptors for antigen. Also, if circulating antibody adheres to the Fc receptors of B cells and then becomes cross-linked by antigen with antibody being produced by that same cell, tolerance occurs. The production of circulating immune complexes may further facilitate immune response to a limited extent by enhancing antigen adherence to presentation cells and beyond this may inhibit further responses in a manner similar to that described for excess antibody. The isotype of the antibody produced is also quite important: IgM is an enhancing type of antibody, whereas IgG acts as a suppressant. This is probably the reason for the effectiveness of RhoGam, a preparation of human IgG specific for the Rh_o erythrocyte antigen that is effective in suppressing an anti-Rh response of an Rh-negative mother giving birth to an Rh + baby.

One of the most intriguing and heuristic concepts in immunology is the matter of idiotypes and their role in regulating immune responses. Any given antibody's hypervariable region is distinctive not only in terms of antigen recognition, it is also distinctive enough to give that particular antibody molecule its own antigenic individuality. Lymphocytes are capable of recognizing the combining site of antibodies as well as their receptors on other lymphocytes as antigens. The antigenic region of the particular hypervariable region is known as an idiotype, and the individual determinants are known as idiotopes. Ordinary antiglobulin sera are produced in a species foreign to the source of that globulin and as such react with a broad range of globulins from that source. Conversely, antiidiotype reactive sera are produced within an individual or if a species is immunized exclusively with an isolated myeloma protein that (having originated from a single lymphocyte clone) is all of one specificity. Although there are many interesting ramifications of the idiotype phenomenon, this discussion is confined to that of antiidiotype down-regulating cells that produce antibodies with this idiotypic specificity. Antiidiotype antibody can accomplish this by (1) cross-linking with B-cell antigen receptors (i.e., the antibodies being produced by that clone). A similar mechanism could also account for T-cell inhibition if the antiidiotype is specific for the variable region of the T-cell antigen receptor (TCR).

Immunologic dogma has long been concerned with the existence of a subpopulation of T cells, the T_s cells, which, when activated, somehow influence immunologic suppression in normal cells. Although there is agreement on the concept of cell-mediated immunosuppression, there is considerable debate on whether the effect is mediated by a distinct population of cells. The molecular nature of the T-cell suppressor factor is speculative, but among those accorded high consideration is a bipartite molecule with an antigen-recognizing chain and another chain with homology similar to a region of a MHC II molecule. If both of these chains react with appropriate receptors on a lymphocyte, suppression results. The production of down-regulating messengers like PGE_2 or transforming growth factor β by lymphocytes or lymphocyte-activated macrophages may be another method. These cells may operate in a circuit whereby antigen-presenting cells stimulate T_s cells under certain conditions to release a factor that activates $CD8^+$ cells. These in turn release suppressor factors that influence effector cell functions.

The debate is further complicated by the postulation that there is yet another distinct population of T cells of contrasuppressor cells (T_{cs}), distinct from T_h cells, that in turn regulates the suppressor cell population. The activation of contrasuppressor cells could then be envisioned to either compete with the T_s cells or control their production of suppressor factors.

The development of immunopharmacology has contributed much to our knowledge of additional influences on immune response controls. External environmental factors, e.g., diet, stress, exercise, even psychological events, are being increasingly recognized as important to a functional immune system. The presence of lymphocyte receptors for endorphins, neuropeptides, catecholamines, corticosteroids, and insulin, among others, exemplifies the myriad possibilities of control by these systems formerly not even considered relevant and often ignored in contemporary cellular immunology. It is known that the immune system even has its "own" hormones in the form of peptides released by the thymus and spleen that affect maturation and differentiation of lymphocytes and may play an important role in their traffic as well. Innervation of lymphoid tissue, vascular smooth muscle, and secretory glands attests to further control of these effector organs other than by cytokines. The nervous system also receives information from the immune system by many afferent autonomic pathways as well as directly to the hypothalamus by important cytokines such as IL-1. Little evidence is available that the central nervous and endocrine systems influence immune responsiveness at the antigen-specific level, but they certainly play a role in influencing the intensity and modality of the various types of responses.

It is important to remember that there are different modes of immune response (antibody, cytotoxic cells, delayed-type hypersensitivity, whether T or B dependent, etc.). These are all subject to special, distinctive controls. The type of antigen-presenting cell depends on anatomic site, and these may be selectively activated depending on the physical and chemical type of antigen, the vehicle and route of its administration, etc. It is also important to realize that individual immunoglobulin responses may be subject to different controls. The regulation of an IgE response is not necessarily the same as that for IgG; in fact, there is considerable information that IgE regulation is highly specialized and distinct. Thus, in assessing the mechanism of action of an immunosuppressive xenobiotic, it would be prudent to keep in mind the great redundancy and variation in types of immune responsiveness, each subject to its own controls.

3. Therapeutic Immunosuppression

Because of the complexity of the immune response, its redundancy, and the number of individual immune response pathways, it is unrealistic to expect that a single drug or agent is going to be totally immunosuppressive for all parameters. If this were true, immunotoxicology would be a daily fact of life resulting from continual contact with numerous xenobiotics. Particular agents are more effective in certain pathways and then perhaps only at definite stages of a target cell population's growth cycle. Uncommitted lymphocytes are much more vulnerable to physical and chemical toxicity then are committed clones or memory cells. This is partly why effective immunosuppression must be carried out at or near the time of initial antigen presentation. Immunosuppressive agents often show little or no activity in presensitized humans or animals but are more effective when introduced at the induction stage of the initial response, i.e., between presentation and effector production during the time when cells are in their maximum proliferative phase. Ablation of immunologic memory is only possible in a practical sense by whole-body irradiation followed by restoration of immune competence with lymphoid cells, a process easily carried out in mice but dangerous and usually impractical in humans. Once again, it is important to distinguish anti-inflammatory or antieffector manifestations of certain agents, (e.g., corticosteroids) from true inhibition of afferent pathways.

Since immunosuppressive agents (including steroids) have widespread functional effects on the immune system, it is not surprising that drawbacks exist in their clinical use. These consist of the induction of iatrogenic (physician-induced) infections and tumors. Subjects on long-term immunosuppressive therapy have a hundredfold greater risk for development of tumors. In studies of transplant patients, increased incidence of carcinomas of the skin and lymphomas of the central nervous system are noticed (Penn 1985).

Although a discussion about the clinical management of transplant patients in anticipating, preventing, and treating rejection crises is beyond the scope of this discussion, such matters are critical adjunctive considerations to be used with immunosuppressive chemotherapy, and the reader is referred to Woodley et al. (1990) for an illuminating discussion. The ideal of achieving immune tolerance to grafts without the need of long-term immunosuppressant therapy is still far from reality, but used together with careful clinical pre- and postoperative management and the monitoring of impending rejection crises, these agents all have a place in clinical immunosuppression. Although various combinations of these agents are used in most individual cases, the following outline discusses only the immunosuppressive properties of them individually.

Corticosteroids

It should be remembered that steroids are really derivatives or synthetic analogs of natural materials, and native substances exert a great deal of influence over the immune response. Many of the immunosuppressive effects of stress can be traced to their action. The suppressive effectiveness of corticosteroids depends on the species in which they are used. The agents are lytic for rat, mouse, and rabbit lymphocytes, yet those from humans, monkeys, and guinea pigs are resistant. Even in the lytic-sensitive species, it is the immature precursor cells that are most affected. Immediately after human administration of steroids there may be an immediate decline in circulating lymphocytes as well as other leukocytes within 4 hr, but this is short-lived and by 24 hr the cells have regained their original numbers. This phenomenon involving T cells (particularly of the T_h subset) more than B cells is not caused by lysis but rather by temporary sequestration (possibly in the bone marrow for lymphocytes, vascular endothelium for neutrophils), followed by later redistribution (Cupps and Fauci 1982).

When steroids are effective in humans, the most likely mechanisms have to do with inhibiting cytokine production, inflammatory cell attraction, and phagocytic functions. Interleukin 1 and IL-6 production are directly reduced, as is that of IL-2 as an indirect consequence. Their effects on inflammatory cells are numerous. Toxic radicals and lysozyme release are inhibited, lysosomal membranes are stabilized, thus slowing release of proteolytic enzymes, intracellular cAMP metabolism is modulated, and chemotactic responses are delayed (Fauci 1979). Because of inhibition of phospholipase A_2 by steroid-induced lipomodulin (Hirata 1981), production of arachidonic acid inflammatory mediators is undoubtedly affected. Corticosteroid therapy affects cell-mediated responses by inhibiting macrophage activation, migration, and adherence, release of lymphokines, lymphocyte–macrophage interactions, and elicitation of skin tests. As a result, corticosteroids are popular for reducing inflammation of both immunoglobulin- and cell-mediated forms of immune injury. The essence of immunosuppression by steroids is thus with the effector arms of the immune response.

Steroids are widely used in treating diseases of immune injury, e.g., hypersensitivity pneumonitis, autoimmune disease, and contact dermatitis, to name a few. They also are employed widely in various combinations with other modalities in blocking transplantation rejection (Woodley et al. 1990). However, this type of therapy, especially if given for long terms, is not to be undertaken lightly in that significant toxicity and morbidity may result. Because macrophage and other phagocytic functions may be inhibited and other inflammatory functions drastically reduced, the body becomes more susceptible to certain types of opportunistic infections. Also, quiescent endogenous infections, e.g., tuberculosis, may become reactivated to progressive disease, and tumor incidence may increase in populations treated in such a manner.

Azathioprine
Azathioprine is the nitroimidazolyl derivative of 6–mercaptopurine, a purine analog that inhibits purine ring synthesis and nucleotide conversions after metabolism, resulting in an inhibition of lymphocyte proliferation.

6-Mercaptopurine (thiol form)   Azathiopurine

It was the immunosuppressive drug of choice from the mid-1960s through the 1970s and is a potent suppressor of cell-mediated immunity without accompanying leukopenia. Azathioprine fell into disfavor once cyclosporine became available but is now under renewed interest in those frequent instances of serious side effects from the latter drug. Although the drug works best if administered at or shortly after primary immunization, it also has been used to treat various autoimmune diseases, permitting the reduced use of corticosteroids. It can be given intravenously as well as orally and is rapidly absorbed from the gut. As with any such cytotoxic drug, long-term use is associated with increased incidences of squamous cell carcinomas and histiocytic lymphomas. Short-term toxicities to other organs are generally reversible (Herrmann and Bicker 1990).

Methotrexate
Methotrexate, an aminomethyl derivative of aminopterin, functions as a folic acid competitor by binding to dihydrofolate reductase.

O   COOH
‖ |
HO-C-(CH₂)₂-CH-NH-C ⟨benzene ring⟩ — N-CH₂ ⟨pteridine ring system⟩
                ‖ |
                O   CH₃

METHOTREXATE

By inhibiting this enzyme, methotrexate depresses purine nucleotide and thymidylate synthesis and is thus a cytotoxic inhibitor of nucleic acid synthesis. Under proper management, patient toxicity is low (Herrmann and Bicker 1990). Although primarily used in tumor chemotherapy, the drug has also had limited use in the treatment of psoriasis and certain autoimmune diseases and to prevent graft-versus-host reactions in bone marrow transplantations.

Cyclophosphamide

Cyclophosphamide is an alkylating agent that is capable of cross-linking DNA strands, leading to direct cytotoxicity during mitosis, but it is active only after being metabolized in the liver.

CYCLOPHOSPHAMIDE

It has been widely used to treat autoimmune disease and is one of the few drugs capable of inhibiting secondary immune responses. Autoantibody titer reductions are a reflection of the observation that the drug has longer-lasting effects against B cells, because of their slower recovery, than T cells (Stevenson and Fauci 1980). Except for high doses used with irradiation prior to bone marrow transplantation, its use in organ transplantation is limited.

Cyclosporin

The favorite immunosuppressive drug of the 1980s was cyclosporin, a cyclic peptide consisting of eleven amino acids. Its popularity was well earned because of the great improvement in facilitating transplant survival, particularly

CYCLOSPORIN A

in cardiac transplantation (Woodley et al. 1990). Although it is essentially an antibiotic in that it is a metabolic by-product of a fungus, it can now be synthesized in the laboratory. Until the advent of cyclosporin, the prototypical immunosuppressants were azathioprine and corticosteroids, which functioned by inhibiting cell division and cytokine production, respectively, and were effective on all elements of the immune system. Although cyclosporin is much more selective in its action, its clinical use is far more complicated because of the wide variety of organ toxicities it incites (Kahan 1989). It first binds to a protein with peptidyl-prolyl *cis–trans* isomerase activity and then becomes converted by isoenzymes of the P-450 group into a more polar and more effective form. Coadministration of drugs that affect these important enzymes will in turn lead to alterations in cyclosporin metabolism with possible attendant changes in effectiveness and harmful side effects. Immunotoxicologists should carefully note this feature with respect to other xenobiotics.

As with many immunosuppressants, most information on the mode of action of cyclosporin emanates from in vitro data that may not necessarily be a reflection of in vivo activity. Cyclosporin reversibly inhibits IL-2, IFN-γ, and other lymphokine production from T_h cells by inhibiting mRNA translation of certain genes (Hess, Tutschka, and Santas 1982; Kronke et al. 1984). Although the cells can be primed by antigen, they cannot complete their activation cascade of effector cells. This specificity is most likely afforded by its known activation of a specific binding protein, cyclophilin (Harding, Handschumacher, and Speicher 1986) as opposed to a more general pinocytotic means of cell access. Cyclophilin probably is very important in signal transduction of T-cell activation and proliferation. Cyclosporin has no effect on events transpiring after gene activation, nor does it have any effect on increasing T_s-cell activity. With these observations in mind, it is readily apparent how subsequent immunologic events, e.g., T-cell recruitment, activation of T-cytotoxic cells, and B-cell responses are going to decrease. The drug has no direct effect on phagocytic and other secondary cells, but any of their functions stimulated by lymphokines or direct lymphocyte-macrophage interaction could be depressed.

With such channeled inhibition of T-helper/inducer cell lymphokine production while sparing any effect on T_s cells, cyclosporin seems a drug too good to be true. It is indeed, in that the drug is accompanied by common and severe side effects, particularly nephrotoxicity. For these reasons, cyclosporin is now combined in several ways with other immunosuppressant drugs to reduce these hazards without compromising effective immunosuppression. Another disadvantage of the drug is that its administration must be continued, since its effects are not antigen specific. Cessation of use often leads to severe, irreversible graft rejection. Beneficial side effects are reduced incidence of bacterial and fungal (but not viral; see Suranyi and Hall 1990) infections accompanying transplantation therapy, no effect on NK-cell activity, and, when it is used by itself, no increase in tumor incidence.

Cyclosporin has also been widely used in treating a number of autoimmune diseases. Often immunosuppressive therapy fails because either profound sensitization has already occurred or, as in the case of type 1 diabetes, so little of the target organ, the pancreatic β cells, remains. However, use of cyclosporin in newly diagnosed diabetics is encouraging, with many properly chosen patients remaining in insulin-free remission for 6 months to a year (Wilson and Eisenbarth 1990). Under the hypothesis that agents can halt autoimmune destruction, but only in patients with adequate β-cell mass, current work is aimed at finding prediabetic markers, identifying individuals among these at high risk for developing overt disease, and aiming immunosuppressive therapy at them. Similarly, although cyclosporin treatment of renal transplant patients certainly facilitates graph acceptance, it is not necessarily effective in inhibiting the glomerulonephritic process that destroyed the original kidneys from subsequently damaging the transplant by the same method (Vincenti et al. 1989).

FK-506

Too new to have its own name, FK-506 is another antibiotic (i.e., a fungal metabolic by-product) that is currently undergoing widespread clinical application. Because of the known IL-2–suppressive effects of cyclosporin, a broad screening program of other microbial fermented broths was undertaken to look for similar activity; it revealed a fungus from which the subsequent active material was isolated (Kino et al. 1987).

The short time from original discovery to actual clinical use was phenomenal (Starzl et al. 1989). The original agent was described as a hundredfold more potent than cyclosporin for similar in vitro activities. In addition, its cytokine inhibition extends to IL-3, IL-4, and IFN-γ (Thomson 1989). One FK-506 property that is different from cyclosporin is the fact that FK-506 interferes with the expression of IL-2 lymphocyte receptors (Woo, Sewell, and Thomson 1990). Such cells would be refractory to exogenous IL-2. It also interacts with a protein-binding receptor that may be important in effecting signal transduction. How this signal relates to inhibition of gene transcription is unclear.

Its advantages are numerous (Macleod and Thomson 1991). Use of the drug suppresses both cell-mediated and humoral immune responses at doses much lower than cyclosporin. It is the drug of choice in many centers for prolonging transplantation

FK-506

acceptance, particularly with livers, and surprisingly is even very effective in reversing transplantation rejection crises. Although it has been used to inhibit experimental autoimmune disease, its use for that purpose in humans has not been evaluated. Because the binding proteins are not unique to lymphocytes, toxicity to other organs can be expected. Reports of toxicity are similar to those on cyclosporin except that with use of FK-506 adjunctive therapy is not needed, and this lowers the total toxic load. Fatal cytomegalovirus infections remain a problem with any type of immunosuppression.

Antibodies

Although modern monoclonal antibody technology has reintroduced the possibility of using specific antibodies to interfere with different pathways of the immune response, it should be recalled that one of the earliest immunosuppressants to be used clinically was antilymphocyte globulin (ALG). The term is used here in the generic sense to include globulins prepared from antisera to thymocytes and lymphoblasts as well. Species such as horses, goats, or rabbits were immunized with various human lymphocyte cell preparations, and the globulins were chemically extracted and purified from the resulting antisera. The ALG was extensively used to depress circulating T cells to manage early rejection crises in renal allograft recipients. Some of the problems encountered using these materials included (1) the lack of standard production protocols leading to variability in preparations, (2) variability in patient response, and (3) ALG contamination with globulins of other specificities (for basement membrane or platelets, for example). At the time of their popularity, there was no specificity toward a particular lymphocyte subset such that there was a general suppression. It was of most value in treating early rejection crises and had no application in treatment of diseases of immunologic injury.

Many of these problems were overcome with the development of monoclonal antibodies specific for particular markers on target cell populations. By definition, monoclonal antibodies are all produced from cells with a single, common ancestor such that their specificities are all narrowly identical. One antibody preparation that has been evaluated, known originally as OKT3, is specific for the CD3 lymphocyte marker of T lymphocytes (Woodley et al. 1990). With this site occluded, signal transduction of MHC II antigen recognition is inhibited; thus, there is no afferent sensitization. However, in vivo administration of this reagent is indeed immunotoxic in that target cells are stimulated to release inflammatory cytokines such as TNF and IL-2, which can account for toxic side effects. Fortunately, these can be modulated pharmacologically. T cells initially decline but soon begin to rise; however, they are devoid of the CD3 marker. This phenomenon of antibody-induced suppression of a phenotypic marker is called antigenic modulation. The development of idiotypic antibodies can complicate treatment with OKT3, rendering it less effective, and results in the reemergence of CD3$^+$ cells (Suranyi and Hall, 1990).

A relatively new approach in using antibodies immunosuppressively has been to prepare anti-IL-2 receptor antibodies (Soulillou et al. 1987). Such a reagent takes advantage of the critical importance of IL-2 signaling in activation, proliferative expansion, and amplification of T-lymphocyte responses. Any cell bearing the IL-2 receptor is capable of responding to one of the cytokines in the afferent pathway, and interference with it in the presence of presented antigen should lead to significant immunosuppression. Mixed clinical results have been reported so far with this approach.

D. CONCLUSION

The distance between the basic understanding of immune responsiveness and purely anecdotal experience in enhancing or depressing the immune response is rapidly closing. The more we learn about the basic features of the immune response, the more capable we will be to undertake intentional control of it for indicated occasions. Similarly, information obtained from the study of such external modulation points the way for immunotoxicologists interested in assessing the modes of actions of many of the substances that may concern them. Therefore, it would greatly profit immunotoxicologists to follow the immunomodulation literature carefully.

References

Allison, A. C., and G. Gregoriadis. 1974. Liposomes as immunological adjuvants. *Nature* 252:252.

Bahr, G. M., and L. Chedid. 1986. Immunological activities of muramyl peptides. *Fed. Proc.* 45:2541–44.

Bardana, E. J., Jr. 1985. Recent developments in immunomodulatory therapy. *J. Allergy Clin. Immunol.* 75:423–36.

Bottomly, K. 1989. A functional dichotomy in CD4$^+$ T lymphocytes. *Immunol. Today* 9:268–73.

Burrell, R. 1988. Immunomodulation by bacterial products. *Clin. Immunol. Newslett.* 9:206–9.

Burrell, R. 1990. Immunomodulation by bacterial endotoxin. *CRC Crit. Rev. Microbiol.* 17:189–208.

Corazza, G. R., G. Zoli, L. Ginaldi, et al. 1991. Tuftsin deficiency in AIDS. *Lancet* 337:12–13.

Cupps, T. R., and A. S. Fauci. 1982. Corticosteroid-mediated immunoregulation in man. *Immunol. Rev.* 65:133–55.

Fauci, A. S. 1979. Mechanisms of the immunosuppressive and anti-inflammatory effects of glucocorticosteroids. *J. Immunopharmacol.* 1:1–15.

Fudenberg, H. H. 1985. "Transfer factor": An update. *Proc. Soc. Exp. Biol. Med.* 178:327–32.

Fudenberg, H. H., and H. D. Whitten. 1984. Immunostimulation: Synthetic and biological modulators of immunity. *Annu. Rev. Pharmacol. Toxicol.* 24:147–74.

Fudenberg, H. H., G. B. Wilson, J. M. Goust, et al. 1980. Dialyzable leukocyte extracts (transfer factor): A review of clinical results and immunological methods for donor selection, evaluation of activities, and patient monitoring. In *Thymus, Thymic Hormones, and T Lymphocytes,* ed. F. A. Aiuti and H. Wigzell, pp. 391–421. London: Academic Press.

Goldstein, D., and J. Laszlo. 1989. The role of interferon in cancer therapy: A current perspective. *Ca-A Cancer J.* 38:258–77.

Gregoriadis, G. 1990. Immunological adjuvants: A role for liposomes. *Immunol. Today* 111:89–97.

Grun, J. L., and P. H. Maurer. 1989. Different T helper cell subsets elicited in mice utilizing two different adjuvant vehicles: The role of endogenous interleukin in proliferative responses. *Cell. Immunol.* 121:134–45.

Hadden, J. W. 1989. Therapeutic immunopharmacology. *Curr. Opin. Immunol.* 2:258–63.

Harding, M. W., R. E. Handschumacher, and D. W. Speicher. 1986. Isolation and amino acid sequence of cyclophilin. *J. Biol. Chem.* 261:8547–55.

Herrmann, D. B. J., and U. Bicker. 1990. Drugs in autoimmune disease. *Klin. Wochenschr.* 68(Suppl. XXI):15–25.

Hess, A. D., P. J. Tutschka, and G. W. Santos. 1982. Effect of cyclosporin A on human lymphocyte responses in vitro. III. CsA inhibits the production of T lymphocyte growth factors in secondary mixed lymphocyte reactions but does not inhibit the response of primed lymphocytes to TCGF. *J. Immunol.* 128:535–39.

Hirata, F. 1981. The regulation of lipomodulin, a phospholipase inhibitory protein in rabbit neutrophils by phosphorylation. *J. Biol. Chem.* 256:7730–35.

Hunter, R. L., and B. Bennett. 1984. The adjuvant activity of nonionic block polymer surfactants. II. Antibody formation and inflammation related to the structure of triblock and octablock copolymers. *J. Immunol.* 133:3167–75.

Hunter, R., F. Strickland, and F. Kezdy. 1981. The adjuvant activity of nonionic block polymer surfactants. I. The role of hydrophile–lipophile balance. *J. Immunol.* 127:1244–50.

Kahan, B. D. 1989. Cyclosporin. *N. Engl. J. Med.* 321:1725–38.

Kino, T., H. Hatanaka, S. Miyata, et al. 1987. FK-506, a novel immunosuppressant isolated from a *Streptomyces.* I. Fermentation, isolation, and physico-chemical and biological characteristics. II. Immunosuppressive effect of FK-506 in vitro. *J. Antibiot.* 40:1249–55, 1256–65.

Kotani, S., H. Takada, M. Tsujimoto, et al. 1984. Immunobiologically active lipid A analogs synthesized according to a revised structural model of natural lipid A. *Infect. Immun.* 45:293–96.

Kotani, S., H. Takada, M. Tsujimoto, et al. 1985. Synthetic lipid A with endotoxic and related biological activities comparable to those of natural lipid A from an *Escherichia coli* re-*mutant. Infect. Immun.* 49:225–37.

Kronke, M., W. J. Leonard, J. M. Depper, et al. 1984. Cyclosporin A inhibits T-cell growth factor gene expression at the level of mRNA transcription. *Proc. Natl. Acad. Sci. U.S.A.* 81:5214–18.

LeClerc, C., D. Juy, E. Bourgeois, and L. Chedid. 1979. In vivo regulation of humoral and cellular immune responses of mice by a synthetic adjuvant, N-acetylmuramyl-L-alanyl-D-isoglutamine, muramyl dipeptide for MDP. *Cell. Immunol.* 45:199–206.

Lee, W. Y., and A. H. Sehon. 1978. Suppression of reaginic antibodies. *Immunol. Rev.* 41:200–47.

Lex, A., K.-H. Wiessmuller, G. Jung, and W. G. Bessler. 1986. A synthetic analogue of *Escherichia coli* lipoprotein, tripalmitoyl pentapeptide, constitutes a potent immune adjuvant. *J. Immunol.* 137:2676–81.

Lise, L. D., and F. Audibert. 1989. Immunoadjuvants and analogs of immunomodulatory bacterial structures. *Curr. Opin. Immunol.* 2:269–74.

Macleod, A. M., and A. W. Thomson. 1991. FK-506: An immunosuppressant for the 1990s? *Lancet* 337:25–27.

Michalek, S. M., N. K. Childers, J. Katz, et al. 1989. Liposomes as oral adjuvants. *Curr. Top. Microbiol. Immunol.* 146:51–58.

Morein, B. 1990. The iscom: A immunostimulating system. *Immunol. Lett.* 25:281–83.

Najjar, V. 1978. Molecular basis of familial and acquired phagocytosis deficiency involving the tetrapeptide, tuftsin. *Exp. Cell. Biol.* 46:114–26.

Penn, I. 1985. Neoplastic consequences of immunosuppression. In *Immunotoxicology and Immunopharmacology,* ed. J. H. Dean, M. I. Luster, A. E. Munson, and H. Amos, pp. 79–90. New York: Raven Press.

Pignol, B., T. Maisonnet, J. M. Menciahuerta, and P. Braquet. 1991. Effect of the double-stranded polynucleotide complex polyadenylate–polyuridylate (poly A–U) on interleukin-6 production by mouse fibroblasts. *Immunopharmacology* 21:33–40.

Ribi, E. 1984. Beneficial modifications of the endotoxin molecule. *J. Biol. Response Modif.* 3:1–9.

Rosenberg, S. A., M. D. Lotze, L. M. Muul, et al. 1985. Observation of the systemic administration of autologous lymphokine-activated killer cells and recombinant interleukin-2. *N. Engl. J. Med.* 313:1485–92.

St. Georgiev, V. 1990. Immunomodulatory activity of small peptides. *Trends Pharmacol. Sci.* 11:373–78.

Sercarz, E., and U. Krzych. 1991. The distinctive specificity of antigen-specific suppressor T cells. *Immunol. Today* 12:111–18.

Soulillou, J. P., P. Peyronnet, B. Le Mauff, et al. 1987. Prevention of rejection of kidney transplants by monoclonal antibody directed against interleukin 2. *Lancet* 1:1339–42.

Starzl, T. E., S. Todo, J. Fung, et al. 1989. FK-506 for liver, kidney, and pancreas transplantation. *Lancet* 1000–0.

Stevenson, H. C., and A. S. Fauci. 1980. Activation of human B lymphocytes. XII. Differential effects of in vitro cyclophosphamide on human lymphocyte subpopulations involved in B cell activation. *Immunology* 39:391–97.

Suranyi, M. G., and B. M. Hall. 1990. Current status of renal transplantation. *West. J. Med.* 152:687–96.

Takada, H., S. Kotani, M. Tsujimoto, et al. 1985. Immunopharmacological activities of a synthetic counterpart of a biosynthetic lipid A precursor molecule and of its analogs. *Infect. Immun.* 48:219–27.

Takayama, K., N. Qureshi, E. Ribi, and J. L. Cantrell. 1984. Separation and characterization of toxic and non-toxic forms of lipid A. *Rev. Infect. Dis.* 6:439–43.

Thomson, A. W. 1989. FK-506—How much potential? *Immunol. Today* 10:6–9.

Umezewa, H., and M. Ishizuka. 1985. Low molecular weight immunomodifiers produced by microorganisms. *Int. J. Clin. Pharmacol. Ther. Toxicol.* 23:S9–S13.

Vincenti, F., C. Biava, S. Tomlanovitch, et al. 1989. Inability of cyclosporin to completely prevent the recurrence of focal glomerulosclerosis after kidney transplantation. *Transplantation* 47:595–98.

Wilson, K., and G. S. Eisenbarth. 1990. Immunopathogenesis and immunotherapy of type 1 diabetes. *Annu. Rev. Med.* 41:497–508.

Woo, J., H. F. Sewell, and A. W. Thomson. 1990. The influence of FK-506 and low concentration of cyclosporin on human lymphocyte activation, antigen expression and blastogenesis: A flow cytometric analysis. *Scand. J. Immunol.* 31:297–304.

Woodley, S. L., D. G. Renlund, J. B. O'Connell, and M. R. Bristow. 1990. Immunosuppression following cardiac transplantation. *Cardiol. Clin.* 8:83–96.

Young, D. B. 1991. The stress of living with people. *Curr. Opin. Biol.* 1:157–58.

9

Assessment of Secondary Immunodeficiencies in Man and Animals

A. INTRODUCTION

Assessment of immunodeficiencies may be made retrospectively or prospectively. In the former, effort is made to determine the nature of the immune defect or injury and, if possible, what caused it. One would necessarily be working with human material with this approach. Prospective studies try to predict possible immune injury in advance and usually require the use of animals or in vitro systems. This chapter discusses the methods of assessment for these two approaches separately although often the same methods are used in each.

Primary immunodeficiencies, i.e., those brought about by genetic or developmental abnormalities, were discussed in Chapter 7. However, the major topic of this text is those secondary immunodeficiencies that are initiated by external and internal forces subsequent to individual development. Therapeutic agents and viruses are major external forces, whereas examples of internal forces include age and metabolic abnormalities.

B. SECONDARY IMMUNODEFICIENCIES ASSOCIATED WITH OTHER DISEASES

Viruses can cause transient or life-threatening immunosuppression. Influenza virus may impair the function of PMNs in peripheral blood, thus increasing the frequency of bacterial infections, e.g., by staphylococci. Infection with the HIV produces profound effects on select cells in the immune system. As part of the acquired immunodeficiency syndrome (AIDS), the virus infects and affects the function of lymphocytes (and other cells) expressing the CD4$^+$ marker. Since the CD4$^+$ cells are the helper/amplifier population, cellular destruction by the virus prevents activation of the immune system.

Occasionally it is necessary to differentiate between viruses as the causal agents of immunosuppression and opportunistic viral infections in previously immunosuppressed patients. In immunocompromised patients, cytomegalovirus infection is the greatest cause of mortality and morbidity (Agnado, Gomez, and Rodriguez 1989). This may be because the virus can be transmitted in blood products, bone marrow, and transplanted organs. Infection with Epstein–Barr (EB) virus may further compromise suppressed individuals. The virus may inhibit the production of antibodies, resulting in hypogammaglobulinemia. The lack of functional antibodies in peripheral blood leads to infections with pneumococci and *Haemophilus*. In addition, the EB virus frequently transforms B cells to create a malignant lymphoma, further reducing B-cell function (Nicolas, Cozum, and Revillard 1988).

Newborns and the elderly may exhibit age-related secondary immunosuppression. Newborns have defects in macrophage migration, chemotaxis, microbial killing, and synthesis of phagocytosis-promoting factors C3 and factor B (Johnson 1988). In older subjects, the nature of the defects suggests that both the antibody and cell-mediated systems are affected (Fox 1984). Many elderly people have an increased frequency of infection with pneumococci and Gram-negative bacteria. Reactivation infections with herpes zoster (shingles) or tuberculosis are also common in this group.

Metabolic disorders and abnormalities may contribute to the immunodeficiency state. Severe malnutrition causes defects in the function of phagocytic cells in addition to T-cell-mediated effector mechanisms. Decreased resistance to streptococci, staphylococci, and measles is often reported. Increased loss of protein or electrolytes can also cause selected immunodeficiencies. In Menetrie's disease there is an excessive loss of protein and immunoglobulin in urine. If the synthetic rate of antibody production does not equal the loss rate, immunodeficiency may occur, resulting in susceptibility to select bacteria. The function of the circulating neutrophil is reduced in diabetics. Although there may be no inherent defect in the cells, they do not respond to chemotactic factors in a normal manner. Occasionally, the use of common therapeutic agents can cause secondary immunodeficiency. As a consequence of the use of diuretics, phosphate may be voided in the urine. In severe hypophosphatemia, the normal function of PMNs may be reduced or inhibited.

The function of monocytes–macrophages may also be impaired in several diseases. One normal function of tissue macrophages is the removal and destruction of aged red cells from circulating blood. In Gaucher's or Niemann–Pick disease, there is a defect in the function of enzymes degrading sphingolipids. As a consequence of the defect, red blood cell debris accumulates within the macrophage (Stanbury, Wyngarten, and Fredrickson 1983). The accumulated lipid inhibits the function of protein kinase C, which is necessary for the membrane transduction of external stimuli that activate or regulate the macrophage. Because the macrophage cannot respond to functional stimuli, resistance to infection can be impaired (Hannun and Bell 1987).

Malignant processes of the hematopoietic system can also induce secondary immunodeficiencies. Leukemia and lymphomas are, essentially, diseases of immunocompetent cells such as monocytes and T and B cells. Although the leukemic cells undergo uncontrolled cellular proliferation, they are arrested in a specific stage of maturation or differentiation. Hence, there may be decreased functional capacity in these cells, resulting in a predisposition to infection with encapsulated microorganisms. Conversely, many lymphomas are of T-cell origin, and the cellular immune system may be impaired. An excellent example of functional impairment of lymphocyte proliferation occurs in Hodgkin's disease. The lack of a proliferative response may allow the activation of latent herpes zoster virus.

The immune system can also be inhibited indirectly by soluble factors released from tumor cells. Although the teleological significance is unclear, products of tumor cell metabolism can essentially simulate microbial virulence factors and inhibit the function of both monocytes and macrophages. A product related to retrovirus structural protein p15(E) inhibits the chemotaxis of monocytes (Cianciolo, Hunter, and Silva 1981). Some tumors also produce soluble factors that suppress the production of cytotoxic free radicals by macrophages (Szuro-Subol and Nathan 1982). Among the most profound immune changes brought about by a tumor product is the inhibition of MHC class II marker expression in macrophages induced by the shedding of membrane vesicles by melanoma cells, by an unknown mechanism (Poutsiaka et al. 1985).

C. DIAGNOSIS OF SECONDARY IMMUNODEFICIENCY

The diagnosis is considered when a patient has a clear history and objective laboratory evidence of recurrent infections or malignancies commonly associated with immune suppression. After exclusion of underlying diseases or confounding factors (e.g., age, malnutrition, infections, or therapeutic agents) as the cause of the problem, the physician will establish a tentative diagnosis of immunodeficiency. Based on the pattern of infection or the type of malignancy, in vivo studies or in vitro laboratory tests can be performed to confirm or negate the diagnostic hypothesis in mechanistic terms.

1. Laboratory Testing

Laboratory tests should be limited solely to supporting the tentative diagnosis in mechanistic terms. Increasing the number of tests performed increases the probability of an abnormal result that may have no relevance to the tentative diagnosis. Testing should proceed, in a logical progression, from commonly available techniques that document the presence of the defect to more sophisticated techniques that explore the cellular and/or functional aspects of the process.

Careful consideration should be given to the design of laboratory studies. All testing should ideally be deferred until the patient is free of infection or medications. This insures that the immune system is homeostatic and not subject to modulation by these agents. In addition to steroids, medications such as cimetidine, insulin, and aspirin can alter the distribution or function of lymphocyte subsets (Chatenoud et al. 1982; Fauci and Dale 1975). The number and function of lymphocytes in peripheral blood are influenced by a number of natural phenomena. Because of diurnal variation, there may be a 50% variation in the numbers of total lymphocytes or subsets at different times of day. Hence, all blood samples should be obtained at the same time of day (Levi et al. 1988). In females, the function of lymphocytes may also be altered during estrus or use of oral contraceptives.

Because the numbers and function of lymphocytes vary in the peripheral blood, there is an essential need to use test and population controls in the testing scheme. Since immune parameters vary with both age and sex, any protocol should include age- and sex-matched controls. All data should be compared to the laboratory historical control values, segregated on the basis of both sex and age. To insure that the immunologic defect is persistent and reproducible, the laboratory tests should be repeated. With the exception of immunodeficiency caused by HIV, most secondary immunosuppression is reversible in a short period of time. For example, if the dose of azathioprine does not damage the ability of the bone marrow to produce immunocompetent cells, the immunotoxic effect is reversed in 7 days. Even the effects of strong alkylating agents (e.g., cyclophosphamide) abate after 2 weeks (Munson 1987).

With the exception of serum immunoglobulin and complement levels in sera, there is no universally acceptable normal range for numbers of lymphocyte subsets or the functional capacity of cells (Anonymous 1981). In the former case, the numbers are influenced by methodology, the counting device, and the method used for data presentation. Functional assays have not been standardized between testing laboratories, as reagents, media supplements, and technical aspects of immunoassays vary extensively. Therefore, each laboratory establishes its own normal ranges by performing the assay under standard conditions with large groups of samples.

2. Antibody-Mediated Immune System

If defects in the antibody-mediated immune system are suspected, there are numerous tests that can determine whether the defect is qualitative or quantitative. Immunoglobulin isotype levels can be ascertained by three different types of assays: radial immunodiffusion assays, where serum samples are allowed to diffuse through agar containing the appropriate antiisotype sera; enzyme-linked immunosorbent assays (ELISA), which use enzyme amplification methods to measure immunoglobulin–antiserum interactions; and measurement of turbidity from antigen–antibody interactions by laser nephelometry.

The presence of normal antibody isotype levels in serum does not exclude the possibility of an antibody-mediated immune defect. Although total levels of serum IgG and IgA may be within normal limits, there may be alterations in specific subclasses of IgG that predispose to select disease process. Also, if the defect is at the level of processing certain antigens (e.g., polysaccharides in Wiskott–Aldrich syndrome) or in phagocytic dysfunction, merely assessing immunoglobulin concentration will be insufficient. Levels of serum IgE are so minute that they are only detectable with radioimmunoassay (RIA) or ELISA technology. The RIA can employ either a competitive or a noncompetitive binding assay. In the competitive assay, radiolabeled IgE is mixed with the test serum, and the amount of label bound to solid-phase anti-IgE is determined (see Fig. 9–1). In this inhibition assay, unlabeled serum IgE competes with the labeled antibody for binding to the solid phase. When there are high levels of IgE in the test sample, a comparatively low level of the labeled IgE binds to the solid phase; low serum IgE levels allow increased binding of the labeled globulin. In the noncompetitive assay, the test serum is first reacted with solid-phase anti-IgE. Following incubation, radiolabeled anti-IgE is added to the mixture. The amount of the radiolabel bound to the solid phase is determined. With increased IgE bound to the solid phase, there is a corresponding increase in reaction with labeled anti-IgE. In some laboratories, enzyme-labeled anti-IgE antibodies have replaced the radiolabeled reagents. Although elevated levels of the IgE isotype have been associated with immediate hypersensitivity reactions, there is little evidence that IgE plays a role in secondary immunodeficiency. Total IgE levels may, however, be helpful in the diagnosis in select diseases involving a dysfunction in the synthesis of IgE (e.g., bronchopulmonary aspergillosis and hyper-IgE syndrome). In these diseases the levels of IgE may approach levels observed in patients with IgE myelomas (de Shazo, Lopez, and Salvaggio 1987).

If total antibody levels are within normal limits, one can determine whether

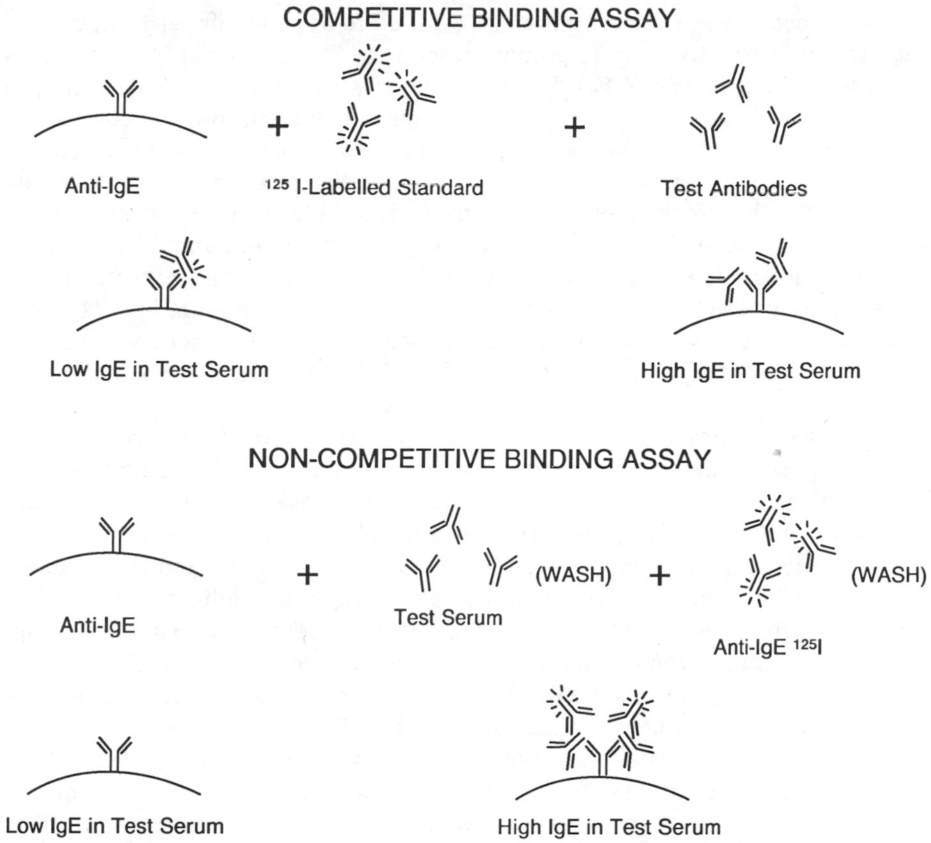

COMPETITIVE BINDING ASSAY

Anti-IgE   125 I-Labelled Standard   Test Antibodies

Low IgE in Test Serum   High IgE in Test Serum

NON-COMPETITIVE BINDING ASSAY

Anti-IgE   Test Serum (WASH)   Anti-IgE 125I (WASH)

Low IgE in Test Serum   High IgE in Test Serum

FIGURE 9–1. Competitive and non-competitive binding radioimmuno assays. In the competitive assay, radiolabeled IgE and unlabeled IgE in the test serum compete for combining sites of anti-IgE attached to the solid phase (curved line). When there are high levels of IgE in the test sample, a comparatively low level of the labeled IgE binds to the solid phase. In the noncompetitive assay, the test serum is first reacted with solid phase anti-IgE. Following incubation, radiolabeled anti-IgE is added to the mixture. The amount of the radiolabel bound to the solid phase is then determined.

the test subject has normal levels of naturally occurring antibodies. A good example would be the presence of normal blood group isohemagglutinins. With the exception of those with AB blood group, all persons above the age of three should have antibodies directed toward A and/or B blood group isoantigens. In the laboratory, serum from the patient can be titered for hemagglutination against red blood cells expressing either the A or B antigen. Failure to find significant levels of appropriate isoantibodies may reflect dysfunction in the B-cell arm of the immune response, failure of IgM production, etc.

The presence of antibodies induced by immunization to common infectious agents may also be useful in the diagnosis of secondary immunodeficiency. In most cases, there should be demonstrable antibodies directed toward common childhood immunogens, e.g., diphtheria and tetanus toxoids. Antibodies directed toward measles and polio viruses would also be expected to be normally present in serum. Solid-phase ELISAs can determine the presence and/or the quantity of each antigen-specific antibody.

In some immunodeficiencies, the patient cannot respond de novo to antigenic stimuli. Since humans are not normally exposed to keyhole limpet hemocyanin, the protein is used to measure primary responses. Some clinical immunologists also use bacteriophage ϕ X 174. Reimmunization with a T-cell-dependent antigen (diphtheria and tetanus toxoid) or a T-cell-regulated antigen (pneumococcus vaccine) can be used to test the secondary or anamnestic antibody response (Baker et al. 1981). It is also possible to modify the immunization protocols to ascertain whether the subject can respond to soluble or insoluble antigens. If the immune system is functional, increases in antigen-specific antibodies should be demonstrable in the serum within 4 to 6 weeks following immunization. It is often useful to ascertain the levels of each IgG subclass within the total population. The antibody response to protein is usually comprised of IgG_1 and IgG_3, whereas the population responding to polysaccharides is IgG_2 (Hammarstrom and Smith 1986).

When reduced levels of immunoglobulin are present in the serum, a search may be taken to determine the mechanism. Generally, the reduction may be caused by increased degradation of antibody or decreased synthesis of immunoglobulin. Antibody levels in the serum are a reflection of three factors: the number of B cells in the circulation, the rate of antibody synthesis, and the catabolic or degradation rate. The degradation rate of immunoglobulin is expressed in terms of antibody half-life ($T/2$). In the peripheral blood, the IgG antibody population persists for a long period of time with an average half-life of 23 days. Of the IgG subclasses, only the IgG_3 subclass has a shorter half-life (8–9 days). The IgM and IgA isotypes have a relatively short half-life of 5–6 days.

Increased antibody catabolism can be easily demonstrated by radiolabeled immunoglobulin tracer studies. When such tracers are injected into the patient, the clearance should follow the pattern shown in Table 9–1. In the interpretation of catabolism data, care must be taken to exclude confounding experimental factors. Loss of immunoglobulin and/or immunocompetent cells occurs in a variety of intestinal disorders affecting the mucosal layer.

Flow cytometry can be used to enumerate B cells in peripheral blood coated with fluorescein-labeled antibodies directed toward specific cellular antigens on lymphocyte subsets (Lovett et al. 1984). A number of fluoresecent antibodies directed toward B-cell markers (CD19–CD21) are commercially available (see Table 9–2 for a list of some common CD antigen markers of circulating lymphocytes). Approximately 30% of normal peripheral blood lymphocytes are B cells, but this ratio can be significantly altered by splenectomy, administration of insulin, active infection, or xenobiotic contact (During, Landman, and Harder 1984). The distribution of B cells secreting IgM, IgA, or IgG and the maturation status of B cells can also be determined by flow cytometry. By using antiimmunoglobulin isotype-specific antisera, it is possible to determine the various isotype-specific

TABLE 9–1.   The Normal Synthesis and Catabolism Rate for Peripheral Blood Antibody Isotypes

	IgG	IgM	IgA
Synthesis rate (mg/kg per day)	33	6.7	24
Catabolism rate (% degraded/day)	6.7	18	25
Half-life (days)	23	5.1	5.8

Source: Modified from Davis et al. (1973).

TABLE 9-2.   Common CD Markers Present on Peripheral Blood Leukocytes

Antigen	Distribution	Specificity
CD2	T cells	Sheep red blood cell receptor
CD3	T cells	Polypeptides signal-transducing unit of CD3/TCR complex
CD4	T-cell subset	Helper/amplifier T cells; HIV receptor
CD5	T cells	Human analog of murine Lyt-1
CD6	Mature T cells, B cells	Crossing linkage induces Ca^{2+} mobilization
CD8	T-cell subset	Cytotoxic/suppressor T cells
CD11b	Monocytes, granulocytes, lymphocytes	Complement III receptor on $CD8^+$ cells
CD16	Granulocytes, lymphocytes	Natural killer cell population
CD19	B cells	B cells
CD21	B cells	B cell complement II receptor
CD23	B cells	Low-affinity receptor for IgE
CD25	Activated T cells	IL-2 receptor
CDw29	T-cell subset	Inducers of help within the $CD4^+$ population
CD35	Granulocytes, monocytes	Complement I receptor
CD45	Leukocytes	Leukocyte common antigen
CD45R	B and T cells	Inducers of suppression within the $CD4^+$ population
CD56/CD57	NK cells	NK cells

B-cell subsets producing antibodies. During the B-cell maturation process different markers are found on the cell surface. In the early B-cell stage, CD10, CD19, CD11b, and HLA-Dr are expressed on the cell's surface. Only CD19, CD20, CD21, CD24, CD11b, and HLA-Dr are found on mature B cells in the peripheral blood (Klinman, Wylie, and Teale 1981). Following stimulation, the numbers of cells expressing T9-transferrin or numbers of HLA-Dr markers can be determined.

Occasionally, B cells may synthesize antibodies but fail to secrete the molecules into the external environment. To document such a defect, the presence of cytoplasmic immunoglobulin in B cells can be determined by immunofluorescent techniques. Fixed cells are stained with anti-heavy chain (μ) specific reagents. Pre-B cells will have synthesized cytoplasmic IgM. Conversely, immature B cells will exhibit only surface IgM, but with further maturation these cells express both IgM and IgD.

The impairment of antibody synthesis can also be documented by in vitro assays using polyclonal B-cell activators. In humans, mitogenic stimulation of B cells by pokeweed mitogen (PWM) requires the interaction of functional T_h cells and B cells (Greaves, Janossy, and Doenhoff 1974; Keightley, Cooper, and Lawton 1976). The majority of B cells responding to PWM are IgD^- B cells, which are considered resting memory cells. Only a small number of uncommitted IgD^+ cells producing IgM are stimulated (Jelinek, Spiawski, and Lipsky 1986). The stimulated cells proliferate rapidly, and intracellular immunoglobulin is demonstrable by day 4. Subpopulations secreting IgG, IgA, and IgM are apparent by days 7-10. Usually, nonstimulated cells produce less than 600 ng/ml of immunoglobulin; PWM-stimulated cells produce approximately 1,600 ng/ml of IgG, 500 ng/ml of IgA, and over 400 ng/ml of IgM.

Bacteria and bacterial products have been used as polyclonal activators, e.g., the polyclonal B-cell activator, *Staphylococcus aureus*-Cowan strain (SAC). Both IgD^- and IgD^+ B cells respond to the SAC with proliferation of IgG, IgA, and IgM antibodies. Although the proliferation of B cells occurs in a T-cell-independent manner, T-cell cytokines are required for B-cell maturation into antibody-producing cells (Falkoff, Zhu, and Fauci 1982). Similar observations have been made with bacterial lipopolysaccharide (LPS).

Coculture experiments with isolated T and B cells from normal subjects can determine the cellular location of the lesion in antibody production. Purified T- and B-lymphocyte subsets from a normal subject and test subjects are cocultured in combinations as shown in Table 9–3. In these experiments, purified T and B cells are incubated in the presence of PWM. Following several days of incubation, the amount of immunoglobulin present in the tissue culture medium is measured. Mixtures of patient's purified $CD8^+$ cells with normal T and B cells can provide information on the functional status of the patient's T_s cells. Similar mixtures can be used to study the effects of T_h cells.

Many different clinical conditions and diseases affect the synthesis of antibodies. Acute and chronic viral infections, especially with Epstein–Barr virus and cytomegalovirus, can alter synthesis. Similar decreases have been reported in subjects with collagen vascular disorders such as systemic lupus erythematosus (SLE). Malignancies affecting the immune system (e.g., leukemia, lymphoma, myeloma, and thymoma) also decrease the numbers or function of antibody-secreting cells.

3. Cell-Mediated Immunity

In this context, cell-mediated immunity encompasses several forms. Both in vitro and in vivo functions of T cells, NK cells, and monocytes/macrophages are included in the coverage that follows.

Enumeration of T Cells

Because the cell-mediated immune response consists of various effector and immunoregulatory cells, more sophisticated assays must be used in vitro or in vivo to define the immune defects. By using flow cytometry and monoclonal antibodies directed toward cellular markers, it is possible to identify and enumerate lymphocyte subsets (Love and Metcalf 1980). However, there is a problem with the nomenclature of these numerous markers and their respective antibodies. Antibodies directed toward cellular epitopes were first produced by two different

TABLE 9–3.   Co-culture Studies to Determine the Nature of the Lesion in Antibody Synthesis

	Antibody Synthesis	Defect
T cell (patient) + B cell (patient)	No	Yes
T cell (normal) + B cell (normal)	Yes	No
T cell (normal) + B cell (patient)	No	B cell
T cell (patient) + B cell (normal)	No	T cell
T_s cell (patient) $\left.\right\}$ + B cell (normal) T_h cell (normal)	No	Increased T_s
T_{h+s} cell (patient) $\left.\right\}$ + B cell (normal) T_h cell (normal)	Yes	Decreased T_h

manufacturers, Ortho and Becton Dickinson. Each manufacturer used a different nomenclature to identify serological reactivity. Ortho used a numerical system with the prefix OKT; the BD system used a different numerical system preceded by Leu. Hence, T cells were OKT 3^+ or Leu 1^+. To simplify the nomenclature, the serological reactivity is now identified by cluster of differentiation or CD (Erber 1990). Following this convention, the OKT 3^+ or Leu 1^+ cells would be identified as CD3 cells. The specificity of certain monoclonal antibodies directed toward human lymphocyte markers is shown in Table 9-2.

Lymphocyte subsets in the peripheral blood can be enumerated using single or dual fluorescent-labeling techniques. For example, all T cells carry the CD2 and CD3 markers, cells of the helper/amplifier T-cell population express CD4, etc. Using two different monoclonal antibodies (separately labeled with different dyes) to stain the same cell, it is clear that, within the CD4 class, there are cells (CD4$^+$, CDw29$^+$) that induce or amplify helper cells and those (CD4$^+$, CD45R$^+$) that evoke suppressor cells. Cells bearing the CD8 marker in the cytotoxic/suppressor T population carry additional markers and can similarly be separated by dual labeling techniques to differentiate cytotoxic and suppressor T cells. It has been reported that T-suppressor cells express complement receptors. When dual labeling techniques are used, the suppressor cells express CD8 and CD11b; cytotoxic T cells carry only the CD8 marker.

Natural killer cells are more difficult to enumerate by flow cytometry because they express markers found on both T and B cells. However, antibodies directed toward the CD16 and CD38 markers have been used to identify the NK-cell population. The subset of NK cells that actually lyse cells from solid tumors are CD16, NKH1 antigen positive (Storkus and Dawson 1991).

Data from flow cytometry studies should be expressed as both percentage of cells and the absolute number per cubic millimeter of blood. The latter determination is a mathematical calculation that considers the total white blood cell count, the percentage of total lymphocytes, and the percentage of each subset. Since each of the three parameters may fluctuate independently of the others, calculation of the absolute numbers reflects the biological relevance. The formula for determination is as follows:

$$\text{Absolute lymphocytes/mm}^3 = (\text{Total white blood cells/mm}^3) \times \left(\frac{\%\ \text{lymphocytes}}{100} \right) \times \left(\frac{\%\ \text{subset}}{100} \right)$$

If one assumes that the cytometry studies have been performed under optimal conditions, statistical analyses should be considered. Because lymphocyte subsets are part of a network and, hence, do not function as separate entities, multivariate statistical analysis is the method of choice.

In the normal state, the immune system is poised to defend the host. The T-helper cells constitute 60–70% of the peripheral blood lymphocytes, of which only 20–25% of the total lymphocytes are cytotoxic/suppressor T cells. Natural killer cells represent the smallest proportion of the total lymphocytes (10–15%). The percentages of some of these subsets vary with disease and age. In the older literature, the helper:suppressor (T4:T8) ratio was often used as an index of immunosuppression. This is particularly true in AIDS patients, who have ratios below 1.0 (normal ratios range between 1.7 to 2.2). It is unclear if a decreased T4:T8 ratio is a generalized phenomenon in immunosuppressed patients. In immunosuppressed renal transplant patients there is great variation in the ratio (Burton 1984; McWhinnie et al. 1985) that has no relationship to episodes of rejection. In these patients a falling T4:T8 ratio correlated only with acute viral infections (Dafoe et al. 1987).

The relationship between altered lymphocyte subset counts and other diseases is less clear. Certainly, decreases in the absolute numbers of CD4[+] lymphocytes herald biologically relevant immunosuppression in patients with AIDS. Similarly, some patients with hypogammaglobulinemia have reduced numbers of CD4[+] cells. In other patients with the same disease, the numbers of CD4[+] cells are normal. Conversely, steroid treatment reduces the number of CD4[+] cells in the peripheral circulation, but the reduction has no effect on antibody synthesis (Grayson et al. 1981). Finally, in some diseases such as Hodgkin's disease there is no alteration in CD4[+] cell numbers (Gupta and Tan 1980). The failure to associate phenotypic changes with disease states may be because individual subsets within the major CD4[+] and CD8[+] populations fluctuate independently. Hence, CD4[+] numbers may be within normal limits, but there may be changes with the subsets that amplify help or suppression. A reduction in the numbers of CD4[+], CD45R[+] cells is associated with active SLE and multiple sclerosis (Morimoto et al. 1987; Schwinzer and Wonigeit 1990).

There may be other reasons why lymphocyte phenotyping does not often correlate with disease. Since there is no standard instrumentation or methodology to phenotype lymphocytes, each laboratory develops its own data. Variations in exposure patterns or concentrations of immunotoxicants may have different immunotoxic effects. Also, the effect of an immunosuppressive agent creates the possibility of subclinical infections in patients. For these reasons, it is difficult to determine whether phenotypic alterations are caused by suppression or infection.

Lymphocyte Transformation

One of the most widely used in vitro assessments for cell-mediated immunity is the lymphocyte transformation test (LTT) in which the ability of lymphocytes to undergo a rapid burst of cellular division is determined after challenge with nonspecific mitogens or antigens. Mononuclear cells (lymphocytes and monocytes) from peripheral blood are incubated with the stimulant over several doses, which encompass both optimal and suboptimal concentrations, for 3–5 days depending on whether mitogen or specific antigen is used. In a number of immunodeficiency states, subjects respond in a normal manner to optimal concentrations of mitogen or antigen; however, decreased reactivity to suboptimal concentrations is often observed (Ziegler, Hansen, and Penny 1975). At the optimal time interval, the cells are pulsed with ^{3}H-thymidine. Because the ^{3}H-thymidine is incorporated into nucleic acid during cellular division, the amount of intracellular radiolabel in counts per minute (CPM) is proportional to the extent of cellular proliferation. By incubating separate sets of cells in autologous serum or pooled human serum, one is able to discern whether defects are caused by inherent cellular defects or serum factors that inhibit proliferation. In inflammatory states the presence of elevated acute-phase reactants in the autologous serum can inhibit mitogen-stimulated proliferation.

Several different mitogens and antigens can be used to stimulate human T-cell proliferation. Purified soluble phytohemagglutinin induces mitosis in most T cells. Depending on the concentration, concanavalin A can stimulate either helper or suppressor cells. Pokeweed mitogen stimulates both B and T cells, whereas bacterial LPS is a B-cell mitogen. Since nonspecific mitogens stimulate lymphocytes in a polyclonal fashion, a greater proportion of them respond, and the incubation time need not be long. Most of the antigens used in skin sensitivity studies can also be used in the LTT, but a longer incubation period is required since far fewer antigen-specific cells are going to respond.

There is variability in the LTT response to mitogens or antigen. The response varies within a population and in the same individual over time. Some of this variability can be attributed to variation in T- and B-cell numbers and/or the functional status of the test cells. Most of the variability can be attributed to culture conditions or media additives used in the culture matrix. Because of the variability in the LTT response, studies should be repeated at several time intervals.

Data from the LTTs can be expressed commonly by the stimulation index (SI), which is simply the ratio between the stimulated and control cultures. Generally, an SI ratio >3.0 is considered a positive response. When one is using the SI method, it is assumed that technical factors influencing the data affected the control and stimulated cultures in an equal manner. However, lymphocytes from patients with AIDS or Wiskott–Aldrich syndrome may have highly activated lymphocytes that incorporate the radiolabel without stimulation; i.e., such cells are already in a state of activation. Often this lowers the SI ratio to abnormal values. In this case, examination and presentation of control and stimulated CPM are a useful tool in data analyses. Of the various methods used to evaluate data, the most reproducible results have been associated with data being expressed as a percentage of normal response (Hosking and Balloch 1983).

Certain clinical states may affect the proliferation of T cells. The ingestion of therapeutic drugs such as prednisolone and cytoxan can cause a decrease in the proliferation of T cells. Similar effects can be induced by viral infections, pregnancy, and old age.

If the LTT data indicate normal lymphocyte proliferation in response to mitogens, additional studies can be undertaken to determine whether the monocytes produce cytokines necessary for chemotaxis of accessory cells or activation of immunocompetent cells. If necessary, studies on the functional capacity of monocytes would be undertaken. The response to chemotactic material, support of T-cell proliferation, and presentation of antigen can be explored further in laboratory studies.

T-Cytotoxic Cells

The functional status of cells involved in defense against cancers or viral-infected cells can be probed in two ways, the mixed lymphocyte reaction (MLR) and the cytotoxic lymphocyte (CTL) assays. The assays take advantage of the fact that in the MLR lymphocytes from one individual will respond to allogeneic lymphocytes in a manner similar to an immunologic response to a mitogen, whereas in the CTL, cytotoxic T cells (T_c) lyse target cells bearing processed antigen. The difference between the two reactions is that lymphocytes, responding to allogeneic cells, interact with class II markers, whereas T_c lymphocytes interacting with tumor or infected cells are already sensitized and will recognize target antigen in context with class I MHC molecules and the CD3/TCR-associated antigen receptor structure. In the MLR assay, stimulator or target lymphocytes are irradiated or treated with mitomycin C to prevent their activation and cellular division. The inability of the stimulator cells to divide is often confirmed by incubation with PHA. Responder lymphocytes to be tested are incubated with the stimulator cells, and, at the optimal time point, ^{3}H-thymidine is added to the culture. Following a defined pulse interval, the cells are harvested, and the amount of intracellular radiolabel incorporation is determined.

Care must be taken in the interpretation of the data from MLR assays. A reduced response in the assay may be caused by a suspected immune defect or by a similarity of MHC markers between the test and responder lymphocytes. To distinguish between the two possibilities, the MHC marker phenotype of both stimulator and test lymphocytes should be determined. Data from MLR assays can be expressed in three different ways. The average CPM for control and test cells is a common method but has a drawback in that it alone does not consider the data from the control measurements. The response can also be expressed as the stimulation ratio (SR). The SR is simply the test value divided by the autologous control for the responding individual. An uncommon data expression method is the comparison of test data to a standard population. Generally, a 50% reduction in the normal response is considered to be abnormal.

The conventional CTL assay is used to study the antigen-specific cytolytic capacity of T cells. After incubation with stimulator cells, the cytotoxic T cells are recovered, washed, and incubated with fresh ^{51}Cr-labeled target cells. As target cells lyse from contact with specific T_c cells, they give up this particular label in proportion to how many cells are dying. After four hours of incubation, the amount of chromium release in the system relative to the spontaneous (i.e., background) and maximum release (100% lysis with acid as a positive control) is determined.

An innovative method to assess polyclonal activation of test cytotoxic T cells involves the use of radiolabeled anti-CD3–producing hybridoma B cells. The anti-CD3 on the B-cell surfaces in effect substitutes for antigen and triggers reactions between the B target cell anti-CD3 and the TCR on the test lymphocytes. The result of T-cell cytolytic action on the B cells is release of the label (Hoffman et al. 1985).

NK Cells

Studies of natural killer (NK)-cell function are undertaken when an individual has a clear history of selective recurrent viral infections or tumors or has been exposed to agents known to depress NK-cell function. The NK cell is the major defense mechanism against herpes and adenoviruses (Biron, Byron, and Sullivan 1989). Also, NK cells play a critical role in defense against sarcomas that metastasize via the blood (Masuyama et al. 1988; Hanna and Fidler 1980), and since the major reservoir of NK cells is in the peripheral blood, their presence and intact function are vital. In humans, LAK cells are simply NK cells that have been activated by either interferon or (usually) interleukin-2 (Grimm et al. 1982; Ortaldo, Mason, and Overton 1966).

Chromium release assays are also used to probe the functional capacity of both NK and LAK cells. Assuming that normal numbers of NK cells are present in peripheral blood (10–15%), mononuclear cells are incubated with ^{51}Cr-labeled K562 erythroleukemia cells to yield several different effector-to-target ratios. During the 4–hr incubation period, the NK cells make close contact with the target cells, trigger the NK cytotoxic apparatus, and deliver a lethal hit to the target cells. It is believed that NK cells recycle and attach to other target cells.

Assays to probe the function of LAK cells are simply modifications of the

NK-cell assay. The major difference in the assays is that the NK cells are preincubated with the activating cytokine. The cells are then incubated for 4 hr with ^{51}Cr-labeled K562 cells (NK and LAK sensitive) or Burkitt's lymphoma-derived Raji cells (NK insensitive and LAK sensitive). Activated LAK cells lyse both the K562 and Raji cells, whereas the NK cells lyse only the K562 cells. Hence, activation of LAK cells by cytokines expands the cytolytic capacity of LAK cells to tumor cells not susceptible to lysis by NK cells. Because of the increase in cytolytic capacity of the stimulated cells, the effector-to-target cell (E : T) ratios are usually lower than that used in NK-cell assays.

The function of NK cells is depressed in lymphoreticular and bladder malignancies. Other diseases with reduced NK activity include collagen vascular diseases, aplastic anemia, and cardiomyopathy. The most severe defect has been reported in subjects with Chediak–Higashi disease. In these patients, NK cells bind to target cells in a normal manner but fail to deliver a lethal hit to the target cell. Usually, NK cells from the blood of these patients have less than 10% of normal NK activity (Roder et al. 1983).

Antibody-Dependent Cellular Cytotoxicity

Although the in vivo relevance of the phenomenon is unproven, monocytes, eosinophils, NK cells, and CD3/Ti-expressing T_c lymphocytes can lyse antibody-coated ^{51}Cr-labeled target cells. All of these cells express Fc receptors that interact with IgG antibody, irrespective of antigen reactivity, bound to target cells (Lanier et al. 1983; Lanier, Kipps, and Phillips 1985). Because of the dependence on antibody and extracellular lysis, the process is termed antibody-dependent cellular cytotoxicity (ADCC).

The effector cell may be dependent on the nature of the target and the source of the antibody. Chicken erythrocytes coated with rabbit antichicken IgG are lysed by monocytes and/or lymphocytes. Conversely, monocytes are the sole effector cells in assays using human red cells coated with anti-ABO isotype antibodies as target cells. Human Chang liver cells coated with rabbit anti-liver-cell antibody are lysed by lymphocytes (Poplack et al. 1976). The reason for the different spectrum of effector cell activity is unclear. In the chicken erythrocyte assay, lysis may be initiated after interaction between the cell-bound antibody and the effector cells. In the case of the Chang liver cells, interaction may require the recognition of MHC marker in addition to the Fc portion of the antibody.

Monocytes

Peripheral blood monocytes constitute approximately 15% of the total mononuclear cell population. Since these cells perform several immunologic functions, several opportunities are afforded for functional assays. In response to chemotactic factors such as C5a and leukotriene B_4, the cells accumulate at the site of inflammation. After recognition of the antigen via Fc receptors that bind antibody–antigen complexes or C3b receptor binding, the antigen is ingested, digested, and presented to the T and B cells in combination with class II markers. Also, monocytes release IL-1 and tumor necrosis factor (Johnson 1988).

By using flow cytometry, it is possible to enumerate monocytes with Fc or complement receptors as well as class II markers. Metabolic and microbicidal capability can be ascertained by assays similar to those described for neutrophils below. To determine whether monocytes can serve as accessory cells that support T-cell proliferation, purified monocytes and T cells are mixed together and stimulated with a polyclonal T-cell activator such as PHA or incubated with allogeneic T cells and stimulator cells in a mixed lymphocyte reaction (Rosenwasser and Rosenthal 1978). The IL-1 and tumor necrosis factor can be measured in assays described in subsequent sections. Although the approach is mainly used for assessment in animals, great potential exists in human immunotoxicology to monitor the expression of MHC class II molecule expression in monocytes or other antigen-presenting cells, as this seems to be an important function capable of being modified by environmental agents.

Skin Testing

When repeated infections suggest a defect in cellular immunity, initial studies are undertaken to determine the status of the patient's delayed hypersensitivity responses to common, "recall" skin test antigens. It is assumed that most persons will have antigen-specific memory lymphocytes directed toward streptokinase-streptodornase, *Candida albicans*, mumps, trichophytin (from a dermophilic fungus), and possibly purified protein derivatives of tubercle bacilli. Following intradermal injection, normal subjects will mount a delayed hypersensitivity response (erythema and induration) within 48 to 72 hr. Normal subjects will respond to two or more of the antigens with skin reactions of greater than 5 mm of induration (swelling).

It is also useful to determine whether the patient can be actively sensitized to a universally sensitizing antigen. In the sensitization protocol, 1–chloro-2,4–dinitrobenzene (DNCB) is painted on the skin several times a week. After resting, the patient is challenged with a dilute antigen. Active sensitization results in a classical skin test reaction.

4. Accessory Functions

The recognition that certain primary immunodeficiency diseases may have adequate antigen-specific functions, but still be defective in protecting the host from opportunistic infections prompted the examination of the effector accessories of immune responses for defects. Similarly, important secondary immunodeficiency diseases exhibit defects in these accessory cells and molecules, and they should not be overlooked in immunotoxicity testing.

Neutrophils

Neutrophils play a critical role in defense against bacterial and fungal infections. The most common test used to study PMN function is the nitroblue tetrazolium test (NBT). Activated PMNs will phagocytize dye–protein complexes and incorporate them into phagosomes. There, in the presence of superoxide, the yellow dye is reduced to an insoluble blue-colored formazan. Dye reduction may be determined either by direct microscopy or spectrophotometrically after extraction of the complexes by dioxan (Hudson and Hay 1989). Since fixed cells can be examined for the presence of the dye, the qualitative method is simple and inexpensive (Baehner and Nathan 1968). A positive NBT does not exclude the possibility of a microbicidal defect. Some patients with severe defects may produce enough superoxide to give a positive NBT but fail to produce additional superoxide when stimulated in stimulation assays (Lew et al. 1981). Hence, additional studies should be considered.

Assays may be undertaken to confirm the bacterial killing capacity of peripheral blood phagocytic cells. Usually, PMNs are incubated with opsonized staphylococci for 60 min. After lysis of extracellular bacteria with lysostaphin, the neutrophils are lysed, and the number of surviving intracellular bacteria is determined. In normal peripheral blood phagocytic cells, the survival rate is less than 5.0% (Metcalf et al. 1986).

If the bacterial killing assays suggest a defect in the functional capacity, additional studies can be undertaken to define the location of the lesion in the metabolic pathways. Although there are numerous pathways required for normal energy production via glucose utilization, this discussion is directed toward the documentation of defects in the sequence of events involved in the killing process. The quantitation of the superoxide radical takes advantage of the fact that the superoxide electrons shift to a higher energy level. When the electron returns to the ground state, light is emitted, resulting in chemiluminescence. The addition of a cyclic hydrazide (luminol) enhances the chemiluminescence, which can be determined in a liquid scintillation counter that has been configured so that its photomultiplier tubes have been taken out of coincident setting. Although not commonly available in the laboratory, electron spin resonance (ESR) with 5,5-dimethyl-1-pyroline-N-oxide as the trap can be used to quantitate hydroxyl radicals produced during phagocytosis (Rosen and Klebanoff 1979). The detection of H_2O_2 is usually done following the indirect oxidation of hydrogen donors such as scopoletin (7-hydrocoumarin). In the first stage of the assay, H_2O_2 reacts with horseradish peroxidase. The reaction products oxidize scopoletin, causing a reduction in the normal fluorescence (Boveris, Martino, and Stoppani 1977).

Occasionally there is a failure to synthesize mediator-containing granules during differentiation and maturation (Gallin et al. 1982). Specialized laboratory techniques are necessary to document defective granule formation. In standard histochemical staining, the azurophilic granules stain with less intensity than controls. In some instances, the cell is devoid of granules. More frequently, the granules appear as clear vesicles (Parmley, Tzeng Baehner, and Boxer 1983).

The neutrophils may also have defects in the synthesis or expression of surface glycoproteins that facilitate adherence to other cells or tissue. Of major importance is the complement CR3 receptor on neutrophils. The CR3 is normally fixed to the bacterial cell surface during complement activation (opsonization). Defects can be documented by flow cytometric or immunofluorescent studies using monoclonal antibodies (e.g., anti-CD11) to the CR3 to ascertain the presence of the receptor.

Other factors may also be important in neutrophil function. Receptors for adhesion factors (LFA-1) may control whether the neutrophils bind to endothelial cells. To probe function defects in adhesion, radiolabeled neutrophils can be incubated with cultured endothelial cells (Hoover, Briggs, and Karnovsky 1978).

Other PMN abnormalities have been described. There are defects in surface protein associated with defective cellular spreading and increased chemotaxis (Springer and Anderson 1986). Defects in cell movement and locomotion can be determined in skin window studies (Addison, Johnson, and Shaw 1982) or modified Boyden chambers (Addison and Babbage 1976). In the skin window assay, the rate of cells accumulating in an abrasion is determined. The evolution of the inflammatory response in the lesion can also be determined. During chemotactic studies using Boyden chambers, phagocytic cells migrate through semipermeable membranes toward a chemotactic agent. However, it is often difficult to differentiate between an increased random movement and directed chemotaxis.

Complement Function

The functional integrity of the complement system is measured in CH_{50} assays. The assay determines the ability of diluted test serum to lyse 50% of a standard sheep red blood cell suspension coated with IgM antibody (hemolysin). The reason for using a 50% endpoint is that a certain percentage of any erythrocyte suspension is extremely resistant to lysis. In addition, the 50% endpoint is more accurately determined by probit analysis than is a 100% endpoint. Since there are several variations of the assay, each laboratory determines its own standard and normal range. A normal value in the CH_{50} assay virtually excludes the possibility of a complement defect.

Immunochemical assays can be implemented to measure levels of C3, C4, C1 esterase inhibitor, and factor B, wherein specific antisera are used to quantitate the unknown. These assays may include single radial immunodiffusion, rocket electrophoresis, and nephelometry. The data may give information concerning the status of both the classical and alternative pathways. A normal C4 level with low C3 suggests activation of the alternative pathway. The activation of the alternative pathway can be confirmed immunoelectrophoretically by demonstrating factor B cleavage. Decrements in C4, C3, and CH_{50} are more associated with activation of the classical complement pathway. Normal C4, C2, and C3 with reduced CH_{50} may suggest defects in the terminal components. Low C3 and CH_{50} levels without particular reference to a specific pathway may be a reflection of continuous complement consumption in subjects with active immune complex diseases such as systemic lupus erythematosus, glomerulonephritis, and selected forms of vasculitis.

Cytokines

Methods used to quantitate cytokines can be broadly separated into immunochemical and biological proliferation assays. ELISA and radioimmunoassays have been attempted to quantitate IL-1, IL-4, and γ-interferon in a variety of biological matrices (Dijkmans and Billiau 1988; Lewis et al. 1988). However, these methods are relatively insensitive for analyses in peripheral blood. Moreover, the antibody methods determine only the total cytokine present in the sample, and functional and nonfunctional forms of the molecule cannot be differentiated in the assay system. Hence, the assay may provide only minimal biologically relevant information (Schumacher et al. 1988). Moreover, there may be false-negative reactions as a result of interference from factors present in the serum samples (Lonneman et al. 1988).

More sensitive methods utilize proliferation assays, which are based on the incorporation of ^{3}H-thymidine into the nucleic acid of dividing indicator cells. Several indicator cells in a costimulation system have been used for IL-1 analyses. Thymocytes from young C3H/HeJ mice proliferate only when incubated with both PHA and IL-1. Cloned albumin-specific T-helper cells (D10.G4.1) have also been substituted for thymocytes. These cells proliferate only when incubated with IL-1 and the antigen presented on the surface of MHC compatible accessory cells (Dinarello and Savage 1989). Costimulation is not necessary for the measurement of other cytokines. A cell line derived from the spleen of C57BL/6 mice can be used in IL-2 assays. This line, CTTL-2, is a cloned cytotoxic T cell that is dependent on IL-2 for growth and proliferation (Cantrell and Smith 1984; Paliard et al. 1988). These cells respond to very low levels of IL-2, making them useful for analyses of IL-2 in blood samples. At the present time quantitation of IL-4 involves using an IL-4–specific monoclonal antibody (11B11) in an inhibition assay. The measurement of IL-5 relies on proliferation of a B-cell (BCL1) hybridoma line (Moller 1988), whereas IL-6 assays use the B9 hybridoma as the indicator cell (Aarden et al. 1987). Measurement of IL-7 involves a more time-consuming and tedious assay. Long-term murine Whitlock–Witte bone marrow cultures are used as a source of pre-B (B220$^+$, cytoplasmic μ chain$^+$) and progenitor B cells (B220$^-$, sIgM$^-$), which are used as IL-7 target cells (Whitlock, Robertson, and Witte 1984; Namen et al. 1988)

Although the proliferation assays are highly sensitive to low concentrations of cytokines, they may not respond in a specific manner. In the IL-1 assay systems, other cytokines present in samples (e.g., tumor necrosis factor, IL-2, IL-6) can induce proliferation of the indicators. The D10.G4.1 cells proliferate vigorously when exposed to IL-2. Hence, there may be false-positive reactions in select assay systems. False-negative reactions are also possible. Nonoptimal concentrations of some cytokines and incorrect stage in cell cycle or even stage of development of the indicator cells can inhibit the proliferation of the indicator cells. These factors should be taken into consideration in the interpretation of data.

The interferons have multiple regulation functions as well as antiviral defense functions that can be explored in different bioassays. γ-Interferon can induce the expression of MHC class II markers on select cells. A cell line (Colo-225) derived from a human colon adenocarcinoma is often used as the target cell. After incubation with fluids containing γ-interferon, cells are reacted with biotinylated antibody directed toward nonpolymorphic epitopes on the human HLA-Dr marker. After amplification with streptavidin–fluorescein isothiocyanate, the cells expressing MHC markers are quantitated by flow cytometric analyses.

The functional capacity of interferons to inhibit viral replication and cell lysis can be explored in tissue culture systems. Cell lines differ in the elicitation of antiviral effects induced by interferon. The trisomy human cell line GM2504 responds to both α- and β-interferon. Assays for IFN-γ use the human lung A549 cell line (Rubenstein, Familetti, and Pestka 1981). The antiviral activity is ascertained as inhibition of the cytopathic effect (CPE) after infection with human encephalomyocarditis virus (Yeh, McBride, and Green 1982). Interferon subtype neutralizing antibodies can also be used to ascertain which interferon is being produced (Vogel, Havell, and Spitalny 1986).

Tumor necrosis factor (TNF) consists of two forms produced primarily by macrophages (TNF-α) or T cells (TNF-β). The observation that TNF lyses sensitive cells can be used as the basis for assay systems. Total TNF can be measured in a simple, highly sensitive assay using TNF-sensitive L929 fibroblast cell lines treated with actinomycin D (Wang et al. 1985). The effect is scored visually after staining with crystal violet. Other assays used to measure TNF are more labor intensive, less sensitive, or require the use of radioisotopes (Chen, McKinnon, and Koren 1985; Espevik and Nissen-Meyer 1986).

D. ASSESSMENT OF IMMUNE FUNCTION IN ANIMALS

Prospective studies are aimed at attempting to assess the immunotoxic potential of selected agents or processes in advance of human contact. In screening for such effects, no single test can comprehensively predict all of the possible effects a given agent might have on something as intricate and complicated as the immune system. For this reason a flexible tier approach to using selective, validated tests in such screening has been developed (Dean et al. 1982). The tier approach is discussed in more detail in Chapter 12. Data from these studies neither establish the biological relevance of any negative or positive effects nor define possible effects in humans and seldom establish mechanisms. Extrapolation of positive or negative immunotoxicity data to the human condition is difficult for reasons discussed in more detail in Chapter 10.

A more suitable approach to animal testing is the problem-solving approach. After careful delineation of the possible effects on humans, mechanistic models are developed in animals. The design of animal toxicology studies should meet certain criteria. The choice of the test should be carefully considered on the basis of adsorption, metabolism, and excretion of the test chemical. These parameters should be similar to those expected in man. In addition, the route of exposure should be similar to that naturally encountered in human exposure and administered over a concentration range where the high dose should cause some kind of overt toxicity without causing mortality in test animals. Generally, the high dose is less than the LD_{10}.

1. Indirect Immunotoxic Effects

In some instances, the immunosuppressive effects may be caused by stress-related or other indirect immunosuppressive effects. Physical, auditory, or sensory stress initiates the release of corticosteroids, which cause alterations in immune function in rodents (Weiss et al. 1981; Monjan and Collector 1977). In high concentrations, corticosteroids can induce lymphoid tissue atrophy and/or functional defects in lymphocytes. The functional defects can be manifested in antibody responses to thymic dependent antigens (Munck, Guire, and Hollbrook 1984). In some species, steroids alter the normal lymphocyte trafficking patterns through the body (Fauci and Dale 1975) which may be responsible for the immunosuppressive effects induced by Oxisuran (van Dijk et al. 1975).

It is often difficult to distinguish between corticosteroid- and test-article induced stress. However, several measurements may be helpful. In normal animals, adrenal weight and morphology can be an indicator of increased steroid activity. Levels of circulating corticosteroid can also be measured. One discriminator of corticosteroid- and treatment-related effects to consider is the use of adrenalectomized animals, but the essential contribution of these endocrines to the normal response is lost.

Other substances can exert indirect effects on lymphocytes. In addition to steroids, most immunocompetent cells have receptors for growth hormones, catecholamines, and acetylcholine, to name but a few. Interaction between ligands and the cellular receptors may either suppress or enhance the function of specific immunocompetent lymphocyte subsets.

Indirect, nonhormonal immunotoxic effects are also possible. Hepatotoxins cause the release of acute-phase inflammatory proteins that are immunosuppressive (Munson 1987). Other suppressive nitrogenous compounds also accumulate in the blood following liver injury. Moreover, in response to test material exposure, animals may fail to ingest proper amounts of food and water. Low body weights combined with deficiencies in amino acids, vitamin B_6, and minerals (e.g., zinc) can cause immunosuppression (Hudson, Saben, and Emslie 1974).

2. Standard Toxicology Endpoints

In most laboratory studies, total and differential blood cell counts are performed as part of a screen for toxic effects. A decrease in the erythrocyte count may be caused by toxic effects on the bone marrow erythrocyte-producing cells or the production of antibodies directed toward the red blood cells. Changes in the total leukocyte count may be caused by a number of toxic factors. Increases in specific subsets suggest inflammatory or malignant (lymphocytes, PMNs) processes or allergic (eosinophils) reactions. Decreased percentages suggest immune dysfunction.

Lymphoid organ weights (e.g., thymus, spleen, lymph node) have often been used as an index of immunotoxicity but at best are very imprecise. From a practical standpoint, accurate and reproducible measurements are difficult. In young animals, the thymus is embedded in a fatty tissue matrix. Because the thymic and fatty tissue closely resemble each other, it is difficult to separate the two. For this reason, thymic weights in normal young animals with no histological abnormalities may vary by 20%. More significant decreases in thymic weight may, however, be an indicator of defective cell-mediated immunity. Secondary lymphoid organs such as lymph nodes are also often weighed. Because of their small size and the difficulty of excision, the lymph node weights vary greatly. Splenic weights may also increase or decrease in relation to external factors. In most species, the spleen is an immunocompetent organ that is also involved in erythropoiesis, myelopoiesis, and removal of aged red blood cells. Therefore, increased splenic weights may reflect increased production or degradation of erythrocytes. Conversely, euthanasia with barbiturates can cause contraction of the spleen, reducing the total weight.

The cellularity (determination of the number of nucleated cells in an organ), viability, and histopathology of lymphoid organs and bone marrow may be useful in the assessment of immunotoxicity when the immune system is the suspected target organ. The methodology is rather insensitive in that more than 30% reduction must be obtained to be biologically relevant.

Viability stains determine the percentage of dead cells in cell populations. The most common vital stain used to determine viability is trypan blue. Living cells do not take up the dye, but dead or dying cells readily internalize the dye. The presence of protein in the media often makes interpretation of data difficult, since the dye binds readily to extracellular protein, preventing it from entering dead cells.

In the normal histological evaluation of lymphoid organs and bone marrow, the tissue structure, types of cells, and cell structure are determined. The thymus is examined because it is involved in the proper development of the T cell and the cell-mediated immune system. Abnormalities would suggest defects in the immune mechanisms involving T cells. In the secondary lymphoid tissue, the T and B cells are segregated in defined areas. T cells are segregated in the paracortical region in lymph nodes, whereas the splenic T cells are localized in the periarteriolar sheath (PALS). The B cells are predominant in lymph node germinal centers and splenic B-cell follicles. Hence, decrements in cell numbers in prescribed regions may suggest immunotoxic effects. Histopathological analyses requires a reduction of approximately 60% of the total cells before an event is considered to be biologically relevant (Irons, 1985).

The normality of the femoral bone marrow can be ascertained by two methods. Generally, a bone marrow smear is used to define cellularity, which is expressed as the myeloid:erythroid (M:E) ratio. In the mouse, the normal ratio is 1.49:1.0 with a standard deviation of 0.47. The ratio in the rat varies with age. In rats less than 1 month of age, the ratio is 0.62:1.0. The ratio in older rats varies from 1.75:1.0 to 1.93:1.0 (Schalm, Jain, and Carroll 1975). The disadvantage of the bone marrow smear is that it is possible to have reduced numbers of total cells with a normal M:E ratio. Occasionally, bone marrow cross sections are used for histopathological analysis. The histology may be compromised by the fact that the bone is decalcified prior to analysis. In spite of the problems associated with analyses, examination of the bone marrow has proven to be a sensitive indicator of TCDD toxicity (Luster et al. 1980).

In assessment of possible immunotoxic effects, the cellularity, viability, and histopathology are compared. A change in the viability may suggest an immunotoxic effect on that organ. When the cellularity and the viability are evaluated concurrently, the data will determine the extent of cell death within the total nucleated cell population. The combination of viability, histopathological data, and cellularity may help determine changes in organ structure suggesting immunotoxicity.

Special immunohistochemistry can be used to identify immunocompetent cells in paraffin-fixed or fresh-frozen samples. Antibody-mediated, immunoperoxidase-amplified stains have been used to identify monocytes and B cells. Attempts have been made to identify T and B cells in formalin-fixed, paraffin-embedded tissue, but the approach has been unsuccessful. Epitopes are altered or deleted from immunocompetent cells following formalin treatment. Antibodies directed toward antigens on unfixed cells will not react in the assay systems. Fresh-frozen tissue, however, can be used in histochemical stains.

Identification and quantification of serum components are often used in screens for immunotoxic events. The albumin:globulin ratio is a common determination. Since albumin is the most abundant protein in serum, fluctuations in levels may indicate altered protein synthesis (e.g., liver damage) or increased excretion (e.g., kidney damage). The globulin fraction consists of various antibody isotypes, and changes may signal a derangement in synthesis (decreases) or neoplastic conditions (increases). Determination of specific immunoglobulin isotype levels may help to confirm the effect on the globulin fractions. Assays similar to those described for human antibody quantitation (radial immunodiffusion, nephelometry, and ELISA) are commonly used in animal studies.

3. Flow Cytometry

Flow cytometric methods can be used to enumerate lymphocyte subsets in both the rat and the mouse. In the mouse, a well-defined battery of antibodies can be used to enumerate all subsets as well as the activation status of the immune system. The technology of enumeration of lymphocyte subsets in the rat is evolving with the generation of antibodies directed toward phenotypic markers (Table 9–4), but care must be taken in that some antirat antibodies have multiple specificities. New dual fluorochrome labeling technology may allow better resolution of lymphocyte subsets and natural killer cells (Woda et al. 1984). This technology has been used to study the effects of bis(tris-n-butyltin) oxide on the rat immune system (Vos et al. 1984).

TABLE 9–4.   Common Monoclonal Antibodies Used to Phenotype Rat and Mouse Lymphocytes

	Cluster Designation	Mouse	Rat
T Cells	CD5	Ly-1	OX19
T helper/amplifier	CD4	Ly-4	W3/25
T suppressor/cytotoxic	CD8	Ly-2,3	OX8
Natural killer cells	CD16	Ly-17	OX19−,OX8+
Complement receptors	CD11b	Ly-6	—
Activated T cells	CD25	TAC	ART-18

4. Antibody-Mediated Immunity

Ex vivo immunologic assays have been the cornerstone in animal immunotoxicology studies. Many of these assays were developed for use in human systems and adapted for use in animal studies. Others were developed specifically for use in animal systems. A unique and commonly used assay in animals is the hemolytic plaque-forming cell (PFC) assay, which permits visualization of the number of antibody-producing cells in the spleen. In mechanistic terms, mice are primed to produce antibodies by immunization with sheep erythrocytes. Four days after a second immunization (the optimal time period for synthesis and secretion of antibody), animals are sacrificed, and isolated splenic cells are mixed with sheep cells and suspended in agarose (Jerne and Nordin 1963; Cunningham and Szenberg 1968). Antibodies diffusing from the B cells react with the immobilized erythrocytes. When guinea pig complement is added to the agarose, the antibody-coated sheep cells are lysed, leaving a clear zone or plaque around the antibody-producing B cells. In the direct assay, B cells producing primarily IgM are enumerated. Under the physical conditions of the assay only IgM antibodies lyse the erythrocytes. The number of IgG- or IgA-producing B cells can be determined by indirect methods wherein anti-IgM is first added to prevent the formation of IgM plaques. Anti-IgG or anti-IgA is then added to the mixture after the synthesized antibody has reacted with the SRBCs. Plaques are scored after the addition of complement, which becomes activated by the antibody complexes on the cell surface.

Although this assay is simple in design and implementation, careful consideration must be given to technical factors that influence it. Animals used as splenic donors must be free of endemic murine viruses. The viruses reduce the ability of the B cells to proliferate in vivo. Second, only selected production lots of fetal calf serum (FCS) will support the ex vivo production of antibody. Moreover, erythrocytes from certain animals will not react with antibodies produced ex vivo by B cells. Hence, reagents must be carefully screened. Third, the guinea pig complement used in the assay must be extensively adsorbed to remove nonspecific reactivity (Mishell and Dutton 1966).

The production of antibody to sheep erythrocytes requires the interactions among T cells, macrophages, and B cells. Hence, the response is T cell dependent. Non-T-cell dependent antigens can also be used in the assay. Trinitrophenol (TNP) linked to Ficoll or *Brucella abortus* can activate B cells in a T-cell-independent manner, but terminal differentiation into antibody-producing B cells is dependent on the presence of interleukins (Mond et al. 1983). These antigens have been designated as T-cell-regulated antigens, type II, to differentiate them from true T-cell-independent antigens, type I. Bacterial LPS is a type I antigen that does not require T cells or T-cell products for activation or terminal differentiation.

Lipopolysaccharide can be used in plaque-forming assays to measure polyclonal antibody responses. Because the antibody produced in these assays has undefined specificity, alternative methods are necessary to develop the plaques. In this context, protein A (which binds the Fc portion of murine IgG) is bound to sheep erythrocytes. Mixtures of B cells and the protein A erythrocytes are combined using the method of Jerne and Nordin (1963). After the newly synthesized antibody has bound to the protein A, antimouse IgG is added to the culture. The antiserum binds to the IgG bound to protein A. This complex activates guinea pig complement, and the erythrocytes are lysed.

Decrements in antibody synthesis only suggest disturbances in humoral immunity. Additional studies must be undertaken to determine which cellular component of the system is defective. Lymphocyte transformation, using lipopolysaccharide, has been used as a probe for B-cell function in mice. The proliferative response is quantified by intracellular incorporation of ^{3}H-thymidine. Data suggest that the assay is not exquisitely sensitive. Moreover, LPS-induced proliferation is not a direct correlate of the PFC response (Luster et al. 1988). This observation is not unexpected, since additional functional and metabolic changes take place before antibody is produced.

The relationship between a decreased proliferative response and disease susceptibility in animals is unclear. However, a decrease in the LPS-induced mitogen response in lymphocytes is associated with increased mortality to influenza virus and increased susceptibility to *Plasmodium* infection.

With flow cytometry techniques, it is possible to ascertain cellular changes that occur immediately after B-cell activation. Increases in calcium concentration and the expression of MHC class II markers can be used as activation markers. In the calcium flux assay, purified B cells are mixed with INDO-1 dye. The B cells are then activated by the addition of anti-IgG, which cross-links cell-bound immunoglobulin. With a flow cytometer, intracellular calcium changes are demonstrable 10 sec after activation (Thompson, Scher, and Schaeffer 1984; Ranson, Morris, and Cambier 1986). Anti-IgG can also be used to activate B cells, which express increased MHC class II markers. After addition of fluorescein-labeled anti-Ia (a mouse MHC designation), cells can be enumerated by flow cytometry (Mond et al. 1981).

Various immunization protocols can be used to ascertain whether animals can mount a de novo antibody response to specific antigens. Commonly, ovalbumin, tetanus toxoid, or *Trichinella spiralis* is used as a T-cell-dependent antigen. For a proper response, functional T_h cells, B cells, and macrophages are necessary in the affector stage of the response. In mice, LPS can be used to directly stimulate antibody from B cells (T-cell-independent antigen, type I). The antigen-specific IgM and/or IgG antibody responses to the T-cell-dependent, type II antigens can be measured. ELISA is the method of choice for the determination of antigen-specific antibodies.

5. Cell-Mediated Immunity

There is a greater range of in vivo and in vitro methods available to study cell-mediated immune responses in animals.

Lymphocyte Transformation

Polyclonal activators can be used to measure the proliferative responses of T cells. The mode of action and the necessity for accessory cells depends on the agent. Phorbol myristate acetate (PMA) plus ionomycin increases the intracellular free calcium and activates protein kinase C. Hence, accessory cells are not needed. Anti-Thy-1 (a universal murine T-cell marker) or CD3 indirectly or directly cross-links the CD3/TCR complex. Both antibodies require the presence of accessory cells for proliferation. Accessory cells are also necessary for proliferation induced by staphylococcal enterotoxins. These toxins react with variable portions of β chains in the TCR. Different toxins (A, B, and E) have diverse specificity. These reagents are useful for activation studies and determining defects in the synthesis of β chains (Marrack and Kappler 1989). Commonly used T-cell mitogens are PHA and Con A. Both mitogens indirectly cross-link the TCR while requiring signals from accessory cells.

Decrements in the proliferative response to PHA have been associated with a susceptibility to infection with *Listeria* and *Plasmodium*. Since both of these organisms evoke a T-cell-mediated response, the correlation is not unexpected. In addition to the T-cell-mediated response, host defense against *Plasmodium* also involves T-cell-dependent antibody synthesis by B cells.

Cytotoxic Cell Assays

As with human assessment, it is important to differentiate the mixed lymphocyte reaction (MLR), used to test the proliferation capacity of T cells recognizing different MHC class II molecules, from the cytolytic lymphocyte reaction (CLR), used to measure the proliferation of T-killer or cytotoxic cells for antigens expressed by target cells in a MHC class I context. The methodology for both is similar to that described for humans; however, in the murine system, irradiated or mitomycin-C-treated allogeneic (H-2 or Mls loci) spleen cells are used as the stimulators. Frequently T cells are removed from this population by treatment with anti-Thy-1 and complement. This increases the ratio of antigen-presenting cells in the assay and reduces the possibility that cytokines produced by treated T cells influence the results.

Rat T cells respond vigorously in the MLR when there is a suitable incompatibility in responder and stimulator MHC markers (Cramer, Shonnard, and Gill 1974). In certain strains of mice, however, it is often difficult to generate a MLR when unfractionated splenic cells are used in the assay. This may be because accessory cell macrophages metabolize arginine to produce citrulline and nitric oxide. The nitric oxide is toxic to other cells in the incubation mixture.

The proliferation of T cells in the MLR should be verified by alternative means. Identification of dividing cells as $CD8^+$ cells is often helpful. Since only activated T cells produce IL-2, the demonstration of increased IL-2 levels in the MLR mixtures often confirms the proliferation of T-cytotoxic cells.

In place of allogeneic lymphocytes, P815 mastocytoma cells are often used as stimulator cells. The nonadherent T cells generated in the MLR can be recovered and used subsequently in chromium release assays with ^{51}Cr-labeled P815 cells to verify functional capability (Brunner, Mauel, and Cerottini 1968; Simpson and Chandler 1986). This assay is similar to that described for humans. Natural killer and lymphokine activated killer (LAK) cells are tested in a manner analogous to the human system. However, the target cells and the target:effector ratios are different. Most assays utilize the murine YAC-1 cells as targets. Since the spleen provides large numbers of cells, E : T ratios from 100 : 1 to 1 : 1 can be used in the assay. Data from murine studies should be interpreted with caution. The murine killer cell population consists of NK cells as well as T cells (Kalland et al. 1987; Ortaldo and Herberman 1984). In mice, definitive studies require the purification or enrichment of the NK-cell population.

In mice, reduced function of NK cells is associated with an increased susceptibility to challenge with B16F10 melanoma or PYB6 sarcoma tumor cells. Functional impairment in the MLR correlated with increased susceptibility to microorganisms evoking T-cell responses and to sarcomas (Luster et al. 1988).

Delayed Hypersensitivity

An in vivo method for evaluating the immunotoxic effect of a xenobiotic on cell-mediated immunity can be performed in animals by administering a xenobiotic concurrently with a potent contact allergen. The ability of the xenobiotic to interfere with the animal's response to this allergen is used as the measure of immunotoxicity. The test exists in many variations, but in one variation, young adult mice are sensitized to 4–ethoxymethene-2–phenoxazol-5–one (oxazolone) by painting both ears with a 3% solution of the oxazolone in 95% ethanol on days 0 and 3 (Sauers et al. 1986). On day 13, the animals are intraperitoneally injected with tritated thymidine. Twenty-four hours later, the left ear of each animal is painted with a 1% solution of the oxazolone in olive oil as a challenge antigen, and the right ear is painted with olive oil alone. Because of the prior sensitization, a delayed hypersensitivity reaction should occur in the left ear in response to the oxazolone, and proliferating cells will take up the label during nucleic acid synthesis. The reaction can be quantitated by removing tissue plugs from each ear and placing them in an appropriate counter. Data are presented as a sensitization index (cpm in the left ear plug/cpm in the right ear plug) and can be compared with indices from animals pretreated with the xenobiotic being tested for immunotoxicity prior to the oxazolone sensitization and/or throughout the development of the response. This test is not routinely performed in the assessment of immunotoxicity, nor is it included in the current tier approaches. Although it is considered too insensitive when compared to other in vitro measures, it may be a more relevant assay.

Macrophage Assays

In animal studies, macrophages are usually recovered from a peritoneal exudate, but it should be kept in mind that certain types of elicitation of these exudates in themselves activate the macrophages to be studied. Several types of macrophages can be elicited by injection with different compounds. Inflammatory macrophages can be elicited by exposure to thioglycollate and proteose–peptone broth (Takemura and Werb 1984). These macrophages have no microbicidal activity, but have enhanced secretion of neutral proteinases such as elastase (Werb, Babda, and Jones 1980). Exposure to certain microorganisms evokes a T-cell-mediated response in most species (Allison, Harington, and Birbeck 1966). The T cells or cytokine products activate the resident peritoneal macrophages. The activated cells usually have little secretory capacity but may have high metabolic activity with release of superoxide anion and hydroxyl radicals (Johnson 1981b). Increased microbicidal and tumoricidal activity is also demonstrable (North 1978; Karnovsky and Lazdins 1978). Often there is an intermediate type of macrophage that is not fully activated. This cell possesses most of the functional attributes of activated cells but lacks the capacity to lyse tumor cells. The term "primed macrophages" has been used for these cells, elicited by injection with pyran copolymer (MV-2).

Activated intraperitoneal macrophages usually demonstrate the entire range of functional capabilities in most laboratory studies. Activated macrophages have decreased Fc receptors for IgG and increased MHC class II markers. The numbers of cells expressing these markers can be determined by flow cytometry (Esekowitz et al. 1981). Several other markers can be used to identify activated cells. Objective markers of activated macrophages include decreased levels of 5'-nucleosidase, increased secretion of plasminogen activator, increased complement- or IgG-mediated phagocytosis, and increased spreading in culture (Johnson et al. 1983).

In addition to the production of superoxide anion and hydroxyl radical, increased utilization of glucose in metabolic pathways is a hallmark of an activated macrophage (Karnovsky and Lazdins 1978). Glucose uptake can be measured by two methods. Activated macrophages oxidize glucose via the hexose monophosphate shunt. Metabolic oxidation of radiolabeled $1-^{14}C$-glucose results in the production of $^{14}CO_2$. The CO_2 can be trapped by the addition of KOH, resulting in a stable compound measurable in a common scintillation counter. The second enzymatic method measures the NADP reduction mediated by hexokinase and glucose-6–phosphate. The quantitation of superoxide anion and hydroxyl radicals utilizes methods described previously.

Select macrophage-derived cytokines can also be measured. When stimulated with LPS, the cells release both IL-1 and tumor necrosis factor α. Both molecules can be measured in proliferation assays described in the discussion of human cytokines.

Macrophages are an integral part of the host defense against tumors. Macrophages activated or primed in vivo and recovered from peritoneal exudates selectively bind tumor cells in vitro (Johnson et al. 1983). However, only the activated macrophages spontaneously secrete a cytolytic protease (Russell, Doe, and McIntosch 1977).

In the laboratory, the macrophages can be tested for their ability to bind and destroy nonadherent tumor cells. The binding of chromium-labeled P815 mastocytoma cells to macrophage monolayers and their destruction can be measured (Marino, Whisnant, and Adams 1981). The secretion of the cytolytic protease into incubation supernates can be measured by testing fluids for the ability to lyse MCA-V cells, a methylcholanthrene-induced sarcoma from C57BL/6J mice (Adams 1980).

Rodent Cytokines

The methods used to measure murine cytokines are similar to those described for humans, although in certain cases, the response of the target cells is less specific than the response to human cytokines. For example, the CTTL-2 cells respond to both murine IL-2 and IL-4 (Hu-Li et al. 1989). To differentiate between the two possibilities, target cell proliferation in the presence or absence of anti-IL-2 or anti-IL-4 is determined. Alternatively, a subline of the CTTL-2 (CTTL-2, CT.4S) can be used directly to measure low levels of murine IL-4 in biological matrices. Different target or indicator cells are also used in the measurement of murine interferons. The assay system consists of interferon sensitive L929 fibroblasts and infection with vesicular stomatitis virus. In the presence of interferon there is little cytopathic effect observed in the assay. To differentiate among various forms of interferon, antibody neutralization of specific interferon classes can be performed.

Host Defense Models

Since most of the ex vivo assays used to assess immunocompetence define only the nature of the defect, additional studies must be undertaken to ascertain the biological relevance of the observation. Host defense models are available to study the effect of xenobiotics on the humoral or cellular immune systems (Fugmann et al. 1983).

The streptococcal model has been used to study the effects on the antibody-mediated immune system. After an intraperitoneal inoculation, the host response involves the production of antibody in a T-cell-independent manner, complement activation, followed by opsonization and phagocytosis by polymorphonuclear leukocytes (Johnson 1981a; Winkelstein 1981). Two species of streptococci have been used as models. *Streptococcus pneumoniae*, which is a human pathogen, is highly lethal to mice in a relatively short period of time (White et al. 1986). The immune response is mediated primarily by activation of the alternative complement pathway and intracellular destruction of bacteria by PMNs. When the less virulent *S. zooepidemicus* is used as the challenge agent, there is a long infection period. In this model, the production of neutralizing antibodies is critical to host survival. Mortality is the endpoint in both streptococcal models. If inhalation exposure is used as the challenge route, the number of viable cells in the lung can be used as the endpoint.

Other viral and protozoan models are also used to study the effects of xenobiotics on the antibody-mediated immune system. The resistance to intranasally administered influenza virus A2/Taiwan H2N2 requires the production of antibody and interferon by the B6C3F1 mouse (Luster et al. 1988). Mortality is observed within 14 days after challenge. Antibodies are the major defense mechanism against the nonlethal, self-limiting mouse malaria organism (*Plasmodium yoelli*). Host resistance is determined by evaluating the number of parasite-infected blood cells 12 days after inoculation. Antibody synthesis and activation of the alternative complement pathway are also important in host resistance to the amoeba, *Naegleria fowleri* (Holbrook et al. 1980; Reilly, Bradley, and Harris 1979). Repeated inoculations of amoebae cause a fatal meningoencephalitis in mice.

Infection with *Listeria monocytogenes* is the most common model used to study delayed hypersensitivity reactions. The immune response involves macrophages and delayed hypersensitivity responses mediated by T cells. Following intraperitoneal or intravenous inoculation, activation of the T-cell-mediated response occurs within 2–3 days. Resistance is determined by mortality or quantitation of bacteria in the liver or the spleen.

In the design of all host defense studies, careful consideration should be given to the nature, viability, and dose of the challenge agent. Some of the xenobiotics are human pathogens (e.g., streptococci and *Listeria*) and should be handled with appropriate caution. Since the animals are inoculated with a concentration of infectious agents producing an LD_{10}–LD_{30} in control mice, the viability of the cells in the inoculum should be standardized. Better experimental results have been obtained by using cells in the log growth phase.

Tumor Models

In the mouse, two tumors are usually studied in model systems. The PYB6 fibro-sarcoma tumor from C57BL/6 mice was developed to screen for host resistance in B6C3F1 mice (Dean et al. 1982). The animals are inoculated subcutaneously in the thigh with an LD_{10}–LD_{30} dose, and the tumor frequency is determined at a later date. Intact cell-mediated immunity and NK-cell function are necessary for tumor resistance (Murray et al. 1985; Urban et al. 1982). The metastatic pulmonary tumor B16F10 was also derived from C57BL/6 mice. The major defense mechanisms are NK cells and macrophages with some T-cell contributions to the response (Luster et al. 1988; Parhar and Lala 1987). In the assay radiolabeled cells are injected via the intraperitoneal route. Pulmonary tumors can be scored visually, and the tumor burden is determined as a reflection of ^{125}I-UdR in the lungs (Murray et al. 1985).

Rat tumor models have been hampered by the lack of defined tumors. Several systems have been described. The Wistar Furth (W/Fu) transplantable tumor (C58NT)D induced by the Gross leukemia virus is highly antigenic and produces only transient tumor growth followed by complete regression within 20 days. The tumor is NK-cell resistant and evokes a CTL response (Oren, Herberman, and Canty 1971; DeLandazuri and Herberman 1972). A suspension of tumor cells (TD10–20) can be administered subcutaneously into the flank of the rats following treatment with the test article for 28 days. The animals should be observed for tumor regression and mortality for 30 days. The mammary adenoma cell line (MADB106) can be used to test the function of NK cells in syngeneic Fischer 344 rats (Barlozzari et al. 1985). A suspension of tumor cells (TD10–20) should be inoculated intravenously into the animals after treatment for 28 days. Animals should be observed for 30 days for mortality and time to death.

References

Aarden, L. A., E. R. DeGroot, O. L. Schaap, and P. M. Lansdorp. 1987. Production of hybridoma growth factor by human monocytes. *Eur. J. Immunol.* 17:1141–46.

Adams, D. O. 1980. Effector mechanisms of cytolytically activated macrophages. I. Secretion of neutral proteases and the effect of protease inhibitors. *J. Immunol.* 124:286–300.

Addison, I. E., and J. W. Babbage. 1976. A raft technique for chemotaxis: A versatile method suitable for clinical studies. *J. Immunol. Methods* 10:385–88.

Addison, I. E., B. Johnson, and M. Shaw. 1982. A human skin window technique using a micropore membrane. *J. Immunol. Methods* 54:129–39.

Agnado, S., E. Gomez, and A. Rodriquez. 1989. A prospective study on a rapid method for diagnosing cytomegalovirus in immunosuppressed patients. *Nephron* 53:322–24.

Allison, A. C., J. S. Harington, and M. Birbeck. 1966. An examination of the cytotoxic effects of silica on macrophages. *J. Exp. Med.* 124:141–53.

Anonymous. 1981. Report of an IUIS/WHO working group. Use and abuse of laboratory tests in clinical immunology: Critical consideration of eight widely used diagnostic procedures. *Clin. Exp. Immunol.* 46:662–74.

Baehner, R., and D. G. Nathan. 1968. Quantitative nitroblue tetrazolium test in chronic granulomatosis disease. *N. Engl. J. Med.* 278:971–76.

Baker, P. J., D. F. Amsbaugh, P. W. Stashak, et al. 1981. Regulation of the antibody response to pneumococcal polysaccharide by thymus derived cells. *Rev. Infect. Dis.* 3:332–41.

Barlozzari, T., J. Leonhardt, R. H. Wiltrout, et al. 1985. Direct evidence for the role of LGL in the inhibition of experimental tumor metastases. *J. Immunol.* 134:2783–89.

Biron, C. A., K. S. Byron, and J. L. Sullivan. 1989, Severe herpes virus infection in an adolescent without NK cells. *N. Engl. J. Med.* 320:1731-33.

Boveris, A., E. Martino, and A. M. Stoppani. 1977. Evaluation of horseradish scopoletin method for measurement of H_2O_2 formation in biological systems. *Anal. Biochem.* 80:145-58.

Brunner, K. T., J. Mauel, and J. C. Cerottini. 1968. Quantitative assay of the lytic action of immune lymphoid cells on ^{51}Cr-labeled allogeneic target cells in vitro: Inhibition by isoantibody and drugs. *Immunology* 14:181-96.

Burton, R. C. 1984. Lymphocyte monitoring in renal transplantation. *Transplantation* 16:983-91.

Cantrell, D. A., and K. A. Smith. 1984. The interleukin-2 T cell system: A new growth model. *Science* 224:1312-16.

Chatenoud, L., S. Berrih, M. C. Bene, et al. 1982. The effect of immunomodulation on peripheral T cell subsets. *J. Clin. Immunol.* 2:61S-66S.

Chen, A. R., K. P. McKinnon, and H. S. Koren. 1985. LPS stimulates fresh human monocytes to lyse actinomycin D-treated WEHI 164 target cells via increased secretion of a monokine similar to human tumor necrosis factor. *J. Immunol.* 135:3979-87.

Cianciolo, G. J., J. Hunter, and J. Silva. 1981. Inhibition of monocyte responses to chemotaxins are present in human cancerous effusions and react with monoclonal antibodies to the P15(E) structural protein of retroviruses. *J. Clin. Invest.* 68:831-44.

Cramer, D. V., J. W. Shonnard, and T. J. Gill. 1974. Genetic studies in inbred rats. II. Relationship between the major histocompatibility complex and mixed lymphocyte reactivity. *J. Immunogenet.* 1:421-28.

Cunningham, A. J., and A. Szenberg. 1968. Further improvements in the plaque technique for detecting single antibody forming cells. *Immunology* 14:599-600.

Dafoe, D. C., L. M. Stoolman, D. A. Campbell, et al. 1987. T cell subset patterns in cyclosporine treated renal transplant patients with primary cytomegalovirus disease. *Transplantation* 43:452-57.

Davis, B. D., R. Dulbecco, H. N. Eisen, et al. 1973. *Microbiology*, p. 446. New York: Harper & Row.

Dean, J. H., M. I. Luster, G. A. Boorman, et al. 1982. Application of tumor, bacterial and parasitic susceptibility assays to study immune alterations induced by environmental chemicals. *Environ. Health Perspect.* 43:81-87.

De Landazuri, M. O., and R. B. Herberman. 1972. Immune response to Gross virus-induced lymphoma III. Characteristics of the cellular immune response. *J. Natl. Cancer Inst.* 49:147-56.

de Shazo, R. D., M. Lopez, and J. E. Salvaggio. 1987. Use and interpretation of diagnostic immunological laboratory tests. *JAMA* 258:3011-31.

Dijkmans, R., and A. Billiau. 1988. Interferon gamma. A master key in the immune system. *Curr. Opin. Immunol.* 1:269-74.

Dinarello, C. A., and N. Savage. 1989. Interleukin-1 and its receptor. *Crit. Rev. Immunol.* 9:1-20.

During, M., R. M. A. Landman, and F. Harder. 1984. Lymphocyte subsets in human peripheral blood after splenectomy and autotransplantation of splenic tissue. *J. Lab. Clin. Med.* 104:110-15.

Erber, W. N. 1990. Human leukocyte differentiation antigens: Review of the CD nomenclature. *Pathology* 22:61-89.

Esekowitz, R. A. B., J.Austyn, P. D. Stahl, and S. Gordon. 1981. Surface properties of bacillus Calmette-Guerin activated mouse macrophage: Reduced expression of mannose specific receptors, endocytosis, Fc receptors and antigen F4/80 accompanies the induction of Ia. *J. Exp. Med.* 154:60-76.

Espevik, M. M., and J. Nissen-Meyer. 1986. A highly sensitive cell line WEHI163 clone 13 for measuring cytotoxic/tumor necrosis factor from human monocytes. 1986. *J. Immunol. Methods* 95:99-105.

Falkoff, R. J. M., L. Zhu, and A. S. Fauci. 1982. Separate signals for human B cell proliferation in response to *Staphylococcus aureus*: Evidence for a two signal model of B cell activation. *J. Immunol.* 129:97–102.

Fauci, A. S., and D. C. Dale. 1975. The effect of hydrocortisone on the kinetics of normal human lymphocytes. *Blood* 46:235–43.

Fox, R. A. 1984. *Immunology and Infection in the Elderly,* p. 44. Edinburgh: Churchill Livinstone.

Fugmann, R. A., C. A. Aranyi, C. Barbera, et al. 1983. The effect of DES as measured by host resistance and tumor susceptibility assays in mice. *J. Toxicol. Environ. Health* 11:827–41.

Gallin, J. I., M. P. Fletcher, B. E. Seligmann, et al. 1982. Human neutrophil specific granule deficiency. A model to assess the role of neutrophil specific granules in the evolution of the inflammatory process. *Blood* 59:1317–29.

Grayson, J., N. J. Dooley, I. R. Koski, et al. 1981. Immunoglobulin production induced in vitro by glucocorticosteroid hormones. *J. Clin. Invest.* 68:1539–47.

Greaves, M., G. Janossy, and H. Doenhoff. 1974. Selective triggering of human T and B cell lymphocytes in vitro by polyclonal mitogens. *J. Exp. Med.* 140:1–18.

Grimm, E. A., A. Mazumder, H. Z. Zhang, and S. A. Rosenberg. 1982. Lymphocyte activated killer cell phenomenon: Lysis of natural killer cell-resistant fresh solid tumor cells by interleukin 2 activated autologous human peripheral blood lymphocytes. *J. Exp. Med.* 115:1823–41.

Gupta, S., and C. Tan. 1980. Subpopulations of human T lymphocytes. XIV. Abnormality of T cell locomotion and of distribution of subpopulations of T and B lymphocytes in peripheral blood and spleen from children with untreated Hodgkins disease. *Clin. Immunol. Immunopathol.* 15:133–43.

Hammarstrom, L., and C. I. E. Smith. 1986. Immunoglobulin diversity and its functional significance. In: *Immunoglobulins in Health and Disease*, ed. M. N. H. French, pp. 31–53. Lancaster: MTP Press.

Hanna, N., and I. J. Fidler. 1980. Role of the natural killer cells in the destruction of circulating tumor emboli. *J. Natl. Cancer Inst.* 65:801–10.

Hannun, Y. A., and R. M. Bell. 1987. Lysosphingolipids inhibit protein kinase C: Implications for sphingolipidosis. *Science* 235:670–74.

Hoffman, R. W., J. A. Bluestone, O. Leo, and S. Shaw. 1985. Lysis of anti-T3 bearing murine hybridoma cells by human allospecific cytotoxic T cell clones and inhibition of that lysis by anti-T3 and anti-LFA-1 antibodies. *J. Immunol.* 135:5–8.

Holbrook, T. W., R. J. Boackle, B. W. Parker, and J. Vessely. 1980. Activation of the alternative complement pathway by *Naegleria fowleri*. *Infect. Immun.* 30:58–61.

Hoover, R. L., R. T. Briggs, and M. J. Karnovsky. 1978. The adhesive interaction between polymorphonuclear leukocytes and endothelial cells in vitro. *Cell* 14:423–26.

Hosking, C. S., and A. Balloch. 1983. A formula to assess lymphocyte responsiveness in vitro. *Birth Defects* 19:21–23.

Hudson, L., and F. C. Hay. 1989. *Practical Immunology*, 3rd ed., pp. 187–90. Oxford: Blackwell Scientific.

Hudson, R. J., H. S. Saben, and D. Emslie. 1974. Physiological and environmental influences on immunity. *Vet. Bull.* 44:119.

Hu-Li, J., J. Ohara, C. Watyson, et al. 1989. Derivation of a T cell line that is highly responsive to IL-4 and IL-2 (CT.4R) and of an IL-2 hyporesponsive mutant of that cell line. *J. Immunol.* 800-7142:800–807.

Irons, R. D. 1985. Histology of the immune system: Structure and function. In *Immunotoxicology and Immunopharmacology*, ed. J. Dean, M. Luster, A. E. Munson, and H. Amos, pp. 11–22. New York: Raven Press.

Jelinek, D. F., J. B. Spiawski, and P. Lipsky. 1986. Human peripheral blood B lymphocyte subpopulations: Functional and phenotypic analyses of surface IgD positive and negative subsets. *J. Immunol.* 136:83–92.

Jerne, N. K., and A. A. Nordin. 1963. Plaque formation in agar by single antibody producing cells. *Science* 140:403–8.

Johnson, R. B. 1988. Monocytes and macrophages. *N. Engl. J. Med.* 318:747–52.

Johnson, R. B. Jr. 1981a. The host response to invasion by *Streptococcus pneumoniae*: Protection and pathogenesis of tissue damage. *Infect. Dis.* 3:282–88.

Johnson, R. B., Jr. 1981b. Enhancement of phagocytosis-associated oxidative metabolism as a manifestation of macrophage activation. *Lymphokine* 3:33–56.

Johnson, W. W., P. A. Marino, R. D. Schreiber, and O. O. Adams. 1983. Sequential activation of murine mononuclear phagocytes for tumor cytolysis: Differential expression of markers by macrophages in several stages of development. *J. Immunol.* 131:1038–43.

Kalland, T., H. Belfrange, P. Bhiladvala, and G. Hedlund. 1987. Analyses of the murine lymphokine activated (LAK) cell phenomenon: Dissection of effectors and progenitors into NK and T-like cells. *J. Immunol.* 138:3640–45.

Karnovsky, M. L., and J. K. Lazdins. 1978. The biochemical criteria for activated macrophages. *J. Immunol.* 121:809–13.

Keightley, R. G., M. D. Cooper, and A. Lawton. 1976. The T cell dependence of B cell differentiation induced by pokeweed mitogen. *J. Immunol.* 117:1538–43.

Klinman, N., D. Wylie, and J. Teale. 1981. B cell development. *Immunol. Today.* 2:212–16.

Lanier, L. L., T. J. Kipps, and J. H. Phillips. 1985. Functional properties of a unique subset of cytotoxic T lymphocytes that express Fc receptors for IgG (CD 16/Leu 11 antigens). *J. Exp. Med.* 162:2089–2106.

Lanier, L. L., A. M. Le, J. H. Phillips, et al. 1983. Subpopulations of human natural killer cells defined by expression of the Leu-7 (HNK-1) and Leu 11 (NK-15) antigens. *J. Immunol.* 131:1789–96.

Levi, F. A., C. Cannon, Y. Touitiou, et al. 1988. Circadian rhythms in circulating T lymphocyte subtypes and plasma testosterone, total and free cortisol in five healthy men. *Clin. Exp. Immunol.* 71:329–35.

Lew, P. D., F. S. Southwick, F. S. Stossel, et al. 1981. A variant of chronic granulomatosis disease: Deficient oxidative metabolism due to low affinity NADPH oxidase. *N. Engl. J. Med.* 305:1329–33.

Lewis, D. B., K. S. Pricket, A. Larsen, et al. 1988. Predicted production of interleukin 4 by activated human T cells. *Proc. Natl. Acad. Sci. U.S.A.* 85:9743–47.

Lonneman, G., S. Endres, J. W. van der Meer, et al. 1988. A radioimmunoassay for human IL-1 alpha: Measurement of IL-1 alpha production in vitro by human blood mononuclear cells stimulated with endotoxin. *Lymphokine Res.* 7:75–84.

Love, L. A., and W. K. Metcalf. 1980. Morphological and histochemical characteristics of density separated lymphocytes in cancer. *Anat. Rec.* 196:A115.

Lovett, E. J., B. Schnitzer, D. F. Keren, et al. 1984. Applications of flow cytometry to diagnostic pathology. *Lab. Invest.* 50:115–40.

Luster, M. I., G. A. Boorman, J. H. Dean, et al. 1980. Examination of bone marow immunological parameters and host susceptibility following pre and post natal exposure to 2,3,7,8-tetrachlorodibenzo-p-dioxin (TCDD). *Int. J. Immunopharmacol.* 2:301–10.

Luster, M. I., A. E. Munson, P. T. Thomas, et al. 1988. Development of a testing battery to assess chemical induced immunotoxicity: National Toxicology Program guidelines for immunotoxic evaluations in mice. *Fund. Appl. Toxicol.* 10:2–19.

Marino, P. A., C. C. Whisnant, and D. O. Adams. 1981. Binding of bacillus Calmette-Guerin-activated macrophage to tumor targets: Selective inhibition by membrane preparations from homologous and heterologous neoplastic cells. *J. Exp. Med.* 154:77–87.

Marrack, P., and J. Kappler. 1989. The staphylococcal enterotoxins and their relatives. *Science* 248:705–11.

Masuyama, K., H. Ochiai, S. Ishizawa, et al. 1988. Relation of H-2 expression on murine

RCT and sarcoma cells to lung colonization and sensitivity to NK cells. *J. Cancer Res. Clin. Oncol.* 114:487–92.

McWhinnie, D. L., N.P Carter, H. M. Taylor, et al. 1985. Is the T4/T8 ratio irrelevant in renal transplantation monitoring? *Transplant. Proc.* 17:2548–49.

Metcalf, J. A., J. I. Gallin, W. M. Nauseef, and R. K. Root. 1986. *Laboratory Manual of Neutrophil Function*, pp. 100–3, 135–43. New York: Raven Press.

Mishell, R. I., and R. W. Dutton. 1966. Immunization of normal spleen preparations in vitro. *Science* 153:1004–6.

Moller, G. 1988. Interleukin 4 and interleukin 5. *Immunol. Rev.* 102:1–350.

Mond, J. W., E. Farar, W. E. Paul, et al. 1983. T cell dependence and factor reconstitution of in vitro antibody responses to *B. abortus* and restoration of depleted responses to chromatographed fractions of a T cell derived factor. *J. Immunol.* 131:633–37.

Mond, J. J., E. Seghal, J. Kung, and F. Finkelman. 1981. Increased expression of I-region antigen (Ia) on B cells after cross-linkage of surface immunoglobulin. *J. Immunol.* 127:881–88.

Monjan, A. A., and M. I. Collector. 1977. Stress induced modulation of the immune response. *Science* 196:307–8.

Morimoto, C., D. A. Hafler, H. L. Weiner, et al. 1987. Selective loss of suppressor-inducer T cell subset in progressing multiple sclerosis. Analysis with anti-2H4 monoclonal antibody. *N. Engl. J. Med.* 316:67–72.

Munck, A., P. M. Guyre, and N. J. Hollbrook. 1984. Physiological functions of glucocorticosteroids in stress and their relationship to pharmacological actions. *Endocrinol. Rev.* 5:25–44.

Munson, A. E. 1987. Immunopathological alterations observed in laboratory animals: Consideration in the choice of experimental animals for evaluation of the immune system. In *Environmental Chemical Exposures and Immune System Integrity*, ed. E. J. Burger, R. G. Tardiff, and J. A. Bellanti, pp. 35–48. Princeton: Princeton Scientific.

Murray, M. J., J. Laver, M. I. Luster, et al. 1985. Correlation of murine susceptibility to tumors, parasitic and bacterial challenge with altered cell mediated immunity following systemic exposure to phorbol myristate acetate. *Int. J. Immunopharmacol.* 7:491–500.

Namen, A. E., S. Lupton, K. Hjerrild, et al. 1988. Stimulation of B cell progenitors by interleukin 7. *Nature* 333:571–73.

Nicolas, J. F., G. Cozum, and J. P. Revillard. 1988. Some viral infections and related disorders associated with long term immunosuppressive treatments. *J. Autoimmun.* 1:559–74.

North, R. J. 1978. The concept of the activated macrophage. *J. Immunol.* 121:806–9.

Oren, M. E., R. B. Herberman, and T. G. Canty. 1971. The immune response to Gross virus-induced lymphoma. II. Kinetics of the cellular immune response. *J. Natl. Cancer Inst.* 46:621–29.

Ortaldo, J. R., and R. B. Herberman. 1984. Heterogeneity of natural killer cells. *Annu. Rev. Immunol.* 2:359–94.

Ortaldo, J. R., A. Mason, and R. Overton. 1966. Lymphokine activated killer cells. Analyses of progenitors and effectors. *J. Exp. Med.* 164:1193–1205.

Paliard, X., R. D. W. Malefijt, H. Yssel, et al. 1988. Simultaneous production of interferon-α by activated human CD4$^+$ and CD8-T cell clones. *J. Immunol.* 141:849–55.

Parhar, R. S., and P. K. Lala. 1987. Amelioration of B16F10 melanoma lung metastasis in mice by a combination therapy with indomethacin and interleukin-2. *J. Exp. Med.* 165:14–28.

Parmley, R. T., R. L. Tzeng Baehner, and C. A. Boxer. 1983. Abnormal distribution of complex carbohydrates in neutrophils of a patient with lactoferrin deficiency. *Blood* 62:538–48.

Poplack, D. G., G. D. Bonnard, B. J. Holman, and R. M. Blaese. 1976. Monocyte-mediated antibody dependent cellular cytotoxicity: A clinical test of monocyte function. *Blood* 48:809–16.

Poutsiaka, D. D., E. W. Schroder, D. D. Taylor, et al. 1985. Membrane vesicles shed by murine melanoma cells selectively inhibit the expression of Ia antigen by macrophages. *J. Immunol.* 134:138–44.

Ranson, J. T., L. K. Morris, and J. C. Cambier. 1986. Anti-IgG induces release of inositol 1,4,5–triphosphate which mediates mobilization of intracellular Ca^{++} stores in B lymphocytes. *J. Immunol.* 137:708–14.

Reilly, M. F., S. Bradley, and L. S. Harris. 1979. Host resistance of mice to *Naegleria fowleri. Infect. Immun.* 42:645–52.

Roder, J. C., R. F. Todd, T. Haliotis, et al. 1983. The Chediak–Higashi gene in humans. III. Studies on the mechanics of NK impairment. *Clin. Exp. Immunol.* 51:359–68.

Rosen, H., and S. J. Klebanoff. 1979. Hydroxyl radical generation by polymorphonuclear leukocytes measured by electron spin resonance spectrospectroscopy. *J. Clin. Invest.* 64:1725–29.

Rosenwasser, L. J., and A. S. Rosenthal. 1978. Adherent cell function in murine T lymphocyte antigen recognition. I. A macrophage dependent T cell proliferation assay in the mouse. *J. Immunol.* 120:1991–98.

Rubenstein, S., P. C. Familetti, and S. Pestka. 1981. Convenient assay for interferons. *J. Virol.* 37:755–58.

Russell, S. W., W. F. Doe, and A. J. McIntosch. 1977. Functional characteristics of a stable, non-cytolytic stage of macrophage activation in tumors. *J. Exp. Med.* 146:1151–65.

Sauers, L. J., D. Wierda, E. R. Walker, and M. J. Reasor. 1986. Morphological and functional changes in mouse splenic lymphocytes following in vivo and in vitro exposure to chlorphentermine. *J. Immunopharmacol.* 8:611–31.

Schalm, O. W., N. C. Jain, and E. J. Carrol. 1975. *Veterinary Hematology*, pp. 244–55. Philadelphia: Lea and Febiger.

Schumacher, J. H., A. O'Garra, B. Schrader, et al. 1988. The characterization of four monoclonal antibodies specific for mouse IL-5 and the development of mouse and human IL-5 enzyme linked immunosorbent assays. *J. Immunol.* 141:1576–81.

Schwinzer, R., and K. Wonigeit. 1990. Genetically determined lack of CD45R-T cells in healthy individuals. Evidence for a regulatory polymorphism of CD45R antigen expression. *J. Exp. Med.* 171:1803–8.

Simpson, E., and P. Chandler. 1986. Analyses of cytotoxic T cell responses. In *Cellular Immunology*, Vol. 2, ed. D. M. Weir, and L. A. Herzenberg, pp. 68.1–68.16. Blackwell: Oxford.

Springer, T. A., and D. C. Anderson. 1986. The importance of MAC-1, LAF-1 glycoprotein family in monocyte and granulocyte adherence. Chemotaxis and migration into inflammatory sites: Insights from experiments of nature. In *Biochemistry of Macrophages,* ed. D. Evered, J. Nugent, and M. O'Conner, pp. 102–26. London: Pitman.

Stanbury, J. B., J. B. Wyngarten, and D. S. Fredrickson. 1983. *The Metabolic Basis of Disease,* 5th ed., pp. 831–56. New York: McGraw-Hill.

Storkus, W. J., and J. R. Dawson. 1991. Target structures involved in natural killing (NK): Characteristics, distribution, and candidate molecules. *Crit. Rev. Immunol.* 10:393–417.

Szuro-Subol, A., and C. F. Nathan. 1982. Suppression of macrophage oxidation metabolism by products of malignant and non-malignant cells. *J. Exp. Med.* 156:945–61.

Takemura, R., and Z. Werb. 1984. Secretory products of macrophages and their physiological functions. *Am. J. Physiol.* 246:C1–C9.

Thompson, C. B., I. Scher, and M. E. Schaeffer. 1984. Size dependent B lymphocyte subpopulations: Relationship of cell volume to surface phenotype, cell cycle, proliferative responses and requirements for antibody production. *J. Immunol.* 133:2333–42.

Urban, J. L., R. C. Burton, M. J. Holland, et al. 1982. Mechansims of syngeneic tumor rejection. Susceptibility of host selected progressor variants to various immunological effector cells. *J. Exp. Med.* 155:557–73.

van Dijk, H., J. A. Bakker, J. Testerink, et al. 1975. Oxisuran and immune reactions: Mediation of oxisuran action by the adrenal glands. *J. Immunol.* 115:1587–91.

Vogel, S. N., E. A. Havell, and G. L. Spitalny. 1986. Monoclonal antibody mediated inhibition of interferon gamma induced macrophage antiviral resistance and surface antigen expression. *J. Immunol.* 136:2917–33.

Vos, J. G., M. J. Van Logten, J. G. Kreeftenberg, and W. Kruizinga. 1984. The effect of triphenytin hydroxide on the immune system of the rat. *Toxicology* 29:325–36.

Wang, A. M., A. A. Creasey, M. B. Ladner, et al. 1985. Molecular cloning of the complementary DNA for human necrosis factor. *Science* 228:149–54.

Weiss, J. M., S. J. Schleifer, N. E. Miller, and M. Stein. 1981. Suppression of immunity by stress: Effect of a graded series of stressors on lymphocyte stimulation in the rat. *Science* 213:1397–99.

Werb, Z., M. J. Babda, and P. A. Jones. 1980. Degradation of connective tissue matrices by macrophages. I. Proteolysis of elastin glycoprotein and collagen by proteinases isolated from macrophages. *J. Exp. Med.* 152:1340–47.

White, K. L., Jr., H. H. Lysy, J. A. McCay, et al. 1986. Modulation of serum complement levels following exposure to polychlorinated dibenzo-p-dioxins. *Toxicol. Appl. Pharmacol.* 84:209–19.

Whitlock, C. A., D. A. Robertson, and O. N. Witte. 1984. Murine B cell lymphopoiesis in long term cultures. *J. Immunol. Methods* 67:333–37.

Winkelstein, J. A. 1981. The role of complement in host defense against *Streptococcus pneumoniae. Rev. Infect. Dis.* 3:289–98.

Woda, B. A., M. L. McFadden, R. M. Welsh, et al. 1984. Separation and isolation of natural killer cells from T cells with monoclonal antibodies. *J. Immunol.* 132:2183–88.

Yeh, T. J., P. T. McBride, and J. A. Green. 1982. Automated quantitative cytopathic reduction assay for interferon. *J. Clin. Microbiol.* 16:413–15.

Ziegler, J. B., P. Hansen, and R. Penny. 1975. Intrinsic lymphocyte defect in Hodgkin's disease: Analysis of the phytohemagglutinin dose response. *Clin. Immunol. Immunopathol.* 3:451–60.

10

Relevance of Immunotoxicologic Findings to Human Immune Competence

A. PROBLEMS IN STUDYING IMMUNOTOXICOLOGY

As with any branch of toxicology or pathology, the most basic problem is defining the normal limits beyond which disease is indicated. Often, as experience accumulates, one finds that the original normality boundaries were set too narrowly, and what constitutes normality is constantly being revised. There is a profusion of laboratory data now available for acceptable limits and values for a variety of immunologic parameters in animals and humans (Coligan et al. 1991; Luster et al. 1988; Rose and Friedman 1980), but these values are only for specific components of the immune system. Few measurements take into consideration the complete response of an intact, functioning system, and none look at the effect in a population. Often the specific values are not comparable between different laboratories because of differences in reagents or techniques, and each laboratory may have to define its own normal limits by screening a suitable number of subjects with no known immunologic defects. We know comparatively little about normal variation of immunologic parameters within an individual, especially diurnal variation.

In classical toxicology, the toxic doses of a given substance are known, and these take into consideration a limited amount of individual variation, so it is reasonable to make predictions concerning the outcome of exposure to known quantities of a given agent. Unfortunately, that same thinking has carried over into immunotoxicology, where matters do not work out so clearly. A major problem with immunotoxicity is in trying to satisfy unrealistic expectations in predicting how humans will respond immunologically to a given agent or exposure.

Chief among these difficulties is trying to be able to predict the allergenicity of a substance. When one considers that a large part of hypersensitivity lies with predisposing factors of the individual exposed to the substance, it almost becomes a futile exercise. Immunotoxic reactions are much more involved than the interaction of an inducing substance with a responsive individual. There are a number of clearly definable risk factors that are used in an attempt to explain why, in a total population all exposed to the same agent, only certain individuals develop allergic or immunotoxic responses. These risk factors may be associated with factors responsible for allergy development, pharmacological disposition of an agent, or a distinctive physiological response mechanism, and all of these factors are initially determined by genetic factors. In addition, there are a number of less well-definable environmental factors that decidedly influence the degree and the incidence of such reactions. Simultaneous or temporally spaced exposure to two or more separate agents or events is becoming recognized as important in synergistically enhancing what would otherwise be an ordinary response if only one of these stimuli were received at a time. The immuntoxicologist must be able to look at the total milieu in which these reactions develop in order to assess them properly. Clearly, much more is involved than the chemical structure of the offending agent.

Linking the incidence of cancer at the present time with carcinogenic stimuli occurring in the past is exceedingly difficult, and the problem linking immunotoxicity with remote events seems even more so. Almost all of what we know about immunotoxic effects stems from studies performed on either people or animals that have undergone recent defined exposures to selected agents. We know next to nothing about what delayed or latent effects may result from an environmental stimulus some time in the past. Complicated environmental diseases such as coalworkers' pneumoconiosis or byssinosis, which may have immunologic components (Burrell 1985), take years to develop, and then not in everyone similarly exposed. Linking these diseases of known exposure with an acceptable immunologic etiopathogenesis has been difficult enough, to say nothing about trying to explain diseases for which the stimuli are unknown.

Perhaps the most vexing problem in immunotoxicology is how to interpret the data obtained from the laboratory in terms of relating them to the possible development of the consequences of loss of immunity, i.e., increased susceptibility to infection or tumor induction. Just exactly what do the abnormal laboratory values mean clinically, and how much damage can the immunologic system sustain before clinical disease results? To answer these questions a variety of studies have been performed. Much has been learned from epidemiologic (e.g., PBBs) and case-account (e.g., phenytoin-induced B-cell toxicity) studies in humans, and there have been numerous studies using experimental animals or in vitro systems with selected xenobiotics. As careful as some of these studies have been, there always remains the problem of extrapolating animal data so obtained to the human experience. Species differences in immune responses are encountered, and what may be true of the mouse or the guinea pig does not necessarily hold true for humans.

B. DEFINITION OF HOW IMMUNOTOXIC ABNORMALITIES ARE REALIZED

Although there exists a wide array of technological means of assessing immune functions in humans as well as in laboratory animals, the most important task is that of attempting to relate abnormal findings to clinical consequences; i.e., (1) does the immunologic abnormality cause or lead to decreased resistance to infections from common, opportunistic microorganisms, or (2) does it lead to an increased susceptibility to cancer? Impairment of functional immunity can be considered in different ways. We purposefully immunize against tetanus, polio, and whooping cough, among others. In addition, many people have naturally acquired immunity to other infectious agents as a result of recovering from once-common childhood diseases, e.g., measles, rubella, and chicken pox (although younger people have been artificially immunized against these latter agents in recent years). The most immediate concern would be whether immune abnormalities would compromise existing immunity to such primary infections, and for this we have very little information.

Rather, most of the results of immune dysfunction have been obtained from studies of patients suffering genetic or developmental anomalies of the immune system, and the results show that most of these individuals sustain repeated infections with a wide variety of common microorganisms of very low virulence. These agents, called opportunists, are seldom seen in primary infections of normal hosts but occur most often when the patient has some predisposing condition affecting the immune system, e.g., patients with one of the aforementioned genetic/developmental immunodeficiencies, patients undergoing long-term immunosuppressive therapy, or those in late stages of a malignancy, especially of the type affecting the lymphoid system. These kinds of opportunistic microorganisms either are part of the normal flora or are found ubiquitously in the environment. Table 10–1 lists a number of opportunistic microorganisms and the clinical condition that is most often associated with them. Some of these infectious agents are of such low virulence that their very presence in an infection is considered a strong reason to look for some kind of a predisposing factor. Indeed, it was this very situation that first alerted physicians to recognize a new disease, now known as AIDS. They noticed the striking incidence of an infection of, at the time, almost inconsequential incidence, *Pneumocystis* pneumonia, often occurring to-

TABLE 10–1.   Common Opportunistic Microorganisms and Clinical Conditions with which They Are Associated

Microorganism	Clinical Condition/Compromised Host Defense
Staphylococcus aureus, *S. epidermidis*	Indwelling IV polyethylene catheters; prosthetic heart valve implants
Streptococcus pneumoniae	Absence of spleen or abnormal splenic function; multiple myeloma
Pseudomonas aeruginosa	Leukopenia associated with malignant tumors, lymphproliferative disorders, or bone marrow failure Cystic fibrosis; severe burns
Serratia marcescens	Extended or permanent urinary catheterization Chronic granulomatous disease
Listeria monocytogenes	Hemoproliferative disorders; pregnancy Newborns or elderly patients; alcoholics
Nocardia asteroides	Immunosuppressed allograft recipient
Mycobacteria	Prolonged use of corticosteroids Immunosuppressed patients
Propionibacterium acnes	Prosthetic heart valve implants
Cryptococcus neoformans	Hodgkin's disease and other lymphomas
Aspergillus spp.	Prosthetic heart valve implants Immunosuppressed patients Patients with old pulmonary abscesses
Candida albicans	Patients on bacterial antibiotics Prosthetic heart valve implants Immunosuppressed patients
Toxoplasma gondii	Pregnancy; immunosuppressed patients
Pneumocystis carinii	Immunosuppressed patients
Herpes simplex virus	Immunosuppressed patients
Varicella–zoster virus	Hodgkin's disease; other lymphproliferative disorders; immunosuppressed patients
Cytomegalovirus	Blood transfusions; immunosuppressed patients

Source: Adapted from Youmans, Peterson, and Sommers (1986).

gether with a rare, benign tumor, Kaposi's sarcoma (Follansbee et al. 1982). The occurrence of only one, let alone both, of these syndromes in an individual was an indication that the immune system was not behaving at a sufficient level. The appearance of such infections as *Pneumocystis carinii* pneumonia, nonpulmonary tuberculosis caused by atypical species of *Mycobacterium*, persistent or disseminated herpes simplex virus, extrapulmonary cryptococcosis, and toxoplasmosis of the brain (in a patient older than 1 month of age) are now recognized as indicator diseases of underlying AIDS. A more extensive list appears in Table 10–2.

Often the type of infection provides a clue to the nature of the immune defect, e.g., cancer, granulocytopenia, depressed cellular immunity, etc. (De Jongh and Schimpff 1988). Repeated infections from Gram-positive, extracellular bacteria indicate dysfunction in B-cell number or function. Repeated intracellular infections with Gram-negative bacteria, mycobacteria, viruses, or fungi indicate similar abnormalities in the T-cell components. Long-standing granulomatous infections involving microorganisms of low virulence in the presence of adequate antibody and lymphocyte function could be an indication of a defect in granulocytes.

Although an increased rate of infection or the incidence of an infection from one of these agents of low virulence is valuable information and something that can be seen in a single individual, the occurrence of a tumor in a single individual is not a remarkable occurrence in itself unless it is an unusual type, like Kaposi's sarcoma. Just as there are opportunistic infective agents of low virulence, there are similar tumors of such low virulence or occurrence in normal populations that their mere appearance in an otherwise healthy adult suggests an underlying predisposing risk. Invasive Kaposi's sarcoma in young adults and lymphoma of the brain in persons under 60 years of age are two examples. Usually, however, the association of an increased incidence of a tumor with exposure to a given agent can be determined only in retrospect by epidemiologic studies.

Epidemiology is of necessity a study often made after the fact (retrospective), and the data are made from observing "experiments of nature," spontaneously

TABLE 10–2.   CDC[a] Surveillance Case Definition Indicator Diseases Associated with AIDS[b]

Candidiasis of esophagus, trachea, bronchi, or lungs
Extrapulmonary cryptococcosis
Cryptosporidiosis with diarrhea persisting >1 month
Cytomegalovirus disease in organs other than liver, spleen, or lymph node in a patient >1 month of age
Herpes simplex causing mucocutaneous ulcer that persists >1 month; or bronchitis, pneumonitis, or esophagitis for any duration in a patient >1 month of age
Kaposi's sarcoma affecting a patient <60 years of age
Lymphoma of the brain (primary) affecting a patient <60 years of age
Lymphoid interstitial pneumonia and/or pulmonary lymphoid hyperplasia affecting a child <13 years of age
Mycobacterium avium complex or *M. kansasii* infections at sites other than lungs, skin, or cervical or hilar lymph nodes
Progressive multifocal leukoencephalopathy
Toxoplasmosis of the brain affecting patient >1 month of age

[a]Center for Disease Control, Atlanta, GA, 1987.
[b]Any of these diseases is regarded as presumptive evidence of AIDS in the absence of laboratory evidence for HIV infection and if all other causes of immunodeficiency disease have been eliminated.

occurring events, as opposed to those designed by scientific planning. Prospective epidemiologic studies are also possible to test a hypothesis of an association of a given agent with a particular disease or abnormality. However, making correlations is difficult because of confounding factors such as smoking, diet, age, and sex. Even with information suggesting the association of a tumor type with a specific substance, the problem remains of deciding if the agent is in itself carcinogenic (or capable of being converted to one, e.g., benz[a]pyrenes) or is an agent that depresses the immune response low enough that tumors arise spontaneously.

Transplantation of most tumors in experimental animals is usually possible only in immunologically immature, congenitally immune deficient, or inbred animals. Otherwise, a tumor will only be initiated if coadministered with an immunosuppressive drug. Among some of the laboratory tumor models that have been studied in conjunction with immunotoxic materials are polyoma virus, SV-40 virus, Lewis lung carcinoma, Moloney sarcoma virus, B16 melanoma, and various transplantable ascites tumors, e.g., L1210 and MOPC-104 (Murray et al. 1985).

Most of the human data have been obtained from long-term studies on patients receiving immunosuppressive therapy in conjunction with receiving a kidney transplant. Spontaneous tumors, primarily those involving the lymphoid system or skin, led to an increasing incidence of cancer the longer the individuals lived, as high as 46% in patients surviving as long as 10 years after transplantation (Penn 1985). These tumors appeared earlier (average of 54 months after contact) than did those appearing after contact with known carcinogens (15–20 years). Other studies showing an association of tumor development with use of immunosuppressants have been obtained from those receiving prolonged therapy for various inflammatory conditions involving hyperreactive immune responses, e.g., rheumatoid arthritis, and from those receiving cytotoxic, antiproliferative drugs for the primary treatment of cancer. It is ironic that drugs that are designed to inhibit rapidly proliferating tumors act similarly on cells of the immune system and that the very drug used for therapy may in itself be immunosuppressive (Katz and Fauci 1988).

But such obvious immunodeficiencies of this degree leading to highly suspicious indicator infections or tumors have not been associated with immunotoxicity of the workplace or environment. Comparatively speaking, these kinds of maladies are the easy ones, and discerning immune impairment of lesser degrees is difficult. A number of factors contribute to the difficulty of linking this sort of infection with an immunotoxic event. The time of onset of infection could be some time after contact with the agent, the contact itself may have been so inapparent that the victim did not realize it, or the infections could occur at such infrequent occasions, be of low virulence, or occur in such few people compared to the number exposed that making the proven connection is very difficult. Often, the only tool definitively capable of linking exposure to an agent with a disease is an epidemiologic study comparing the incidence of a given disease in large groups of people exposed or not exposed to the agent in question. The link between cigarette smoking and lung cancer could only be established by such studies, for example, and similar studies have shown that smokers also experience increased numbers and durations of respiratory infections.

Thus, identifying immunotoxic abnormalities in the laboratory is much easier than defining them clinically, but the biggest problem is relating how the former leads to the latter. Even this cause-effect relationship is not straight forward because of the existence of many confounding factors such as genetic predisposition and the presence of synergistic environmental conditions at the time of exposure to the xenobiotic.

C. RISK FACTORS: ALLERGY

Unfortunately, the great discovery of IgE in relation to immediate hypersensitivity has also had its down side. In spite of the wealth of very useful information it has provided, there has been the tendency to view all adverse immunologic reactions strictly in terms of an external stimulus generating an internal response. Close examination reveals many other participating factors in addition to the external antigen and the allergic responses induced. In assessing the question of why not all individuals exposed to a toxic substance become affected, one must consider a number of alternatives in addition to the obvious one of immunotoxicity for a variety of reasons additional to being exposed to an agent. Chief among these factors are genetic predisposition and environmental enhancing factors.

Clinical hypersensitivity in certain pulmonary diseases has been studied most regarding the contribution of a genetic trait in influencing subsequent exposure to a toxic agent. Exposure to various industrial inhalants such as silica is coupled with a number of pathological entities, but that leading to emphysema (progressive destruction of the connective tissue that constitutes the air space walls) is coupled with another genetic factor, the inability to synthesize the proteolytic enzyme inhibitor α_1-antitrypsin (Janoff 1985). Normally, this material holds proteolytic enzymes like elastase in balance. Without it, substances that induce inflammatory reactions cause unregulated proteolysis, thus contributing to the destruction of alveolar tissue. Similar genetic bases could account for the differential ability of individuals to produce anti-inflammatory factors (acute-phase reactants) that greatly influence how a given individual would respond to an offensive agent. Similarly, genetic factors could determine a wide differential range in metabolic activity expressed in a population such that immunotoxicants are degraded or rapidly cleared in some, whereas in others they either remain undegraded or are altered into more toxic analogs.

Of the different types of immunotoxicity, the human IgE-mediated type of allergy has been studied in most detail from the genetic standpoint. Although almost anyone may develop a hypersensitivity to a given substance, there is a distinct segment of a population that is clinically atopic, i.e., individuals who are abnormally hyperreactive to a variety of environmental agents. These people have increased incidence of allergic rhinitis, bronchial asthma, atopic dermatitis, or food allergy. Those with allergic rhinitis exhibit with almost constant sinus congestion, runny nose, and eye irritation in the absence of infections and irritants. Those who suffer from bronchial asthma have increased airway sensitivity to a variety of physical and chemical agents that results in increased narrowing of the airways. This condition is not entirely caused by antigen-mediated sensitivity. Clinically, the airways hyperreactivity in these predisposed people can be detected by pulmonary function studies following inhalation challenge with a pharmacological agent, acetylmethylcholine (Woolcock 1988).

Several non-MHC genes have been identified that influence the allergic state in various ways (Marsh and Bias 1988). The total amount of human IgE produced is under at least two levels of gene control. The most agreed-on is a recessive allele governing "high" IgE production, arbitrarily defined as > 230 ng/ml; i.e., levels higher than this tend to be found only in those with the homozygous recessive genotype. There also appear to be significant polygenic factors involved in regulation of total IgE.

Another major genetic component involved in IgE-mediated allergy is the MHC-determined immune response (Ir) genes. Although most studies of such genetic control of specific immune response have been conducted in inbred strains of rats and mice, numerous studies have been made comparing the gene frequency of certain identifiable human MHC products with responsiveness to certain well-characterized antigens (e.g., the protein Amb V isolated from ragweed pollen). These data show distinct relationships between presence or absence of a gene and the ability to mount immune responses to the given antigen. Perhaps most important is the significance of how these MHC-related genes interact with those controlling the amount of IgE responsiveness, but information is available for only a few allergens.

To illustrate further how allergic manifestations are affected by much more than possession of antigen-specific IgE, it is becoming clear that additional factors for promoting histamine release from basophils are necessary. Chief among these is a family of cytokines collectively known as histamine-releasing factor (HRF). These molecules can be produced from a wide variety of cells, including monocytes and B and T lymphocytes (MacDonald and Lichtenstein 1990). The release of these cytokines appears to be dependent on the presence of a particular type of IgE, but not just any IgE. Everyone has IgE, but only a minority experience allergic symptoms. One reason is that IgE is heterogeneous, differing substantially in its degree of glycosylation. Only a certain kind of IgE, termed IgE^+, interacts with the HRF, whereas another type (IgE^-) does not (MacDonald and Lichtenstein 1990). How this interaction takes place must await further physical studies on the differences between IgE^+ and IgE^-. Presumably, this IgE heterogenity is genetically determined, but this has not been substantiated as yet.

In addition to these sets of genes, release of pharmacologically active mediators, at least in the case of histamine release from basophils, seems to be gene controlled. Moreover, responsiveness to a mediator might well have a genetic component. Thus, should the "wrong" combination of genes from these different systems occur in one individual, the atopic state would be clearly defined. Further, the degree of responsiveness, as well as clinical manifestations, all appear to be related to sex, race, and age. For example, the atopic child or young adult tends to grow out of individual clinical manifestations with age.

D. RISK FACTORS: PHARMACOLOGICAL

Explaining individual idiosyncrasies that are not allergy based is more difficult because of the dearth of studies on other possible explanations. Pharmacologists recognize idiosyncratic reactions to drugs but formerly considered many of them to be allergic in nature. There is an increasing realization that there is a difference between allergy and idiosyncratic reactions. If we exclude all of the many immunologic responses to drugs that could account for abnormal reactions, there remain a number of physiological or pharmacological host factors that determine reactivity to such agents. Vincent (1986) points out that the terms "idiosyncratic" and "unpredictable" are often erroneously used interchangeably. An idiosyncratic reaction should be predictable in a small susceptible population, but the major problem toxicologists have is in defining that population. Idiosyncratic drug reactions are those occurring in a minority of any population at the lowest end of the frequency distribution of a dose–response curve, i.e., that small number of individuals reacting to the smallest test doses.

These people who manifest hyperreactive responses to low dose levels without preimmunization have a genetic component that is responsible either for how the drug is metabolized or for how that person's cellular/molecular mechanisms respond. These pharmacogenetic bases are further complicated by the numerous types of environmental factors that affect gene expression or the occurrence of the clinical manifestation. Genes could affect how a drug is metabolized. If the drug itself is toxic, and if there is a gene responsible for a derangement or absence of its main degrading enzyme, then that agent's effects will be prolonged. Such is the case where reduced plasma cholinesterase is responsible for the prolonged action of succinylcholine in anesthesia (Nebert and Weber 1990). Because this short-acting drug, which is used to relax skeletal muscle, cannot be quickly cleared, a prolonged relaxation of muscles involved in breathing may be so severe as to result in apnea.

Fever and rashes within 1 to 2 weeks of onset of sulfonamide therapy occur in up to 5% of patients receiving the drug. By far most of the patients experiencing such reactions in one study were found to acetylate the oxidative products of initial metabolism more slowly, thereby allowing intermediates to be present longer (Rieder et al. 1991). These intermediate products may participate as major inducers of the adverse reactions, as evidenced by direct lymphocyte toxicity studies.

In other instances there could be a great deal of genetic variation resulting in polymorphic gene products. An individual with an abnormal gene product would never be noticed unless that person becomes exposed to an agent that interacts with that product. In these instances, only a certain subset of the population is going to metabolize the drug in such a way as to result in toxic by-products. When an environmental stimulus is additionally required to express the abnormal gene action, clinical manifestations might be erroneously considered immune in origin. Such is the case in certain types of porphyria, a situation in which abnormal pigments are deposited in the skin and, when subjected to sunlight, undergo photooxidation that results in skin toxicity resembling allergic reactions.

Although decreased sensitivity might occasionally be explained in immunologic terms, in other instances genetic abnormalities account for such alterations. A number of drug idiosyncrasies that have been traced to genetic mechanisms are presented in Table 10–3. In addition to genetic factors, other conditions that are known to alter pharmacological reactivity to substances are age, presence of concurrent disease, nutritional status, hormone levels, diurnal variation in drug disposition or sensitivity, environmental factors that induce or inhibit drug metabolism, and efficiency of repair mechanisms (Nebert and Weber 1990). Although a fair amount is known about pharmacogenetics, much less is known about genetic factors that affect physiological responsiveness. Some of the host factors that definitely have genetic bases contributing to the way individuals hyperrespond to environmental agents are airway hyperresponsiveness to methylcholine challenge, increased propensity of basophils to release histamine, dermatographism, and hyperreactivity to histamine. Hyperreactivity to cholinergic stimuli (i.e., bronchial smooth muscle constrictors) may prove to be ex-

TABLE 10-3.   Representative Human Pharmacogenetic Disorders

Enzyme deficiency or defective protein
  Succinylcholine apnea
  Acetylation polymorphism
    Isoniazid-induced neurotoxicity
    Drug-induced lupus erythamatosus
  Increased susceptibility to drug-induced hemolysis
    Glucose-6-phosphate dehydrogenase deficiency
  P450 monooxygenase polymorphism
    Debrisoquine 4-hydroxylase deficiency
  Hyperbilirubinemia
Increased resistance to drugs (nonimmune)
  Inability to taste phenylthiourea
  Coumarin resistance
  Possibility of defective receptor
    Steroid hormone resistance
    Cystic fibrosis
    Trisomy 21
  Defective absorption
    Juvenile pernicious anemia
  Increased metabolism
    Succinylcholine resistance
    Atypical aldehyde dehydrogenase
Changes in drug response caused by enzyme induction
  Porphyrias
Abnormal drug distribution
  Thyroxine (hyper- or hypothyroidism)
Disorders of unknown etiology
  Chloramphenicol-induced aplastic anemia
  Phenytoin-induced B-cell toxicity
  Halothane-induced hepatitis

Source: Adapted from Nebert and Weber (1990).

plained by something as simple as a diminution in the type of cholinergic autoreceptors that are responsible for negative feedback inhibition of the effector neurotransmitters (Ayala and Ahmed 1989).

E. RISK FACTORS: ENVIRONMENTAL

Given the fact that a proportion of a population is clinically atopic (variously estimated as 15–20%; see Smith 1978), the key question in considering one who is exposed to an antigen, even the atopics, is: why is it that only some of the exposed population develop hypersensitivity? This same question may be extended to other types of immune injury or toxicity. Farmers, coal miners, chemical workers, etc. are all exposed to certain agents in the course of their occupations, but only some of them will develop hypersensitivity pneumonitis, pneumoconiosis, or TDI asthma, respectively. A genetic predisposition must be there, but perhaps external risk factors other than the offending agent are also important.

In an epidemiologic study of drug-induced aplastic anemia and agranulocytosis, a great disparity in risk was found regarding the use of the analgesic sodium metamizole. The rate ratio estimate for Ulm (West Germany), West Berlin, and Barcelona was 23.7, compared with Budapest and Israel, where the ratio was only 0.8 (Anonymous 1986). Only two known factors were associated with this great difference. The drug was used very commonly in the latter locations, very uncommonly in the former. The other difference was the obvious geographic one, which in itself implies that there may be some important environmental factor that additionally is responsible for the development of this toxicity.

The presence of damp, moldy conditions in the home contributes greatly to the prevalence of lower respiratory symptoms, even taking into account those with existing allergic or asthmatic conditions (Dales, Burnett, and Zwanenburg 1991). Not only do these conditions promote the aerosolization of aeroallergens such as fungi and mites, these agents may also be the source of inherently inflammatory or priming substances, and their heightened presence may be an indication of inadequate ventilation that allows other toxicants to accumulate.

One of the most important external personal risk factors (and one that can be controlled) for the development of pulmonary disease following exposure to additional environmental insults is smoking. Smoking has been shown epidemiologically to increase the risk substantially of developing disabling pulmonary disease to a variety of airborne materials including cotton dust (Selikoff and Hammond 1979), coal mine dust (Morgan 1984), and asbestos (Heyden and Pratt 1980).

Perinatal environmental factors may influence the subsequent development of allergy in an individual (Björkstén and Kjellman 1990) and smoking is one of these. Although umbilical cord levels of IgE may also be genetically determined, there is a relationship between cord IgE levels and increased risk of development of allergic disease during infancy and childhood (Croner and Kjellman 1990). Thus, this association reflects a genetic predisposition, subsequently influenced by exposure of the fetus/infant to environmental agents. Most of this IgE seems to be polyclonal in origin and does not necessarily imply intrauterine sensitization to specific antigens. Maternal smoking during pregnancy has been associated with a greater than threefold rise in cord IgE and more than a fourfold risk of developing atopic disease before the age of 18 months in infants born of nonallergic parents (Magnusson 1986). However, there are negative studies as well (e.g., Oryszczyn et al. 1991), and the results may possibly be explained by the amount of smoking, a variable not yet considered. Parental smoking is not only associated with more evident development of subsequent allergy, but maternal smoking has also been correlated with increased mortality and morbidity to pulmonary infectious diseases (Rantakallio 1978; Cogswell, Mitchell, and Alexander 1987).

Another possible enhancing risk factor that is recognized but cannot be controlled is the occurrence of infection prior to the time of exposure. The association of viral (but not bacterial) infection with triggering development of bronchial asthma, particularly in children and to some extent in adults, has long been recognized (Busse 1990). But even in these instances, other factors are also required, e.g., the type of virus causing the infection, the age at which the infection first takes place, the presence of certain constitutional symptoms at the time of infection, genetic predisposition, preexisting airway hyperreactivity, and sex. When one considers the number of mechanisms by which viral infection can induce airway hyperreactivity for which there is evidence, the multifactorial nature of a seemingly simple event becomes more evident. Busse (1990) has recently reviewed such mechanisms and among those proposed is that certain viruses, notably respiratory syncytial virus, may enhance B-cell IgE synthesis and mediator release from basophils, either directly or through the action of interferon from virus-stimulated lymphocytes.

The viruses may also interfere with β-adrenergic function by directly inhibiting such function, by passively allowing the mast cell to promote more mediator release, or by enhancing cholinergic stimulation of airways smooth muscle. Finally, the virus may also desquamate epithelium, thus exposing afferent neurons to stimulation and decreasing the amount of an endopeptidase that normally degrades the peptidergic smooth muscle contractant substance P. The ultimate response is most likely to be a combination of several of these events. It is hypothesized that should viral infection occur in a genetically predisposed worker who is simultaneously being exposed to an industrial substance, an enhanced late-phase reaction to that substance might possibly take place (Lemanske et al. 1989). Aside from the matter of asthma, the inflammation produced during an infection possibly facilitates sensitization to environmental antigens, and the infectious agents could also function as immunologic adjuvants (Björkstén and Kjellman 1990).

Additionally, there is an increase in occurrence of iatrogenic (physician-induced) diseases stemming from various therapeutic regimens associated with modern medicine. Long-term treatment with drugs that depress or alter the immune system may play a role in how humans respond to environmental agents. The effect of drugs taken by the mother during pregnancy on subsequent allergy has not been extensively studied, but in one small study of mothers taking β blockers (metroprolol), increased neonatal IgE levels and subsequent development of allergic disease were noted (Björkstén, Finnstrom, and Wichman 1988).

In children with an innate or environmentally induced increased propensity to develop allergy, the simultaneous occurrence of allergens or additional adjuvant factors at this time is, of course, important. The presence of allergens such as pollens, house dust mites, cat proteins, etc. at the time of the infant's birth has been shown to increase risk to these agents at a later time. The allergy-preventing results of breast feeding versus cow's milk feeding have recently been reviewed, and information suggests that there is merit to manipulating the diet of a lactating mother of an infant in families with genetic predisposition to allergies (Björkstén and Kjellman 1990). Various external enhancing or adjuvant effects have also been noted. Smoking has been mentioned previously. The development of infants in the presence of environmental/industrial pollutions or inadequately ventilated residences has not been looked at with any degree of certainty but deserves the same sort of intense scrutiny that has been given to smoking.

F. NON-ANTIGEN-SPECIFIC IMMUNOLOGIC ENHANCEMENT

Another reason certain individuals might be excessively responsive at a given time might be that primary incidental stimuli may serve to prime inflammatory mediators that temporarily render that individual more responsive to a second, unrelated stimulus. The coincidental exposure to two or more stimuli within a given time may induce synergistically altered responses, whereas if these same two unrelated stimuli were received at separate times further apart, there would be no abnormal reaction. Much of what we know about this kind of exaggerated responsiveness has been learned from the study of host response to bacterial endotoxin, and the prototype of this type of response is the Shwartzman reaction (Shwartzman 1928). The endotoxin-induced Shwartzman reaction can be manifest in either a dermal or a systemic form. In the dermal form, a sensitizing dose of endotoxin or whole Gram-negative bacteria is injected intradermally into the skin of a rabbit. Twenty-four hours later, the same animal is given an intravenous dose of endotoxin, which need not be antigenically related to that of the sensitizing dose. A severe hemorrhagic dermal reaction leading to necrosis will occur within 24 hr of the second or provoking dose. In the generalized form (sometimes referred to as the Shwartzman–Sanarelli reaction), both sensitizing and provoking doses are given intravenously and induce generalized intravascular coagulation as well as bilateral renal necrosis accompanied by fibrin deposition and a precipitous drop in leukocytes and platelets. This is not an antigen-specific reaction because the two doses do not need to be antigenically related, the time between sensitization and provocation is too short to induce antigen-specific reactivity, and the increased sensitivity does not last more than a few days.

It is now felt that this type of temporal increased reactivity may result from several mediator systems being turned on to such an extent by various types of priming stimuli that occur prior to exposure to a further stimulant. Much attention has been directed to the idea of endotoxin-initiated "second signals" wherein endotoxin primes target cells for subsequent enhanced reactivity. This is an exceedingly complex area and could involve several different types of systems including calcium ion channel triggering, activation of cyclic nucleotide synthesis, increased toxic oxygen radical formation, and enhanced cytokine production, e.g., TNF and IFN-γ (Heremans 1990). This relates to immunotoxicity in that if an individual encounters an immunomodulating agent at near the same time he encounters a potentially immunotoxic substance, the combined effects of mediators from the two stimuli may synergistically cause an exaggerated reaction.

Several microbial products are known immunomodulators (Burrell 1988), and the possibility exists that these kinds of mechanisms might account for some of the enhancement of immune injury that is known to follow certain types of infectious disease. Streptococcal pyrogenic exotoxin is known to enhance the development of delayed-type hypersensitivity to simultaneously administered antigens and even enhances many of the biological activities of bacterial endotoxin on host mediation systems, particularly those of macrophages (Bohach et al. 1990). The microbial immunomodulator about which the most is known is bacterial endotoxin (Burrell 1990). This complex lipopolysaccharide associated with outer membrane proteins is a major structural unit of Gram-negative bacteria, which in themselves are very common in the environment and a major cause of infectious disease.

Although all of these examples of double signals employing a known microbial immunomodulator can be viewed as enhanced immunologic activity, most are accompanied by inflammation. The main point is that if an infection were present at the same time the host receives a second signal in the form of a xenobiotic, altered reactivity may be expected even in the face of no prior exposure to that specific xenobiotic. The presence of an immunomodulator at such a time might even *down*-regulate a response. The T-cell cytokine IL-2, which is known to regulate NK-cell activity, is depressed in burn patients, and NK cells from such patients have a lowered response to IL-2. It is also well known that these patients are in a way immunosuppressed in that they are particularly susceptible to systemic infections with Gram-negative bacteria. It has been shown that sera from burn patients suppress NK-cell activity from normal control donors, but this inhibitory activity can be removed by first removing the endotoxin from the sera by affinity chromatography (Bender et al. 1988). If the patients are treated 5 days with the antibiotic polymyxin B (to prevent the emergence of opportunistic Gram-negative bacterial infections), no decline in NK activity or IL-2 responsiveness is seen. This is a clear case of two insults (the burn and the presence of the Gram-negative bacteria) synergistically combining to depress an important immune function.

Thus, a close look at the etiopathogenesis of a disease as seemingly straightforward as IgE-mediated allergy to a well-recognized allergen reveals a multiplicity of additional extrinsic as well as intrinsic factors that could be present, often at critical times in reference to the allergen exposure, in order for clinical disease to be realized. The major conclusion from these discussions is that even in the case of a single idiosyncratic reaction to a definable extrinsic substance, clinical responsiveness, as well as detectable characteristics measured in the laboratory, are complex multifactorial events, and certainly one cannot place the blame of causality solely on the inducing agent.

G. PROBLEMS WITH PREDICTING AND INTERPRETING IMMUNOTOXICITY

Thus, from the kinds of data available, we tend to think of agents capable of exerting an immunotoxic effect as potentially dangerous in terms of increased risk for infection or tumor. Obviously, it takes a long time to learn of a given agent's potential carcinogenicity risk, and then only in retrospect. Since hindsight is so expensive and dangerous, i.e., there is much time lost while people are still being exposed to dangerous substances, the question comes up, can immunotoxicity be predicted? Under experimental enhancing conditions and using animals with unique sensitizing characteristics such as the guinea pig, one can induce hypersensitivity to almost any substance. There are some approaches used in industry to help weed out the most potent contact sensitins for delayed-type hypersensitivity, which presumably is based on molecular properties, but there are no comparable procedures for identifying human immediate-type allergens. Identifying such potent human allergens is usually a matter of either skin testing a panel of volunteers in advance or gaining accumulated experience from actual use. The problem of predicting immunotoxicity other than allergy in humans is even more complicated because it occurs at two levels; i.e., does exposure to the agent alter an immunologic laboratory value, or does it lead to an increase in clinical infection/tumor incidence?

Since pretesting unknown substances on humans at a range of doses, including very high ones, is out of the question, we are left with the following approaches in attempting to predict immunotoxic or hypersensitivity consequences ahead of time: (1) the use of experimental animals; (2) various in vitro procedures using materials obtained from humans, including measuring various parameters on humans who have been exposed to the substance in question; and (3) testing new materials on panels of human volunteers. The first problem is encountered from the various in vitro assays that immunologists use. Whether the samples being tested are from experimental animals exposed to controlled doses or from humans exposed to varying conditions of the substance, the problem comes up of how to interpret a value out of the normal range; i.e., how much outside the normal range does a value have to be to indicate a significant aberration? The bottom line with so many human studies is that, in spite of all of the data linking depressed laboratory values in specific immune parameters, few examples exist where one can directly relate "bad numbers" to a specific clinical effect, e.g., increased infection. We know for example that a T-helper/T-suppressor ratio is normally around 2:1, but when it drops to as low 1:5, as happens in AIDS, the immunologic consequence is profound. Where we need information is in determining at what point there is a crossover from normal, no adverse affect to abnormal, significant impairment.

There are a number of immune response pathways, both antigen-specific and non-specific, many of them redundant. Even in a given pathway there may occur various shunt mechanisms so that if a given pathway is blocked, the reaction may still proceed to completion by an alternate route. Because the immune system is charged with defense against infectious agents and tumors, it is unlikely that minor perturbations of the immune system would result in increased mortality. Although the concept is controversial, data suggest that there is tremendous functional reserve in the immune system in individual animals and humans. Biologically relevant effects occur only after the functional reserve capacity has been exceeded. Animal studies have suggested that the antibody-producing cells (e.g., plaque-forming cells) must be reduced by 40% before the animal is susceptible to select viral infections. A reduction of 40–60% in both NK and cytotoxic T cells is associated with a susceptibility to development of certain tumors (Dean et al. 1987). It follows that small but statistically significant changes in ex vivo assays would not be biologically relevant.

Our knowledge of just how much reserve we have and how much injury we can sustain is very imprecise at the present time and is an area deserving more research (Trizio et al. 1988). An excellent example of how immunologic effector redundancy serves to cushion the total immune response if one part is adversely modified may be found in the relationship of T_c cells and NK cells. Both cell types are major defense mechanisms against viral-infected cells, but by different mechanisms. Infection with certain viruses (e.g., herpes and adenoviruses) reduces the expression of MHC class I markers on the surface of infected cells, thus impairing the ability of T_c cells to recognize and destroy virus-carrying cells (Anderssen et al. 1985; Jennings et al. 1985). Since NK cells do not require recognition of viral antigen in MHC context, they serve to maintain protection.

In addition, there are multiple redundant defense mechanisms within the system. Failure or impairment of a single effector circuit may be compensated for by other effectors. For example, exposure to dimethylnitrosamine reduces T- and B-cell function in the mouse. However, host resistance to *Listeria* is not diminished because of increased macrophage activity (Holsapple, Bick, and Duke 1985).

With these problems, it can be seen that setting exposure standards or even calculating risk factors for any known immunotoxic substance is impossible at the moment and will be very difficult in the future. We first need to define concisely what is meant by immunotoxic, and for each substance tested, we will need to have dose–response information available from longitudinal studies (i.e., the effect of graded doses over a long period of time). In humans, such information is necessarily anecdotal and epidemiologic. We further need to have more basic science information on the extent of reserves of the immune system in both animals and man to know how much injury it can sustain. We need to have more information on intrinsic and external synergistic factors that influence or modify immune injury or hypersensitivity induction.

Finally, there are many questions in risk analysis that lie outside the realm of scientific endeavor. Aside from the etiology of milk intolerance and celiac sprue, where there is obvious clinical impairment to easily identified agents, the question comes up, if wheat and milk were only occupationally related agents or chemically manufactured products instead of essential foods, would these agents be considered toxic for the general population, and would exposure limits be prescribed? Many useful therapeutic agents are extremely beneficial yet are known to carry significant immunotoxic risk (e.g., chloramphenicol, methyldopa, steroids). Serious allergic reactions have been triggered by administration of such drugs as sulfas, penicillin, and chymopapain. Are the benefits of these agents to be denied to those who require them? If a given drug or chemical is known to carry a low, measurable risk toward developing a specified immunologic abnormality, including clinical reactions as serious as fatal anaphylaxis, just how low must that risk be before it is considered acceptable? Clearly, such decisions are not in the realm of the laboratory.

H. PROBLEMS IN EXTRAPOLATING EXPERIMENTAL ANIMAL DATA TO HUMANS

There is an enormous literature available detailing alterations in selected immune components to given agents in a variety of animal species, but except for hypersensitization, few of these details have been observed in humans (Trizio et al. 1988; Thomas, Busse, and Kerkvliet 1988). No single species of experimental animal completely duplicates the human situation; each has its advantages and disadvantages. Therefore, drawing conclusions about human allergy/immunotoxicity from experimental animal data is always fraught with a degree of uncertainty. Added to this are the use of inappropriate dosages, routes, and durations of exposures of xenobiotic as well as the use of only selected parameters for study and one becomes understandably confused when trying to make meaningful conclusions from the data relative to human experience (Sharma and Zeeman 1980; Trizio et al. 1988). Animal results do not inevitably predict human adverse reactivity, nor do humans inevitably experience the same toxicity as do animals (Davies 1984).

For example, a test material is usually used at high concentrations for short periods of time, but acute or chronic doses at high or low concentrations may have different effects on the immune system. Acute doses of dichloroethane suppress the immune response, but chronic doses of the same material have no immunotoxic effects (Munson et al. 1982). Second, the age or the maturity of the test animal may influence the results of the study. Compounds such as diethylstilbestrol affect neonates but have little effect on adults. Hence, studies performed in adult animals would give a false-negative immunotoxic effect. Third, similar false, negative results can be demonstrated when there are species-dependent effects in immunotoxicology studies. For example, hexachlorobenzene suppresses immune function in the rat but stimulates the murine immune system (Vos et al.

1986). Fourth, the pharmacology, metabolism, and toxicological profile of the chemical is usually unknown. Since these parameters may be significantly different in man, it is possible that effects in animals may not be duplicated. Finally, many of the immunologic endpoints have not been evaluated for predictive effects. Thus, the toxicological significance of the data cannot be established, and additional testing must be employed to establish the biological significance.

Animal species differ in regard to numerous details in immunologic sensitization, to the ways in which their individual immunologic components respond to environmental materials, and to how they express immunologic injury. Immunologists favor rabbits for their ability to produce precipitating antibody, and as such they are the animal of choice for inducing precipitin-dependent reactions such as Arthus reactions and immune complex glomerulonephritis. Delayed-type hypersensitivity (DTH) is easily induced in them, and they exhibit good skin reactions. They are the species of choice for studying alveolar macrophages and other cells obtainable by bronchoalveolar lavage. Comparatively little is known about their MHC systems, but they have served as models for allotypic immunoglobulin markers.

Guinea pigs are favored for both immediate and delayed-type hypersensitivities and exhibit well-defined skin and pulmonary reactions on challenge. They produce non-IgE cytophilic antibodies, which really are relevant to human antibodies. This quality has facilitated the use of smooth muscle strips from sensitized animals in various immunopharmacological assays, e.g., the Shultz–Dale and the passive cutaneous anaphylaxis assays. The pharmacology of their lungs is distinctly different, and it is very difficult to subject them to bronchoalveolar lavage because of their susceptibility to endemic, easily transmissible infections. Because the guinea pig has enormous levels of serum complement, it remains the animal of choice to study the complement system. There are many parallels between guinea pig and human complement except for the matter of quantity, i.e., the guinea pig has an enormous amount in comparison.

Mice are easily the most commonly used animal for the study of efferent immunologic pathways. Indeed, much of what is known about T–B-cell cooperation, antigen presentation, MHC restriction, and interleukin biology has been learned from the mouse. They have also been the favored species to produce both B- and T-cell hybridomas. Mice can readily be inbred to produce isogenic and congenic strains, which have greatly facilitated such immunologic studies as adoptive transfer and immune reconstitution. Although the murine MHC class I and II loci differ in many ways from humans and reside on different chromosomes, there is enough similarity that an enormous amount of fundamental immunology has been learned from their use (e.g., generation of immunoglobulin diversity, efferent pathways). However, these similarities do not extend to the efferent immunologic pathways, and, indeed, data from mouse studies have even misled investigators. Mouse complement is very low, and because of this, the role of cytotoxic antibody in graft rejection was long underestimated. The DTH reactions in mice differ substantially from those in rabbits, guinea pigs, and man, and there could be serious question about the human relevance of any study of this kind done with mice.

Rats have long been a favored species among toxicologists but have not been used nearly as much by immunologists. Their DTH effector mechanisms also differ substantially, but their IgE responses are more nearly like those of man. In this respect, much about IgE control has been learned from the rat. More is being learned about their MHC systems, and they have been used for hybridoma production.

In trying to draw conclusions from data obtained from animals subjected to xenobiotics for immunotoxicity testing, one should remember how greatly a selected immune parameter, e.g., lymphocyte responses, can vary to a given test substance, e.g., corticosteroids. Lymphoid cells of rats, mice, and rabbits are very susceptible to steroid-induced lysis, in contrast to those of monkeys, guinea pigs, and humans. Because of this, treating these species with comparable doses will yield quite different results, and it is reasonable to expect similar species differences to other agents (Webb and Winkelstein 1984). Trizio et al. (1988) have reviewed in detail many of the disparities of data obtained from various species used to study the same xenobiotics, particularly in reference to humans. But as long ago as 1980, Sharma and Zeeman reviewed the difficulty in trying to compare the results of different animal studies to the same agent. Although the warning was sounded over a decade ago, their admonitions still stand. They selected DDT as an example and compiled a table of the studies done on this substance at that time. An adaptation of that comparison is given in Table 10–4 and well illustrates the problem. Not only are different species being used to evaluate DDT, but also different doses and regimens, different antigen challenges, and different means of assessment. Depending on what one is looking for, almost any kind of response may be obtained. If we cannot confidently compare results

TABLE 10–4.   Varying Effects of DDT on Antibody Levels[a]

Test Species	Dose and Regimen	Antigen Used	Effect[b]
Goldfish	10 or 50 mg/kg, IP 2 days preimmuniz	SRBC	−
	10 or 50 mg/kg, IP 1 wk preimmuniz 4 wk postimmuniz	BSA	0, −
Chicken	100 ppm feed, 40 days	SRBC	0
	10–100 ppm feed, 11 mo	SRBC	+, then −
	500–800 ppm feed, 6 wks	BSA	0
	5–625 ppm feed, 2 wks	BSA	0
	5–900 ppm feed, 2 wks	S. pullorum	0, + at med. doses
	100 ppm feed, 146 days	Newcastle vaccine	+
Duck	10/100 ppm feed, 2 wks	SRBC	First +, then −
Rat	40 mg/kg, oral 60 days	BSA	+
	20/200 ppm feed, 31 days	Diphtheria toxoid	?, −, 0
	200 ppm water, 7 wks	Ovalbumin	−
Guinea pig	15 mg/kg, IP, every other day, 2 wks	Diphtheria toxoid	0
Rabbit	4–150 mg/kg feed, 8 wks	SRBC	0
	200 ppm water, 38 days	SRBC	−
	200 ppm water, 38 days	S. typhi	−
	10 mg/kg, oral, 10 days	S. typhi	+
	10/20 mg/kg, oral	S. typhi	−
	2 ml, oral	Brucella vaccine	−
Human	5 mg/day oral, 20 days	S. typhi	+
	Related to ambient DDT levels	Diphtheria toxoid	0
	?	Typhoid vaccine	−

[a]All data compiled prior to 1980.
[b]Abbreviations used: 0, No effect; +, enhancement; −, depression.

Source: Adapted from Sharma and Zeeman (1980).

from different animal studies, how then may we expect to extrapolate these data to human relevance?

Many of the difficulties and contradictory results encountered in trying to evaluate and compare different animal studies stems from the nonuniformity of approaches. The matter of species selection has been detailed earlier, but the matter of age should be given more attention. Individual species mature immunologically at different ages, and then not all at once to all antigens. Hematopoietic tissues may be much more susceptible to xenobiotics, and this may be important if one is interested in the various perinatal factors that influence subsequent immunity. Otherwise it is dangerous to compare results with those from mature animals. As we learn more about the effects of glucocorticoids and neurological regulation on the immune response, more attention will need to be given to the matter of sex selection and to the stress to which the animals are subjected. (Is the room of barking dogs next door to the one housing rabbits in the animal quarters?) Since many studies have shown diurnal variation effects on immune parameters, more attention will need to be paid to the time of day procedures are carried out and to seeing that procedures are carried out at the same hour each time they are repeated.

Regarding the use of xenobiotics, the matter of unrealistic dose levels, routes, and regimens has received much criticism, and deservedly so. Toxicologists should be familiar with dose–response curves, but this is a new concept for many immunologists. As with other areas of toxicology, a given agent can be either inhibitory or stimulatory depending on dose (see Table 10-4; compare responses for sheep erythrocytes versus *Salmonella typhi*). Even when one uses the same species and controls the dose of the xenobiotic administered, difficulty will be encountered in comparing responses obtained if different antigen challenges are used. The matter of investigating different doses of the same antigen has been given insufficient attention. In view of the fact that the timing of administration of immunosuppressive drugs given for the prevention of organ transplant rejection is so critical (Webb and Winkelstein 1984), more attention needs to be paid to similar considerations in immunotoxicology. Some agents are more immunosuppressive when given prior to antigen administration, but others are most effective when given at or near the time of antigen.

The more involved or complicated the assay, e.g., measuring survival against a challenge infectious agent in experimental animals exposed to a test xenobiotic, the more probable it is that there will be interlaboratory variation in results. Some years ago the National Toxicology Program at the NIEHS undertook a validation study of a battery of immunologic tests to be applied to immunotoxicity testing. Although the experimental design and methodology were all the same, there was enough interlaboratory variation in execution to affect the results. Although all laboratories agreed that the test agent did induce depressed resistance to the challenge agent, there was a variation of >35% in how much.

There are those, even among the medical science profession, who state that animal models have little relevance to the human situation; however, immunologists have learned an enormous amount from their study that has indeed proved highly relevant to humans. The lesson to keep in mind is to understand that there are species differences and one should not be a captive of the experimental results if they conflict with the human experience. The alternative of not using animal testing is irresponsibility in assuring the safety of those exposed to the material or in trying to learn in what manner a given material is immunotoxic. By under-

standing mechanisms of immunotoxicity, one can help avoid inducing immunotoxicity by similar agents and pathways in the future.

References

Anderssen, M., S. Paab, T. Nilsson, and P. A. Peterson. 1985. Impaired intracellular
    transport of class I MHC antigen as a possible means for adenovirus to evade immune
    surveillance. *Cell* 43:215–22.
Anonymous. 1986. Risks of agranulocytosis and aplastic anemia. A first report of their
    relation to drug use with special reference to analgesics. *J.A.M.A.* 256:1749–57.
Anonymous. 1987. Revision of the CDC surveillance case definition for acquired immuno-
    deficiency syndrome. *Morbid. Mortal. Weekly Rep.* 36:3S–15S.
Ayala, L. E., and T. Ahmed. 1989. Is there loss of a protective muscarinic receptor mecha-
    nism in asthma? *Chest* 96:1285–91.
Bender, B. S., A. Winchurch, J. N. Thupari, et al. 1988. Depressed natural killer cell
    function in thermally injured adults: Successful in vivo and in vitro immunomodulation
    and the role of endotoxin. *Clin. Exp. Immunol.* 71:120–25.
Björkstén, B., O. Finnstrom, and K. Wichman. 1988. Intrauterine exposure to the beta-
    adrenergic receptor-blocking agent metoprolol and allergy. *Int. Arch. Allergy Appl.
    Immunol.* 87:59–62.
Björkstén, B., and N.-I. M. Kjellman. 1990. Perinatal environmental factors influencing
    the development of allergy. *Clin. Exp. Allergy* 20(Suppl. 3):3–8.
Bohach, G. A., D. J. Fast, R. D. Nelson, and P. M. Schlievert. 1990. Staphylococcal and
    streptococcal pyrogenic toxins involved in toxic shock syndrome and related illnesses.
    CRC Crit. Rev. Microbiol. 17:251–72.
Burrell, R. 1985. Immune system. In *Environmental Pathology*, ed. N. K. Mottet,
    pp. 320–43. New York: Oxford University Press.
Burrell, R. 1988. Immunomodulation by bacterial products. *Clin. Immunol. Newslett.*
    9:206–9.
Burrell, R. 1990. Immunomodulation by bacterial endotoxin. *CRC Crit. Rev. Microbiol.*
    17:189–208.
Busse, W. W. 1990. Respiratory infections: Their role in airway responsiveness and the
    pathogenesis of diseases and asthma. *J. Allergy Clin. Immunol.* 85:671–83.
Cogswell, J. J., E. B. Mitchell, and J. Alexander. 1987. Parental smoking, breast feeding,
    and respiratory infection in development of allergic diseases. *Arch. Dis. Child.* 62:338–
    44.
Coligan, J. E., A. M. Kruisbeek, D. H. Margulies, et al. 1991. *Current Protocols in
    Immunology.* New York: John Wiley & Sons.
Croner, S., and N.-I. M. Kjellman. 1990. Development of atopic disease in relation to
    family history and cord blood IgE levels—eleven years' follow-up in 1654 children.
    Pediatr. Allergy Immunol. 1:3–9.
Dales, R. E., R. Burnett, and H. Zwanenburg. 1991. Adverse health effects among adults
    exposed to home dampness and molds. *Am. Rev. Respir. Dis.* 143:505–9.
Davies, G. E. 1984. Immunotoxicology: The viewpoint of an industrial immunologist. In
    Immunotoxicology: A Current Perspective of Principles and Practices, ed. P. W. Mul-
    len, pp. 151–61. Berlin: Springer-Verlag.
Dean, J. H., L. M. Thurmond, L. D. Lauer, and R. V. House. 1987. Comparative toxicol-
    ogy and correlative immunotoxicology. In *Environmental Chemical Exposures and Im-
    mune System Integrity*, ed. E. J. Burger, R. G. Tardiff, and J. A. Bellanti, pp. 85–
    100. Princeton: Princeton Scientific.
De Jongh, C. A., and S. C. Schimpff. 1988. Infection in the compromised host. In *Immu-
    nological Diseases*, 4th ed., ed. M. Samter, D. W. Talmage, M. M. Frank, et al.,
    pp. 963–78. Boston: Little, Brown.
Follansbee, S. E., D. F. Busch, C. B. Wofsy, et al. 1982. An outbreak of *Pneumocystis
    carinii* pneumonia in homosexual men. *Ann. Intern. Med.* 96:705–13.

Heremans, H., J. Vandamme, C. Dillen, et al. 1990. Interferon-gamma, a mediator of lethal lipopolysaccharide-induced Shwartzman-like shock reactions in mice. *J. Exp. Med.* 171:1853–69.

Heyden, S., and P. Pratt. 1980. Exposure to cotton dust and respiratory disease. Textile workers, "brown lung," and lung cancer. *J.A.M.A.* 244:1797–98.

Holsapple, M. P., P. H. Bick, and S. C. Duke. 1985. Effects of N-nitrosodimethylamine on cell mediated immunity. *J. Leuk. Biol.* 37:367–81.

Janoff, A. 1985. Elastases and emphysema. Current assessment of the protease–antiprotease hypothesis. *Am. Rev. Respir. Dis.* 132:417–33.

Jennings, S. R., P. L. Rice, E. D. Kloszewski, et al. 1985. Effect of herpes simplex virus types 1 and 2 on surface expression of class I major histocompatibility complex antigens on infected cells. *J. Virol.* 56:757–66.

Katz, P., and A. S. Fauci. 1988. Immunosuppressives and immunoadjuvants. In *Immunological Diseases*, 4th ed., ed. M. Samter, D. W. Talage, M. M. Frank, et al., pp. 675–98. Boston: Little, Brown.

Lemanske, R. F., E. C. Dick, C. A. Swenson, et al. 1989. Rhinovirus upper respiratory infection increases airway reactivity in late asthmatic reactions. *J. Clin. Invest.* 83:1–10.

Luster, M. I., A. E. Munson, P. T. Thomas, et al. 1988. Development of a testing battery to assess chemical-induced immunotoxicity: National Toxicology Program's guidelines for immunotoxicity evaluation in mice. *Fund. Appl. Toxicol.* 10:2–19.

MacDonald, S. M., and L. M. Lichtenstein. 1990. Histamine-releasing factors and heterogeneity of IgE. *Spring. Semin. Immunopathol.* 12:415–28.

Magnusson, C. G. M. 1986. Maternal smoking influences cord serum IgE and IgD levels and increases the risk for subsequent infant allergy. *J. Allergy Clin. Immunol.* 78:898–904.

Marsh, D. G., and W. B. Bias. 1988. The genetics of atopic allergy. In *Immunological Diseases*, 4th ed., ed. M. Samter, D. W. Talmage, M. M. Frank, et al., pp. 1027–46. Boston: Little, Brown.

Morgan, W. K. C. 1984. Coal workers' pneumoconiosis. In *Occupational Respiratory Diseases*, ed. W. K. C. Morgan and A. Seaton, pp. 377–448. Philadelphia: W. B. Saunders.

Munson, A. E., L. S. Sain, V. M. Sanders, et al. 1982. Toxicology of organic drinking water contaminants trichloromethane, bromodichloromethane, dibromochloromethane and tribromomethane, *Environ. Health. Perspect.* 46:117–26.

Murray, M. J., N. I. Kerkvliet, E. C. Ward, and J. H. Dean. 1985. Models for the evaluation of tumor resistance following chemical or drug exposure. In *Immunotoxicology and Immunopharmacology*, ed. J. H. Dean, M. I. Luster, A. E. Munson, and H. Amos, pp. 113–22. New York: Raven Press.

Nebert, D. W., and W. W. Weber. 1990. Pharmacogenetics. In *Principles of Drug Action*, ed. W. B. Pratt and P. Taylor, pp. 469–531. New York: Churchill Livingstone.

Oryszczyn, M.-P., J. Godin, I. Annesi, et al. 1991. In utero exposure to parental smoking, cotinine measurements, and cord blood IgE. *J. Allergy Clin. Immunol.* 87:1169–74.

Penn, I. 1985. Neoplastic consequences of immunosuppression. In *Immunotoxicology and Immunopharmacology*, ed. J. H. Dean, M. I. Luster, A. E. Munson, and H. Amos, pp. 79–90. New York: Raven Press.

Rantakallio, P. 1978. Relationship of maternal smoking to morbidity and mortality of the child up to the age of five. *Acta Paediatr. Scand.* 67:621–31.

Rieder, M. J., N. H. Shear, A. Kanee, et al. 1991. Prominence of slow acetylator phenotype among patients with sulfonamide hypersensitivity reactions. *Clin. Pharmacol. Ther.* 49:13–17.

Rose, N. R., and H. Friedman. 1980. *Manual of Clinical Immunology*, 2nd ed. Washington: American Society for Microbiology.

Selikoff, I. J., and E. C. Hammond. 1979. Asbestos and smoking. *J.A.M.A.* 242:458–59.

Sharma, R. P., and M. G. Zeeman. 1980. Immunologic alterations by environmental chemicals: Relevance of studying mechanisms versus effects. *J. Immunopharmacol.* 2:285-307.

Shwartzman, G. 1928. A new phenomenon of local skin reactivity to *B. typhosus* culture filtrate. *Proc. Soc. Exp. Biol. Med.* 25:560-61.

Smith, J. S. 1978. Epidemiology and natural history of asthma, allergic rhinitis, and atopic dermatitis (eczema). In *Allergy: Principles and Practice*, ed. E. Middleton, Jr., C. E. Reed, and E. E. Ellis, pp. 891-929. St. Louis: C.V. Mosby.

Thomas, P. T., W. W. Busse, and N. I. Kerkvliet. 1988. Immunologic effects of pesticides. In *The Effects of Pesticides on Human Health*, ed. S. B. Baker and C. F. Wilkinson, pp. 261-95. New York: Princeton Scientific.

Trizio, D., D. A. Basketter, P. A. Botham, et al. 1988. Identification of immunotoxic effects of chemicals and assessment of their relevance to man. *Fund. Chem. Toxicol.* 26:527-39.

Vincent, P. C. 1986. Drug-induced aplastic anemia and agranulocytosis. Incidence and mechanisms. *Drugs* 31:52-63.

Vos, J. G., G. M. J. Brouwer, F. X. R. van Leeuwen, and S. Wagenaar. 1986. Toxicity of hexachlorobenzene in the rat following combined pre and post natal exposure: Comparison of effects on immune system, liver and lung. In *International Symposium on Immunotoxicology*, ed. G. Gibson, R. Hubbard, and D. V. Parke, pp. 219-35. London: Academic Press.

Webb, D. R., and A. Winkelstein. 1984. Immunosuppression, immunopotentiation, and anti-inflammatory drugs. In *Basic and Clinical Immunology*, 5th ed., ed. D. P. Stites, J. D. Stobo, H. H. Fudenberg, and J. V. Wells, pp. 271-87. Los Altos: Lange.

Woolcock, A. J. 1988. Asthma. In *Textbook of Respiratory Medicine*, ed. J. F. Murray and J. A. Nadel, pp. 1030-68. Philadelphia: W. B. Saunders.

Youmans, G. P., P. Y. Paterson, and H. M. Sommers. 1986. *The Biologic and Clinical Basis of Infectious Diseases*, 3rd ed., p. 739. Philadelphia: W. B. Saunders.

11

Agents and Effects
of Immunotoxicity

A. INTRODUCTION

Information concerning human immunotoxicology can be organized according to whether one looks at who is being affected, by what kind of agent, how it is caused, or what type of effect is produced. One way is to study the types of people who are affected by responsible agents epidemiologically, but this science has had few successes in uncovering new incidents unreported previously. Rather, epidemiology is most often useful in looking backwards (retrospectively) or forwards (prospectively) from a point where a cause–effect relationship is either already known or highly suspected. Most of our initial information concerning possible cause–effect relationships has come from anecdotal reporting on cluster-case incidents (Fleming, Ducatman, and Shalat 1991). Unfortunately, there can be many reasons for clusters of incidents to occur together, many circumstantial or by coincidence, and cluster-case incidents per se do not prove etiology. They raise the initial suspicion, but it remains for the epidemiologist and experimental biologist to prove the relationship.

Reliable epidemiologic data have been largely obtained from three general types of populations at risk. One of the largest groups from which much data are available is that of occupationally exposed workers who are either involved in manufacturing synthetic products, extracting or working with natural products, or who are using manufactured chemicals in some kind of a process. Patients and consumers of therapeutics or cosmetics comprise a second population inasmuch as both groups are exposed to known amounts and types of foreign substances, and any reactions that ensue may be studied closely. What is of most concern to the public is how people might be exposed to substances in the ambient environment (air, food, and water) about them. News accounts of places like the Love Canal and Times Beach raise the incidence of suspicion of being poisoned among the populace, but very little useful data have been obtained from such accounts, and that which has is often subject to opprobrium. We need to know objectively just what kinds of immunotoxicity, if any, has resulted in people living in these areas.

A second way information concerning immunotoxicology can be organized is according to the type of agent, usually chemical, that has been incriminated in the toxicity. This method is a favorite of laboratory scientists who look for structure–function relationships and who like to work with isolated systems to discover links between cause and effect. Virtually all experimental animal data have been obtained in this manner. As useful as this approach is, it neither realistically duplicates human exposure nor is it often applied to exposures to complex substances. A further drawback is that animal models infrequently duplicate the signs and symptoms of patient complaints. This sort of approach naturally leads to studying immunotoxicology from the type of injury produced or the mechanism of toxicity. This is a useful procedure that has many benefits including learning ways to inhibit progress of the toxicity or to restore immune competence, but it has the disadvantage in that too often human disease is of mixed etiopathogenic type of complex exposures.

Immunotoxicology can most relevantly be studied by viewing the types of clinical illnesses associated with exposure to these agents. In order for either the epidemiologist or the laboratory scientist to provide meaningful data, pertinent knowledge concerning the clinical course and pathology of adverse reactions occurring in humans exposed to agents under natural conditions is first necessary.

B. CLINICAL EFFECTS OF IMMUNOTOXICOLOGY

Human disease suspected of immunotoxic origin can be grouped according to the organ system most often affected. Each organ system may be a route of sensitization on exposure as well as a target of immunologic manifestations.

1. Skin Manifestations

The skin can be an excellent route for agents to enter the body and exert other types of immunotoxic effects. The amount of absorption of a material varies not only with the individual but also with the anatomic area of skin in contact with the agent (Webster and Maibach 1985). For example, the absorption of either toxins or antigens is more than threefold greater from the axilla or scalp than from the forearm.

One dramatic example of the skin as a target organ is urticaria (hives), which consists of an eruption of short-lived edematous swellings of the skin associated with intense itching. Lesions resemble large mosquito bites, appearing with alarming suddenness, and antigen-induced urticaria may last 4 hr or longer. Angioedema is a similar manifestation involving the subcutaneous tissues and mucous membranes and may last longer. The two manifestations often coexist. Much of urticaria and angioedema arise from a mixture of genetic, immunologic, and physical stimuli or origins. All forms share a common inflammatory pathway for inducing the characteristic lesions. Some may be incited by physical factors affecting cholinergic receptors in the genetically susceptible, e.g., pressure, cold. A genetic disease affecting the complement system known as hereditary angioedema (Chapter 5) may be quite serious and life threatening. In those types with a more pronounced immune etiology, antigen interaction with IgE bound to mast cells in the skin leads to the manifestation. Many of these incidents are triggered by eating certain allergens associated with a high incidence of reactions, e.g., shellfish, strawberries and other soft fruits, nuts, and oral penicillin. A papular type of urticaria more often follows biting or stinging by venomous arthropods. Any agent that can nonspecifically degranulate mast cells might trigger a similar episode if opportunity for mast cell contact in the skin is available.

One must be careful in assigning an immunologic cause to any of the many types of occupational dermatoses. It has been variously estimated that only 20–30% of these conditions may show evidence of patch test reactivity, indicating cell-mediated-type hypersensitivity; the rest are caused by primary irritants or toxic effects. Toxic manifestations, e.g., rash, itching, scaling, exclusive of any immunologic component may resemble those from IgE- or lymphocyte-mediated reactions. Workers engaged in leather tanning and finishing, poultry/egg processing, manufacturing sealants, adhesives, or abrasives, fish packing, boat building and repairing, and landscaping are the groups most at risk for true, immune-induced skin manifestations. The oil uroshiol, which is an environmental contact sensitin from the plant popularly known as poison ivy, also belongs in this category. The synthetic chemicals dinitrochlorobenzene and dinitrofluorobenzene are universal sensitins capable of inciting the contact sensitivity in anyone coming in contact with them. So universal is their sensitizing ability, these agents are often used in assessing immunodeficiency states. Table 11–1 lists a number of agents known to induce contact cell-mediated sensitivity. Some of these agents are associated with higher degrees of risk, but others are based on isolated reports involving few individuals. Humans undoubtedly have unique effector mechanisms in their skin to account for the unique vesicular type of eruption with erythema that is not produced by any of the commonly used laboratory animals.

A rather common skin disease of partial immunologic significance is atopic dermatitis. This disease is a chronic, periodic skin disorder, primarily of infants and children, that depends on a complex interrelationship of genetic predisposition and an imbalance of immunologic and pharmacological mediators in the skin. The disease is characterized by marked pruritus, varied and continually changing morphology of skin lesions, increased serum IgE levels in most individuals, increased susceptibility to certain skin infections, and fluctuating abnormalities in cell-mediated immunity and β-adrenergic responsiveness (Leung, Rhodes, and Geha 1987). A complicated hypothesis to explain the pathogenesis of this baffling disease has been offered. Briefly, all of these manifestations occur in people who have a predisposing genetic cutaneous hyperreactivity. In one type of this disease, environmental agents may provoke attacks by interacting with IgE on effector cell surfaces. If such agents can be identified, steps can be taken to avoid such stimuli. Individuals with the other general type of this disease do not display elevated IgE levels but do possess the same lowered "itch" threshold. Regardless of the type of trigger, the response is also affected by vascular permeability change, release of mast cell or macrophage cytokines, or an imbalance of

TABLE 11–1.   Common Contact Sensitins

Plant	Synthetic Compounds	Minerals
Poison ivy	Benzocaine	Beryllium
European primrose	Epoxy resins	Nickel
Perfumes	Mercaptans	Cadmium
Rosin	Picric acid derivatives	Chromates
	Chlorinated hydrocarbons	Silver
	Ethylenediamine	Zirconium
	Paraphenylenediamine	Cutting oils
	Thimerosal	
	Neomycin	
	Dinitrochlorobenzene	
	Dinitrofluorobenzene	

drenergic and cholinergic receptors. If the manifestation is severe enough to break the skin, additional antigens may gain entry. Inflammatory lymphokines might then be liberated during antigen processing, which would attract more lymphocytes and activated macrophages, which, in turn, could lead to epidermal proliferation, fibroblast proliferation, and basophil granule release. An imbalance of immunoregulatory cells, the relative proportion of autonomic neural receptors, and the various quantities and types of mediators released could account for the many faces this disease presents during its course in a given individual. Given the importance of genetic components in this disease (nearly 70% of patients with this disease exhibit a family history of this disease: Rajka 1960), one must use caution in condemning a given etiologic agent.

A number of therapeutic and cosmetic materials provoke a range of skin reactions. Oils used as bases in many ointments for either medical or cosmetic purposes may induce contact sensitivity. Not only is the skin an excellent route to induce such reactions, when the ingredients are dissolved in solvents (e.g., in perfumes), cutaneous absorption is greatly facilitated. One short-lived disease was called the "underarm antiperspirant granuloma," and because of the inclusion of sodium zirconium lactate in the deodorant formulation that induced cell-mediated hypersensitivity and, over a long period of application, led to granuloma formation developed. Once the key ingredient was incriminated, the compound was either eliminated or modified in such a way that this is no longer a problem. It does illustrate, however, how new technology or commercial products transmitted to hundreds of thousands of people may quickly produce new medical problems.

2. Manifestations of the Respiratory Tract

The respiratory system shares with the skin and the gastrointestinal tract those surfaces most in contact with the external environment and antigen load. Not only is the lung being constantly bathed in large volumes of air in which particulates, gases, and vapors are suspended, but it receives virtually the entire cardiac output in the circulation. The anatomy of the lung is constructed to clear effectively both the exterior (the air) and the internal environment (the blood) of foreign matter. Distal airways of the lung are lined with alveolar macrophages and type II epithelial cells capable of expressing MHC class II molecules (Schneeberger et al. 1986). Depending on species, lymphocytes might also normally be present on the surfaces of distal airways. Clearance from the circulation is effected by access of lymphoid aggregates adjacent to the pulmonary microcirculation. The linings of the upper airways are underlaid with IgA- and IgE-secreting lymphocytes, and various complement components are released onto the surfaces as well. Because of these structures and anatomic location, the lung represents an excellent route of immunization, but it is also the target of many types of immune injury.

Although the lung may be a site of infection or tumor initiation in any individual, those with immune dysfunction tend to develop only certain types. Bacterial pneumonia, a process of infection-inducing exudate in the terminal airways, might be considered evidence of lowered resistance, either locally in the lung or as a result of general systemic stress. Epidemics of pneumonia tend to occur in crowded, stressed populations, and individual pneumonia may develop following inhalation of toxic substances in those with a variety of predisposing immune dysfunctions, e.g., immunologic immaturity, depression in antibody-synthesizing ability. Pneumonia caused by agents of extremely low virulence, e.g., *Pneumocystis*, are a certain signal of serious underlying immune dysfunction. The unusual severity of the *Legionella* in the original 1976 epidemic that gave that microbe its name was most likely related to the age of the affected population (Fraser et al. 1977). Older individuals are more likely to have a variety of underlying pulmonary and cardiovascular ailments that stress their local tissue resistance to enhanced infection by pathogens of only low virulence. Finally, the course of certain types of pulmonary infection as well as the type of pathology produced may be largely the result from immune events. Infections by the tubercle bacilli are complicated by the fact that the individual develops delayed-type hypersensitivity to tuberculoproteins present in the microbe, which greatly enhances inflammation and granuloma formation in the developing lesion. Conversely, poor resistance to this microbe is associated with an extremely rapid and overwhelming infection.

The upper respiratory system is a common target for the effects of immediate-type hypersensitivity to airborne allergens leading to allergic rhinitis, which may be seasonal or perennial, depending on the type of allergen. Table 11–2 lists many of the well-known respiratory allergens. For a more extensive discussion of allergens in atopic workers, see Terr (1986). Many of these same allergens may also trigger both immediate and late-phase types of asthma affecting the airways, as discussed in Chapter 6. Other types of immune or immune-like injury include (1) lung connective tissue serving as a target of both cytotoxic antibody and lymphocytes; (2) deposition of intravascular immune complexes possibly leading to fibrosis; (3) much bystander tissue injury occurring as a result of lymphocyte toxicity to foreign antigens; (4) nonspecific complement activation and/or mediator release occurring as a result of inhalation of noxious particles; and (5) inhalation of substances interfering with adrenergic/cholinergic balance possibly inducing asthma reactions.

3. Ocular Manifestations

Generally speaking, the eye is very resistant to infections. The constant winking and flushing activities of the tears, which are laden with secretory IgA and certain innate antimicrobial substances, help keep the eye free of microbes. Although the conjunctiva may become inflamed with a variety of microbes, the keratinized

TABLE 11–2.   Representative Antigens That May Cause Respiratory Allergy

Pollen	Organic Dusts	Animal Sources	Molds
Timothy	Coffee	Horse dander	*Alternaria*
Orchard grass	Sawdust	Pet danders	*Aspergillus*
June grass	Seed meals	Avian dander	*Hormodendrum*
Maples	Flour	Cockroach exoskeleta, eggs, etc.	*Rhizopus*
Birches	Enzymes	Human dander mites	*Helminth* sp.
Oaks	Pyrethrum	Cat saliva	*Penicillium*
Ragweed		Rodent urine	*Cladosporium*
Lamb's quarters			
Pigweed			
Plantain			
Sheep sorrel			

cornea is highly resistant to infection so that when that part of the eye becomes infected, particularly by fungi, it is often a signal that the immune system is functioning below normal level. Immunosuppressed patients or those with underlying disabilities, e.g., leukemia, are most likely to develop this kind of infection.

The eye is sensitive to a variety of immunologic injuries, particularly to immediate-type allergens, either airborne or introduced by splashing accidents, association with contact lenses, or rubbing from the hands (Greiner, Ross, and Allansmith 1988). The most common manifestation is conjunctivitis, often associated with hay fever, in which the eye is responding to the same allergens present in the air that affect the respiratory system. In the past, the eye has even been used as a sensitive indicator for determination of immediate-type hypersensitivity. A dilute drop of suspected antigen was placed in the eye and observed for evidence of local inflammation. Immediate types of allergy may range from mild conjunctivitis and tearing to angioedema.

A number of ocular conditions associated with wearing contact lenses are known, e.g., a bothersome condition known as contact-lens-associated giant papillar conjunctivitis. Although it affects both hard and soft lens wearers, the condition is much more common in the latter. Signs include giant papilla formation on the conjunctiva underneath the eyelid, excessive mucus secretion, itching, and inability to continue wearing the lens. Ocular infiltration of mast cells and eosinophils seem to indicate the basis for pharmacological treatment and suggest an immune etiology. It is possible that an abrasive action of the artificial lens affords entry of environmental antigens attached to the lens and enhances irritation. Although it is recommended to clean the lenses more frequently in enzyme (papain)-based detergents, this procedure may lead to the induction of an IgE-mediated conjunctivitis to the papain (Bernstein et al. 1984). Thimerosal, a lens disinfectant, has induced cell-mediated types of sensitivity expressed as conjunctival hyperemia and intolerance to lens wear.

A more serious ocular disease of autoimmune origin is sympathetic ophthalmia, characterized by the immunologic destruction of the uveal pigment. Physical trauma, which could include severe toxic accidents to the eye, is a prerequisite. Apparently, such physical trauma exposes the uveal tissue to the immune system, from which it is normally sequestered. Immune effectors (most likely cell-mediated elements with antiuveal pigment sensitivity) formed in the process then may have a chance to react with the tissue in both the injured and noninjured (sympathasizing) eye with eventual resultant loss of sight. The lens of the eye may also be an immunologic target made antigenic by microbial (e.g., staphylococcal) toxins, and the unproven possibility exists that environmental toxicants introduced under inflammatory conditions might also initiate this destructive process.

4. Gastrointestinal Manifestations

The most commonly thought of immunologic manifestation of the gastrointestinal tract is so-called food allergy. The term has met with much controversy because of overuse by both lay and professional people. There had been a tendency in the past to carelessly assign this diagnosis on the basis of very little clinical or laboratory evidence. The popular conception still is that food allergy is very common when in fact in those studies that have attempted to detect immune causation, the incidence among infants was found to be between 4% and 6%, decreasing to only 1–2% in older children and less than 1% in adult populations (reviewed in Sampson 1988). Part of the confusion stems from failure to differentiate food intolerance from food allergy. Food intolerance may be caused by enzyme deficiencies, physiological reactions to food additives or preservatives (e.g., sulfites or monosodium glutamate), contaminating toxins from microorganisms, disturbances from incorporated antibiotics, reactions to pharmacological agents present (e.g., caffeine), as well as psychological reactions to the taste, texture, or the knowledge of the nature of what is being eaten (Zwetchkenbaum 1990). What may be taken as an allergy to certain types of fish may in fact really result from biochemical changes produced by *Pseudomonas* bacteria that decarboxylate histidine into histamine, which causes the adverse reactions.

On the one hand, the gastrointestinal tract is exposed to the largest antigen load of any organ system. Yet, in those types of reactions that are immune mediated, the list of foods containing putatively allergic heat- and acid-resistant glycoprotein antigens is rather short. Peanuts and other nuts, eggs, milk, fish and shellfish, soy, and wheat together account for over 90% of the positive reactions. After digestion, some minimal peptide resists hydrolysis and must be absorbed intact in order to be antigenically effective. Many types of immunoglobulin response, primarily IgA, can be generated, most of which are probably effective in clearing the peptides from the circulation. The problem comes when IgE responses are generated in susceptible individuals. Abnormalities such as achlorhydria or immunologic immaturity seem to contribute to the incidence of sensitization. Symptoms may appear immediately after ingestion but usually after about 2 hr and range from general anaphylaxis in rare cases to cutaneous (urticaria, atopic dermatitis), respiratory (asthma), gastrointestinal (vomiting, diarrhea, colic, etc.), or neurological (migraine) manifestations. The explanation for the variety of organ system effects is unknown.

Evaluation of populations must be carried out by double-blind, placebo-controlled studies in order for a foodstuff to be properly incriminated as an offending agent (Bock et al. 1988). Skin testing may be of help, particularly in eliminating suspected agents, because there is excellent correlation between negative skin tests and absence of associated clinical signs (Sampson 1988). Positive skin tests may be helpful but do not necessarily correlate with provocation of symptoms. For example, it is estimated that over 50% of the population is skin test sensitive to egg white, yet fewer than 1% of adults are bothered by ingestion of it. When allergies/intolerances are known, it is easy to recommend avoidance, but often the offending agent (e.g., antibiotics or egg white) may be present in unknown quantities in processed foods. Diet manipulation that carefully eliminates one item at a time and compares the results is a very time-consuming and laborious process that may be needed to identify the offending agent.

There are also delayed-in-time responses to food allergens that take place hours to days after ingestion. One syndrome known as food-protein-induced gastroenteropathy, usually associated with cow's milk or soy, is reliably evaluated only by biopsy demonstrating infiltrates of lymphocytes, eosinophils, and plasma cells. Its etiology is obscure, but continued inflammation may lead to villous atrophy, malabsorption, and anemia. The offending agent should induce a reaction within 48 hr, and elimination from the diet usually resolves the matter.

Care must be taken in merely associating an eosinophilia with an allergic etiology. A comparatively new disease of modern technology recently appeared that is known as the eosinophilia–myalgia syndrome (EMS) and results from the ingestion of a product variously marketed as a dietary supplement or tranquilizer, L-tryptophan. In the United States there have been at least 23 deaths and over 1,500 cases (Selman, Rissenberg, and Melius 1991). Although many organ systems in this chronic illness are seriously affected, and many symptoms are present, a marked increase in circulating eosinophils is a universal finding. The effect carries over to newborn infants of mothers who are users. The first cases were found by the case-cluster incident method, but subsequent epidemiologic studies indicated that those affected seemed largely to be users of one particular brand, one that had been made from a bacterium genetically engineered to produce increased amounts of the amino acid (Raphals 1990).

Whether the toxicity was caused by a contaminant in the product resulting from the genetic manipulation or from the manufacturing process is unknown at the present. The severity and occurrence of signs and symptoms do not seem to be dose related. Although a toxic syndrome can be reproduced in rats with the agent from the specific company (but not from a USP-grade product) at dose levels comparable to those used by humans, no eosinophilia was noted (Crofford et al. 1990). Muscle biopsies from humans have been analyzed by quantitative immunocytochemical analysis and were characterized by a marked increase in $CD8^+$ T cells and macrophages infiltrating affected tissues (Emslie-Smith et al. 1991). There were few B and NK cells, and the number of eosinophils was either erratic or very low. There was no evidence of complement membrane attack complex deposition. The authors concluded that the tissue pattern suggested a cell-mediated reaction against a widespread antigen present on fascia, perimysium, and blood vessels.

The gastrointestinal tract is also a target of immune effectors and often exhibits pathology if immunodeficiency diseases are also present. Frequently malabsorption and diarrhea accompany these immune disturbances. The gut of the immunodeficient person will have increased susceptibility to a number of low-virulence pathogens, e.g., *Giardia*. Other types of infection tend to be more chronic, e.g., those caused by *Campylobacter*. The gut of the AIDS patient is a common target of HIV indicator infections, e.g., cryptosporidiosis and cytomegalovirus. Autoimmune diseases such as pernicious anemia with chronic atrophic gastritis accompany each other in that chronic inflammation, possibly initiated by a microbial process that destroys the epithelial cells that also secrete intrinsic factor that is needed for intact erythrocyte development. In addition to the inflammation, antibodies are also produced that combine with circulating intrinsic factor and block intestinal uptake of the intrinsic factor–vitamin B_{12} complex.

Two serious inflammatory diseases of the bowel, chronic ulcerative colitis and Crohn's disease, have histopathology and circulating lymphocyte subset patterns suggestive of an immune etiology. The pattern suggests an initial lymphocyte infiltrate that evokes macrophage- and neutrophil-mediated damage. There is demonstrated reactivity to bacterial as well as mucosal tissue antigens. That the incidence of these diseases is higher in industrialized countries implies a possible environmental link, but no definitive agent has yet been identified.

C. SELECTED AGENTS OF IMMUNOTOXICITY

Most of the discussion in previous sources of information in the immunotoxicology literature is arranged by chemical type or class of agent, and most of this has been limited to in vitro or experimental animal studies. The intent of the present coverage is to select examples of those agents that have been studied mostly with respect to the principles of relevance outlined in Chapter 10, especially in reference to human applications. Where possible, discussion of each agent begins with the cluster-case incident. The coverage is not intended to be exhaustive, merely illustrative, so that the reader may grasp an idea of the state of knowledge regarding each agent.

1. Polybrominated–Polychlorinated Biphenyls and Toxic Oils

Occasionally notorious accidents occur and thus present "experiments of nature" to study. Since there is little time for planning and humans, not animals, are affected, severe restrictions in design of what can be done are imposed on those making the studies. Often these accidents are realized only in retrospect (polybrominated biphenyl poisoning in Michigan) or in locations of the globe difficult to access quickly (Bhopal, Chernobyl, etc.). Although the results of investigations into such incidents are open to many criticisms, these should be tempered by the understanding of the reactionary conditions in which results had to be obtained.

Polybrominated Biphenyls

The Michigan polybrominated biphenyl (PBB) example is discussed in some detail because it illustrates so well some of the problems in assessing human immunotoxicity. In this instance, a commercial preparation of PBB was accidentally used in place of an inorganic ingredient in preparing a feed supplement for lactating cows (Fries 1986). This material was used throughout Michigan in 1973 and 1974. Toxic manifestations in the cattle were reduced milk production, joint swelling, hyperkeratosis, persistent mastitis, cutaneous and subcutaneous infections, abscess formation on back legs and udder, and various reproductive anomalies, but not necessarily anything related to infection. The agent contaminated not only beef and dairy cow products but also poultry and eggs. Identification of the toxic ingredient did not occur until 9 months after the contamination, by which time the PBB had become widely distributed throughout the state. Ingestion of contaminated products by humans extended beyond the farm residents. The PBB could be demonstrated in serum and adipose tissues of these individuals at least through 1980 (Bekesi et al. 1983). Clinical signs and symptoms included fatigue, a striking decrease in the ability to do physical or mental work, and an unusual need for sleep. Memory impairments and reduced energy were noted. Arthritic changes and other symptoms affecting the hepatic, neurological, and musculoskeletal systems were also noteworthy. Of most interest to the present discussion was that there was little that was related to increased susceptibility to infections or tumors.

A unique opportunity to study these farm residents immunologically in 1977 and later in 1980 was afforded Bekesi et al. (1983, 1985). Those in the exposed population were compared with age-matched controls, dairy farm residents living in the nearby environmentally similar state of Wisconsin who had not been exposed to the contaminated products, and with some New York City residents where the in vitro laboratory work was done. Total T- and B-lymphocyte counts, functional mitogenic assays, immunoglobulin content, and abnormalities in the

TABLE 11-3.   Cellular Data from Michigan PBB Exposure Accident Studies

Subjects	T Cells[a]	PHA[b]	CON A[b]	B Cells[a]	PWM[b]
New York City	1,986	102,226	98,151	521	95,130
Wisconsin Dairy	1,473	97,662	96,662	487	90,636
PPB–Michigan, normal[c]	1,341	92,272	94,634	467	93,199
PPB–Michigan, abnormal[c]	917	28,457	36,177	331	39,159

[a]T and B cells refer to the absolute numbers of cells per unit volume.
[b]All mitogen proliferation data are recorded in terms of counts per minute tritiated thymidine uptake in lymphocyte proliferation assays.
[c]The authors divided their exposed subjects into two groups depending on whether they gave values within normal or abnormal limits. They did not statistically compare all of the exposed group with either control population.

Source: Data from Bekesi et al. (1983).

number and percentage of what were then called "null cells" were studied. At the time the study was done, a null cell was so called because it did not express typical markers of either B cells (i.e., immunoglobulin staining by immunofluorescence) or T cells (then determined by rosette formation with sheep erythrocytes). Although considered to be an immature cell at the time of the study, these cells would now be considered mature NK cells and not necessarily related to either B or T lymphocytes.

Although the original study has serious statistical flaws, the authors concluded that in at least 18 of 45 Michigan residents sampled, a statistically significant decrease in absolute number of T cells as well as a decreased mitogenic response to standard T-cell mitogens was demonstrated. Although the absolute number of B cells was not changed, these T-cell-depressed subjects also evinced decreased mitogenic responses to a B-cell mitogen (see Table 11-3). It should be pointed out that these authors did not evaluate all of the exposed population statistically as one numerical group, and we have no data to compare the two exposed Michigan groups from the standpoint of level and duration of exposure, serum level of PBB, etc. Had they done so, their results might well have been insignificant, but the fact remains that they could identify a subset of 18 people with markedly abnormal laboratory values. Of greatest immunologic interest was the finding of a persistent *increase* in NK cells in many of the same subjects (19/40) when retested 5 years later. This seems to indicate that the PPB exposure has resulted in a permanent increase in NK cells, but whether because of a stem cell effect or continual stimulation from residual PPB is unknown. In a further study by this same group, elevated levels of IgG, IgA, and IgM as seen in Table 11-4 were reported (Bekesi et al. 1985). Taken together with the data indicating reduced mitogen responsiveness, one might conclude that secretion, not proliferation, was affected.

The most difficult thing about these studies is how to interpret the obviously

TABLE 11-4.   Immunoglobulin Data (mg/dl) from Michigan PPB Exposure Accident Studies

Subjects	IgG	IgA	IgM	Total Ig
Wisconsin dairy	877	202	98	1,192
Michigan, general population	1,286	271	129	1,686
PPB–Michigan dairy	1,606	288	142	2,039
PPB–chemical workers	1,188	275	112	1,577

Source: Data from Bekesi et al. (1985).

abnormal laboratory findings because, as yet, the exposed people do not seem to be affected by unusual numbers of infections or tumor incidence; i.e., how can there be abnormal B-cell function and T_h-cell number and function on the one hand and immunoglobulin hypersecretion on the other? A toxicologist would consider such changes merely adaptive, not toxic, responses. Certainly, by this time, any reduced resistance to infectious diseases by opportunists would have been realized. Increased tumor incidence can only be recognized after long-term retrospective studies, but it has been nearly 20 years since the incident occurred.

Experience gained from the use of combinations of immunosuppressants in transplantation surgery showed increases in tumor incidence in a much shorter time than this, and although the incubation period of HIV can be quite long, the immunologic defects are also clinically realized much earlier. On the other hand, the relationship of exposure to crocidolite asbestos fibers and development of mesotheliomas may take 20–40 years or more (Seaton 1984). There is no question that PBB can be toxic for many organ systems (Fries 1986). When one considers the generally agreed-on importance of NK cells against tumors, it may be ironic that the PBB actually *enhanced* tumor resistance by increasing NK-cell number. In an epidemiologic study of over 2,500 industrial workers exposed to PBB, a lower than expected mortality from all causes was found, and except for the incidence of two types of cancer, neither of which was statistically significant, all cancer mortality was also lower than expected (Brown and Jones 1981).

Yet, even these results are controversial because two other studies on exposed Michigan residents failed to find significant differences in immune parameters. In one study (Landrigan et al. 1979), significantly higher levels of circulating lymphocytes were found in a high-PBB concentration exposure group of their study population when tested in 1976–1977, but no demonstration of depressions in absolute numbers of T or B cells could be found in the same subjects. Another study (Stross et al. 1981) found no significant differences in B or T cells among exposed Michigan residents, PBB workers, or unexposed controls. Although statistically significant depressions in lymphocyte responses to certain lymphocyte mitogens in the exposed groups were seen compared with the unexposed, these values were considered within the normal range of the reporting laboratory, and thus no significance was attached to the finding. A possible explanation for altered lymphocyte responsiveness to mitogens was provided by the demonstration of an increase in very-low-density serum lipoproteins in sera from swine fed PBB, which suggests that altered lipid metabolism in the liver indirectly affected the composition of lymphocyte cell membranes (Howard, Werner, and Sleight 1980).

Polychlorinated Biphenyls

Similarly, an outbreak of poisoning broke out in Taiwan in 1979 involving over 2,000 persons. The source of poisoning was a particular brand of rice-bran oil that was accidentally contaminated by polychlorinated biphenyls (PCB). It was detectable in the oil samples at concentrations of from 4.8 to 204.9 ppm and in the blood of poisoned patients from 3 to 1,156 ppb. Although there were intitial significant depressions in the percentage of total T cells, active T cells, and T_h cells when measured 1 year after exposure, when remeasured 3 years later, there was partial recovery of the T_h cells and an increase in CD8$^+$ cells (Lü and Wu 1985). Signs and symptoms ranged from headache, ocular disturbances, and general malaise to diarrhea, myalgia, and arthritis. A similar disease outbreak was reported from Japan in 1968 and is now given the name of yu-cheng, which means oil disease. It was characterized mostly by acneiform eruptions and pigmentation as well as several other signs and symptoms involving many organ systems. Infections per se were not detailed but were largely confined to superficial skin infections, e.g., tinea versicolor, pyoderma, dermatophytosis, and warts, diseases not usually associated with immunodeficiency.

In almost all instances, in vitro lymphocyte mitogenesis assays using lymphocytes from exposed individuals and PWM, Con-A, PHA, or PPD showed *enhanced* stimulation indices. The most noteworthy findings were depressions in T-cell number, particularly in the T_h subset, and of delayed-type skin hypersensitivity to tuberculin and streptococcal enzymes, which in the case of tuberculin seemed to persist into the fourth year. Loss of delayed skin test sensitivity (anergy) is considered a measure of immune suppression. That these people were probably tuberculin sensitive before the accident (as seen from the high incidence of reactivity in the controls) indicates widespread exposure to the tubercle bacillus. Such a finding is usually interpreted to mean that the reactors are carrying these bacteria in an inactive but viable form. Reactivation tuberculosis might possibly become more widespread as this group ages, but so far it has not.

In general, laboratory studies in rodents with either agent have been unhelpful. One relevant study was performed with oral feeding of PCB to monkeys in graded doses (5–80 µg/kg per day) and evaluated beginning at 55 months after initiation of exposure (Tryphonas et al. 1991). Decreased anamnestic responses (IgG and IgM) to a T-cell-dependent antigen (but not to a T-cell-independent one) were obtained, but with equivocal dose–response relationships. There were significant dose related decreases in lymphoproliferative responses to PHA and Con A but not PWM mitogens. Although there seemed to be no effect at any dose level in the percentage of $CD4^+$, $CD8^+$, or $CD20^+$ (a B-cell marker) cells, there was a lower mean percentage of CD2 cells (taken as a measure of total T cells).

It should be noted that practically all of the animal studies have been made with the highly chlorinated biphenyl compound known as Aroclor 1260. There seems to be a greater risk of carcinogenicity in rodents with the more highly chlorinated species of PCB, yet these comprise only 12% of the total sold in the United States (Abelson 1991). Few immunotoxic studies have been done with the more abundant, less carcinogenic compounds with lower chlorination.

Toxic Oil Syndrome

In 1981 another technological accident that involved thousands of cases and hundreds of deaths (nearly a 0.16% mortality) occurred in Spain among people using a cooking oil prepared from olive oil adulterated with an industrial grade of rapeseed oil (Kilbourne et al. 1983). Chief findings were an explosive pneumonitis characterized by no particular infectious agent, severe gastrointestinal upsets, rash, and a striking eosinophilia. Some subjects developed progressive disease; advanced neuromuscular disease occurred some months later in 20–30% of these patients. Death was from failure of the respiratory musculature and infectious complications. Various clinical evidence suggested autoimmune reactions in some patients, e.g., vasculitis and scleroderma skin lesions.

The imported rapeseed oil had been denatured with 2% aniline for industrial use, and its low cost may have contributed to its clandestine mixture and sale as a cooking oil. Subsequent gas–liquid chromatography and multivariate analyses made on blind-coded recalled samples identified a marked dose–response correlation between contamination with free aniline and various fatty acid anilides with increasing risk of illness (Kilbourne et al. 1988). Another subsequent investigation was carried out on histopathology sections immunofluorescently-stained for eosinophilic major basic protein (MBP) and on serum MBP levels in samples obtained from patients (Ten et al. 1990). The results indicated a high incidence of eosinophil infiltration coincident with the peak of acute disease. Serum MBP levels remained elevated throughout the disease. Significant deposits and circulating levels of MBP would certainly have been inflammatory.

Eosinophils may have been preferentially attracted chemotactically by the anilides or one of their many possible metabolic intermediates and, once activated, could have degranulated, releasing MBP as well as other inflammatory mediators including eosinophil-derived neurotoxin. The latter produces characteristic patterns of neuromuscular weakness when injected into animals. Some of these mediators could have amplified the response by inducing mast cell degranulation and by modulating leukotrienes. There are certain similarities in mechanism between this and the eosinophilia–myalgia syndrome discussed above.

2. Pesticides

Pesticides represent a possible immunotoxic threat not only to those involved in manufacture and application but to consumers of products contaminated with these agents as well. Their widespread use, manner of application, ability of some to cross the placental barrier, and their tendency to be concentrated and unchanged in the food chain are contributing factors to great concern. Except for substances like DDT, an organochloride, and organophosphates like malathion, which exert effects in lab animals within narrow limits; few have been studied systematically. Often, pesticides are effective only at high concentrations or heavy exposure. At other times, it is difficult to compare doses given to the animals with realistic levels humans might encounter. Many agents do not show the same sort of metabolism or pharmacokinetics in experimental animals as they do in man. An additional problem encountered in assessing agricultural chemicals for allergenic or immunotoxic effects is that these products are seldom in pure form, and the offending agent has often proved to be a contaminating substance in the technical-grade formulations. For example, technical-grade (86% pure) pentachlorophenol has been shown to depress T-cell cytolysis in vitro and enhance tumor formation in vivo in murine systems whereas the 99% pure form was without effect (Kerkvliet, Baecher-Steppan, and Schmitz 1982). Similarly, alleged malathion contact sensitivity has been traced to contaminating diethyl fumarate (Thomas et al. 1988). Yet, pesticides should be considered presumptively immunotoxic from the limited animal and human data available and for the potential related to their widespread use.

The animal data have previously been reviewed by Dean, Luster, and their colleagues (see Chapter 1 for references) and summarized by Thomas et al. (1988), so they are not repeated here except to point out those studies with most human application. Since some of these agents pass the placental barrier in unmodified form, and there is a greater risk of toxic effects on developing systems, perhaps more attention should be placed on perinatal exposure. For example, some pesticides/defoliants are contaminated with 2,3,7,8–tetrachlorodibenzo-p-dioxin (TCDD), which has been shown to induce greater immune dysfunction in newborn rodents than in adults (Thomas and Faith 1985). Although most studies suggest that the carbamate class of insecticides, e.g., carbaryl (Sevin), are fairly nontoxic immunologically (Street 1981), one study of women chronically exposed to aldicarb-contaminated ground water (<61 ppb) demonstrated increased numbers and percentages of $CD8^+$ T cells and decreased ratios of CD4/CD8 cells (mean of 1.88 versus 2.54 in unexposed controls). However, no self-reported adverse personal or reproductive health effects were noted (Fiore et al. 1986). In this case, animal studies would not have predicted the human result, because mice given environmentally relevant graded doses of aldicarb in drinking water over a 34-day period exhibited no change in number, percentage, or function of T, B, or NK cells (Thomas et al. 1987, 1990).

Documenting any actual reduced immunity in humans induced by pesticides has been difficult. Although changes in various hematological and immune parameters have been recorded in some workers exposed to these agents, there is no evidence to indicate that there is any change in infectious disease resistance in them. Changes in serum immunoglobulins and C3 in workers exposed to chlorinated hydrocarbons were unaccompanied by any change in resistance (Wysocki, Kalina, and Owczarzy 1985), although an increase in upper respiratory infections did accompany demonstrable impairment in neutrophil chemotaxis in workers exposed to organophosphates (Hermanowicz and Kossman 1984). Thus, more attention should be directed to the type of immune parameter selected for study instead of concentrating on those that are easiest to measure.

In addition to possible damage these agents may cause the immune system, certain pesticides are common incitants of both skin contact and IgE-mediated respiratory hypersensitivities. Often in trying to assess the potential of pesticides to induce contact sensitivity, not only is there poor agreement between the guinea pig maximization and human maximization tests, both have proven to be poor predictors of actual clinical incidence of dermatitis caused by many agents, e.g., malathion, captan, maneb (Thomas et al. 1988). Although the incidence of contact dermatitis among these workers is undoubtedly underreported, the actual incidence of verified disease is very low considering the extent and manner of usage of the products.

Evaluating immediate-type hypersensitivities has also been difficult. Certain organic pesticides that have anticholinesterase activity will induce reactions resembling immediate-type inhalant hypersensitivity because of the unopposed cholinergic stimulation they cause (Corbett 1974). One must also dissociate irritant effects produced in atopic individuals or in those with hyperreactive airways. The documentation that IgE antibodies are responsible for any pesticide-induced bronchial reactions seems to be rare (Thomas et al. 1988). The possibility exists that pesticides could induce autoimmune reactions by becoming haptenic in vivo and inducing IgG antibodies, which in turn would react with the haptens attached to blood cells. At least one incident of immune-induced autohemolytic anemia associated with dieldrin use has been documented (Hamilton, Morgan, and Simmons 1978), although it is more likely that many of these agents may induce aplastic anemia by becoming absorbed by the bone marrow.

A workshop sponsored by the Task Force of Environmental Cancer and Heart and Lung Disease, devoted to evaluating the human relevance of the immunologic effects of pesticides, made several conclusions (Thomas et al. 1988). Excluding contact hypersensitivity, it was concluded "that the data are insufficient to conclude that chronic exposure to pesticides at environmentally relevant levels results in interactions with the immune system which adversely influence human health.'' Several reasons for the differences seen between experimental animal and human studies were given and included: (1) the exposure levels used in animal studies may not be achieved in humans; (2) currently used routine tests for human parameters may not detect any changes if they do exist; (3) difficulty in defining and measuring adverse human health effects; and (4) results in immune dysfunction may be latent and require longer periods for observation or further immuno-modulation by other events in order to be realized.

3. Polycyclic Aromatic Hydrocarbons

Polycylic aromatic hydrocarbons (PAH) are well-known toxicants and carcinogens resulting from the combustion of various fossil fuels, wood, and tobacco. Moreover, exposure to these products is more widespread than just in the chemical industry. One of the most studied combustion products has been 7,12–dimethylbenz[a]anthracene (DMBA). The first evidence demonstrating the carcinogenic potential of these materials was obtained in the late eighteenth century from chimney sweeps with a high incidence of scrotal cancer related to their exposure to soot and coal tar.

It is of interest that those PAHs that are carcinogenic, including DMBA, also possess potent immunosuppressive properties. Except for epidemiologic data, most of the available information stems from animal studies. The problem with interpreting the animal data from PAH exposure is that one cannot be sure that the increased tumors seen in experimental animals treated with PAHs are caused by its immunosuppression or its direct carcinogen-inducing activity.

DMBA has been shown to inhibit several aspects of cell-mediated immunity both in vivo in experimental animals and in vitro. It suppresses the lymphoproliferative response to PHA, Con A, and alloantigens, along with tumor cytolysis mediated by NK cells and the generation of cytotoxic T lymphocytes. DMBA also causes a decrease in the number and percentage of splenic lymphocytes expressing the murine T-cell markers Thy 1.2, Lyt-1, and Lyt-2 (Burchiel et al. 1988). The Lyt-1 cells appear more sensitive to DMBA than other T-cell subsets, suggesting that the T-helper cell is a primary target. In addition, depressions in cell-mediated host resistance to PYB6 tumor cells and *Listeria monocytogenes* have been reported. In some of these studies, immunosuppression was observed at doses that did not alter splenic cellularity or weight, which demonstrates that the inhibition is functional and not from generalized lymphotoxicity.

DMBA has also been shown to inhibit humoral immunity (Ward et al. 1986). Both IgG and IgM antibody responses to T-dependent (SRBC) and T-independent (TNP-Ficoll and TNP-LPS) antigens were suppressed, demonstrating that both mature and immature B cells are affected. In addition, DMBA suppressed the lymphoproliferative response to LPS in vitro and decreased the total number and percentage of splenic cells expressing B-cell markers (Burchiel et al. 1988).

It is well documented that DMBA is metabolized by the cytochrome-P450–dependent enzyme system and that these metabolites are responsible for the carcinogenic response. In the in vitro studies cited above, DMBA was added directly to the cultures. If metabolites were also responsible for the immunotoxic effects, then the lymphocytes or adherent cells should be generating them. This is plausible since these cells possess inducible cytochrome-P450 activity. Although conflicting results have been reported, studies conducted using labeled DMBA with a higher specific activity and P450 enzyme inhibition studies indicated that the effects were attributable to the metabolites (Kawabata and White, 1989; Ladics, Kawabata, and White 1991).

The mechanism of DMBA-induced immune suppression is not fully understood. Based on the results of the numerous screening assays cited above, most cells of the immune system are affected. Mechanistic studies have shown that antigen-pulsed macrophages from DMBA-treated mice were not able to activate fully antigen-primed T cells from normal mice (Yamashita and Hamaoka 1982). The authors speculated that DMBA induced its immunosuppression by impairing the antigen-presenting activity of macrophages.

Investigations have also demonstrated that DMBA could suppress the production of IL-2, and addition of exogenous IL-2 could restore the suppressed cytotoxic T-cell activity (House et al. 1987). These data suggest that the effect of DMBA occurs at the level of the T-helper cell as opposed to an end-stage effector cell. Recent studies have carried this one step further and have suggested that the DMBA-induced lesion may be a dysfunction of the T-cell antigen receptor in its role of either antigen recognition or transmembrane signaling. Monoclonal antibodies directed at the CD3 receptor can induce T-cytotoxic-cell activity in the presence of lymphokines (Crispe, Bevan, and Staerz 1985). DMBA can suppress this induction, which supports the hypothesis that the effect of DMBA is on antigen-specific activation mediated by the CD3 receptor.

4. Dioxins

Dioxin (2,3,7,8–tetrachlorodibenzo-p-dioxin or TCDD) is another substance clouded in controversy, partly because it was found to be a contaminant of the defoliant known as Agent Orange used in the Vietnam War. Discussions of the human effects of TCDD have unfortunately become emotionally entangled with medical compensation claims made by veterans returning with various illnesses from this unpopular war, and this controversy continues. There is no question that TCDD is extremely toxic in experimental animals, including monkeys, and is a potent carcinogen or, more likely, a promoter or cocarcinogen in most species. Nearly all experimental studies agree that TCDD severely affects the developing thymic epithelia of perinatal rodents, with most changes seen in the prothymocyte, and subsequent seeding of T cells from there to secondary-level organs (Fine, Gasiewicz, and Silverstone 1989). The effect is more severe and extensive than that seen in adults exposed to similar concentrations. Avian studies indicate that prehatching TCDD exposure also inhibits B-stem-cell development in the bursa of Fabricius (Nikolaidis et al. 1990). It is one of the few agents that has been studied from the standpoint of the host resistance of laboratory animal offspring of mothers exposed to the agent (reviewed in Vos 1977; Spreafico et al. 1983). But objectively, the question remains just how toxic is the material for humans, and what, if any, effects does it have on the human immune system? Although the data are meager, the evidence seems to indicate that humans are much more resistant to the toxic effects than most animal species studied.

The best available studies of TCDD immunotoxicity have come from two particular accidents. An industrial explosion occurring in 1976 that caused a massive exposure of the town of Seveso, Italy (Garattini 1977) serves as the best example of an acute exposure. Several kilograms of TCDD were spread over a 700–acre area, making this incident the best studied, and it could well represent the worst-case scenario in terms of acute human exposure. Within a few days, several children were hospitalized with chloracne, a severe skin eruption seen in those exposed to certain chemicals including the polyhalogenated biphenyls reviewed above. Interestingly, a number of small animals began dying at about the same time. Later more children developed chloracne, and larger animals such as dogs, horses, sheep, and cows began dying. The number of people exposed around the site ranged, depending on degree of exposure, from 750 individuals with high exposure to 32,000 for minimal exposure. Approximately 150 women were in the first trimester of pregnancy, but the rate of spontaneous abortions and the number of congenital anomalies in infants coming to term was no greater than normally expected. Very little residual skin disfiguration remained in the children with chloracne, and as yet no reports of increased incidence of infection or tumors have been received. From these acute data, TCDD does not appear to have nearly the same toxic effects in humans as those seen in animals.

Homes and soils in the area have received only minimal clean-up since that time, and although some families moved away from the area, many have returned. Not only are the people living there continuing to receive exposure from residual TCDD, but also the chemical is known to reside in significant levels in serum lipids for many years, as much as 37 in one study (Fingerhut et al. 1991). Studies performed on 22 victims soon after the accident reported the circulating complement levels, immunoglobulin concentrations, and proliferative responses of T and B cells to mitogens were all within normal limits, but unfortunately the data were not shown (Reggiani 1980).

Unlike the Seveso incident, residents in the Times Beach-Quail Run area of Missouri (U.S.A.) were chronically exposed from months to years to soils sprayed with dust-suppressing oils contaminated with significant amounts of TCDD. The contamination occurred in 1971, but epidemiologic studies were not initiated until 1983 and revealed little of immunologic interest. More extensive studies of a population subset exposed to soil containing an average of 2,200 ppb TCDD and interior dust samples containing approximately 1 ppb was carried out later (Hoffman et al. 1986). Although certain laboratory parameters of immune function were altered in the exposed population, some in a statistically nonsignificant manner, no documentation of clinical immune disorders or excessive infection has yet been found. Decreased percentages of T3, T4, and T11 markers were found in the exposed group, but the mean number of T-cell subsets was comparable between groups. Non-T peripheral lymphocytes were significantly greater in the exposed group, and T4/T8 ratios < 1.0 were significantly decreased.

Because of the dearth of immunologic data obtainable from humans, consideration of cancer morbidity and mortality data on individuals exposed to high levels of TCDD may be helpful. In a retrospective cohort study in over 5,000 workers exposed to TCDD, the incidence of cancers previously thought to be associated with TCDD was not found to be elevated (Hodgkin's, stomach, liver, and nasal cancers, and non-Hodgkin's lymphoma), but in one subgroup with exposure greater than 1 year and a greater than 20–year latency since initial exposure, the mortality was significantly increased for soft tissue sarcomas and for respiratory system cancers (Fingerhut et al. 1991). Also, there was a slight but statistically significant increased mortality from all types of cancer combined, although the increase was not proportional to the duration of exposure. The increase for this parameter was even greater in the 1/20–year subgroup. Important confounders that were not evaluated as being enhancers of the TCDD exposure were smoking and exposure to other chemicals. For example, disagreement with results from previous epidemiologic studies may have arisen because many workers are simultaneously exposed to chlorophenolic and phenoxy herbicides along with the contaminating TCDD. Although contamination of synthesized chemicals no longer is significant, and regulatory limits are extremely conservative (based on the animal data), so that contemporary workers are no longer exposed to TCDD, there still remains a chance that humans may inadvertently become exposed to TCDD-contaminated products at toxic waste sites, etc. For such people, we really have very little definitive immunologic data.

This is an ideal example of experimental immunologists and clinicians needing to interchange their information more often. The experimentalists have two very important findings. One is that early thymic events are the prime immunologic targets of TCDD toxicity in animals. Clinicians, although able to show significant changes in various immunologic laboratory markers, have been unable to discern any pattern of immunosuppression or lasting patterns of clinical disease in exposed adults possessing residual levels of TCDD in their serum lipids (reviewed in Stehr-Green, Naylor, and Hoffman 1989). However, all clinical studies have been in those who have been exposed as adults, not perinatally. Although these adults have shown significantly decreased levels of circulating thymosin$_{\alpha-1}$ (Stehr-Green, Naylor, and Hoffman 1989), a clinical and immunologic survey of the infants (who are now young adults) exposed prenatally at Seveso would be very useful.

The second important finding from the experimental laboratories is that there seem to be at least two receptors to which TCDD binding can occur (an aryl hydrocarbon hydroxylase receptor and a steroid hormone receptor) that account for much, but not all of the toxicity (Kerkvliet et al. 1990; Wilhemsson et al. 1990). But why is it that humans are not as severely affected as animals? Is there something different in quality or density of these human receptors? Do heat shock protein responses that are known to occur following TCDD exposure (Wilhemsson et al. 1990) differ significantly in humans from that of animals, or is the modulatory activity of these proteins different in humans? The animal studies have given the human immunologists a number of good leads to follow.

5. Drugs

Drugs might be considered on the basis of the type of immunotoxic reaction with which they are associated. The most potent types of immunotoxic drugs in this regard are those given purposely for immunosuppression or immunopotentiation (Chapter 8). A second, very large group consists of those drugs that induce various types of immediate or contact-type hypersensitivities. Slightly related to these are those drugs that induce other types of immune injury or are associated with the induction of autoimmune disorders. Finally, there could be a group of drugs that inadvertently cause damage to the immune system, e.g., phenytoin or α-methyldopa and lead to secondary infections.

But even this classification may be oversimplified for one trying to assess which drug might be the cause of an adverse reaction under study. Patients often undergo therapy with more than one drug, which presents the problem of identifying one out of several possible agents, as well as the additional consideration of the possibility of synergistic or additive drug interactions. An additional, difficult problem is the identification of sweeteners, coloring, and other additives used in drug manufacture that may be allergenic or immunotoxic. Recently, a compendium of these additives used in the formulation of antibiotics has been published (Kumar, Weatherly, and Beaman 1991).

Drug Allergy

A large proportion of iatrogenic (physician-induced) illness is caused by adverse drug reactions. Incidence rates in hospitals range from 0.3%–15%, depending on type of medical service, but very few adverse drug reactions from outpatient populations are reported to pharmaceutical companies or national registries. Because modern therapeutic strategies may apply several drugs to one patient, and since adverse drug reactions often mimic other diseases, ascribing an immunotoxic event to a specific drug is often impossible. Of all adverse drug reactions, 6–10% are primarily concerned with allergic reactions, but separating the truly allergic from pharmacological intolerance or drug idiosyncrasy is often difficult (Mathews 1984). The main way allergic reactions differ from these other types is that the patient's history often elicits information that the particular drug had previously been tolerated by the patient at the dosage used. Some drugs, e.g., opiates and polymyxin B, may induce reactions that mimic allergies because of their propensity to cause nonspecific release of pharmacological mediators from mast cells.

The most alarming, unpredictable drug reaction is systemic anaphylaxis (discussed in more detail below). Less severe allergic reactions are also induced by these same agents, and the most vexing question concerns why there is such a vast spectrum of physiological responses. Although many of these drugs have only rarely been reported to cause such serious reactions, penicillin, various sulfa drugs, and quinolone derivatives are more commonly associated with them. Other agents causing significant morbidity are L-asparaginase in cancer chemotherapy and various intravenously administered muscle relaxants, especially those containing tertiary or quarternary ammonium groups (de Weck 1990).

Penicillin and its analogs may not only induce anaphylaxis, urticaria, and other forms of IgE-mediated reactions, they may also induce a serum-sickness-like syndrome characterized by delayed onset of rash, fever, joint inflammation, and lymphadenopathy. It only develops 10–14 days after initial administration of the agent and after immunization has been induced, only if there is still enough of the agent remaining in the circulation to react with the immune effectors. The reaction is likely of mixed etiology involving IgE, circulating immune complexes, and complement activation. Circulating immune complexes may also induce vasculitis by localizing in arterioles of the skin and initiating complement-dependent inflammation. In addition to penicillin, other drugs inducing such reactions are sulfas, thiouracils, hydantoins, and allopurinol.

The causes of dermal eruptions following drug administration are very difficult to sort out, but comparatively few are mediated by truly allergic mechanisms. Although IgE mediation most likely accounts for urticaria and angioedema, the mechanisms of vesicular or papular eruptions are obscure. Respiratory manifestations of drug allergy include those symptoms that are part of the anaphylactic syndrome as well as asthma, bronchospasm, eosinophilic infiltrates, and occasionally chronic pulmonary fibrosis. Pulmonary hyperreactivity induced by aspirin and other nonsteroidal anti-inflammatory agents is particularly bothersome but apparently not mediated by IgE reactivity. It has been suggested that these patients manifest a cyclooxygenase blockade of arachidonic acid metabolism, leading to preferential production of leukotrienes from the lipoxygenase pathway, but this remains unproven and controversial. Pulmonary reactions are likely to be provoked in asthmatics by the irritant effect on already hyperreactive nerve endings from various food additives, e.g., food coloring dyes and preservatives, especially parabenzoates and sulfites. Ironically, the latter was formerly used as a preservative in the bronchodilator inhalers asthmatics were using for relief.

Contact dermatitis, i.e., reactions from cell-mediated immunity, is limited largely to topically applied medications, but occasionally skin manifestations may appear in one given the agent by injection who had previously been sensitized by having it applied topically. Not only can reactions be induced by prescription medications but also by any number of patent medicines, lotions, hair sprays, etc. Topicals containing certain mercurials and sulfonamides have been largely abandoned because of their high rate of contact dermatitis induction. Table 11–1 lists some drugs and other agents most often associated with the induction of contact dermatitis.

In order for a drug to induce an allergy, it must be antigenic. Few drugs are large or complex enough to be complete antigens; rather, most are small-molecular-weight haptens that complex in vivo with carrier proteins or cell membranes to become complete antigens capable of inducing immune responses. In some cases, the drug becomes reactive with carrier molecules only after becoming converted to a metabolic intermediate. In these instances, studies of skin test reactivity or IgE reactivity to the native molecule may give false-negative results. Structure-function relationships are sometimes helpful in explaining the basis for or predicting allergy. The most frequently studied class of drugs in this respect has been the penicillins, but several problems are encountered in trying to interpret the data. Many of the antibody studies have been done in rodents, and of those done in humans, many studies were concerned with antibodies of the IgG type; in other words, studies have concentrated on penicillin antigens, not allergens (Baldo and Harle 1990). Although several structural variants of the penicillin family have been described as minor antigens, only IgE antibodies to the penicilloyl moiety have been considered to be associated with clinical sensitivity (Baldo and Harle 1990). Within this group, the four-member β-lactam ring and various R- side chains have been shown to interact more frequently with human IgE antibodies.

Tertiary or quarternary ammonium groups have been identified as IgE-reactive groups on many muscle relaxants (Baldo and Harle 1990). These molecules, as well as certain others like chlorhexidine, are of interest because they are bivalent and can directly cross-link two adjacent IgE molecules without further conjugation. Other molecules that have been studied to identify the immmunochemical determinants are morphine, thiopental, trimethoprim, and sulfamethoxazole (Baldo and Harle 1990). An important consideration in the laboratory study of molecules is making sure that the reactive antigenic group is stereochemically available to react with the antibodies and not hidden within the molecule or occluded by attachment to the solid-phase support systems used in the assays.

Drug-Induced Immune Injury and Autoimmunity

Chapter 6 discussed the immunologic mechanisms of the many other types of host damage brought about by harmful reactions of the immune system. Purpura, erythema multiforme (a drug-induced disease of obscure origin, possibly involving immune complexes), asthma, pulmonary infiltrative disease with eosinophilic infiltrates, and adverse effects on the liver and kidney are a few of the reactions or diseases that may be associated with specific drugs in certain individuals. Unfortunately, the list is long on examples and short on explanations, for in fact, the precise etiopathogenesis of many of these reactions is unknown, and immune events may only be involved peripherally.

Many drug reactions are considered to be autoimmune in origin. Drug-induced lupus (discussed in Chapter 6) is a familiar example. For some reason, taking a particular drug triggers in some individuals the ability to initiate antibody formation to nuclear histones but seems unrelated to the chemical structure of the drug. Among the array of drugs associated with this form of lupus are various antibiotics, antiinflammatory agents, psychotropic drugs, antiarrhythmics, and antihypertensives (Rubin and Burlingame 1991). Various forms of drug-induced hemolytic anemia and agranulocytosis (see Table 6–2 in Chapter 6) are also common and are related to a variety of mechanisms. Other examples are more guilt-by-association affairs and include development of several types of autoimmune reactions after D-penicillamine, Sjögren's syndrome after practolol, tubular nephropathy after sodium methicillin, and anti-factor-VIII antibodies after penicillin. Table 6–5 in Chapter 6 listed a number of drugs associated with, but not proven as causative of, various autoimmune reactions. No single, common mechanism is available to explain how such a wide variety of effects can be induced by these unrelated agents. Various aspects of polyclonal B-cell activation, elevated serum levels of IgE, cytotoxic T-cell–cell reactions to drug fixed to antigen-presenting cell membranes, deposition of circulating immune complexes, and emergence of antiself MHC class II clones are among the many possibilities with more than one likely to be present at once.

Drug-Induced Modulation of the Immune System

Other than for those drugs intentionally given for immunosuppression or immunopotentiation and those with which allergic or immune injury is associated, there is comparatively little information available on drugs that damage the immune system. It is rather surprising there is so much concern for environmental agents that might cause changes of questionable significance such as increased serum immunoglobulin levels or changes in T_h/T_s ratios but so little interest in what prescription or proprietary drugs do in this regard. Of the drugs that should be most closely evaluated would be those used over a continuous time. Perhaps the two drugs that have induced the best-known immunotoxic changes are phenytoin (discussed in detail in Chapter 7) and methyldopa.

One common drug used by thousands of asthmatics is theophylline, a profound cAMP phosphodiesterase inhibitor. Not only did theophylline inhibit normal human NK-cell activity in vitro, it also induced impaired NK-cell function in volunteers given therapeutic dosages for only 7 days (Yokoyama et al. 1990). Of most interest was that the serum concentration of the drug induced by this regimen was lower than that yielding the same degree of inhibition in vitro. Although the effect of such activity has not been clinically evaluated, one could speculate that increased opportunistic infections of the airways would be associated with more asthmatic attacks.

A certain class of antihypertensive drugs, most exemplified by α-methyldopa, seems to cause aberrations in the immune system sufficient enough to lead to autoimmune disease. It is one of the drugs that can cause the drug-induced lupus syndrome (see Chapter 6) and has sometimes been associated with chronic autoimmune hepatitis but is most known for its induction of drug-induced hemolytic anemia. Although 15% of patients taking the drug develop antinuclear antibodies, and up to 25% develop a positive indirect Coombs test for IgG (i.e., the serum contains antibodies capable of reacting with erythrocytes), only a minority (<1%) produce erythrocytes coated with a sufficient amount of low-avidity, antierythrocyte antibody to lead to clinical hemolytic anemia (Worlledge 1973). Somehow this drug (as well as certain others) stimulates the production of IgG antierythrocyte antibodies, usually with specificity for the Rh isoantigen. This reaction is unique in that the chemical structure of the drug is not involved in the antigenic reactivity of the antibody to itself but to a third party. Moreover, the antibodies can remain detectable up to 2 years after withdrawal from the drug. Although it is unknown how the drug induces this phenomenon, there is some evidence that the drug inhibits suppressor activity, possibly by causing an accumulation of cAMP in T-regulatory cells, leading to unregulated B-cell proliferation (Kirtland, Mohler, and Horwitz 1980).

Interesting immunomodulating side effects of the 2–aminothiazolyl cephalosporin derivative cefodizime have been described (Labro 1990). This antibiotic was synthetically altered to resist β-lactamase degradation by penicillin-resistant bacteria, but in the process, several beneficial in vivo and in vitro properties were coincidentally conferred on the molecule. These include the induction of several enhanced neutrophil and monocyte phagocytic functions in patients being treated with the drug.

6. Anesthetics

A troublesome potential source of immunotoxicants may be the various types of anesthetics, particularly inhalants, used in modern surgery. Substances like halothane, nitrous oxide, and cyclopropane are among those that have been demonstrated to cause temporary human effects on immune parameters (Finlayson 1989). With many types of modern surgery lasting 12 hr or more, such prolonged contact of these agents with already debilitated patients may possibly be important in contributing to postsurgical sepsis. There are several confounding variables that make interpretation of data from patient studies difficult. The depression observed could be caused by (1) existing infectious, renal, or traumatic disability, (2) the endocrine stress imposed by the rigors of prolonged surgery, (3) the physical stresses on cell membranes caused by the shearing and turbulent forces that cells are exposed to in the bypass oxygenators, or (4) the anesthetics, relaxants, transfusions, and other medications used during surgery.

Leukopenia associated with prolonged nitrous oxide administration has been known for over 45 years. In one study (which removed the confounder of existing disability from concern), lymphocytes from normal renal transplant donors were obtained during surgery and at various times postoperatively for immunologic characterization (Slade, Simmons, and Yunis 1975). All values of samples taken during surgery or immediately after, including total lymphocyte, T-cell, and B-cell counts, mitogen responsiveness, and mixed lymphocyte reactivity (even if the study cells were the stimulator cells), showed marked immediate depressions. Some values reached only 10% of the normal, preoperative levels. All in vitro values gradually returned to normal between 1 and 5 days, depending on the parameter. Skin test reactivity to common bacterial antigens declined slowly and returned to normal over even longer times. The type of anesthetics and relaxants used varied, and the study made no attempt to correlate decrements with a particular agent.

At this point the question concerns whether these depressions were caused by the anesthetic or by the endocrine stress of surgery. One laboratory animal study was designed to address this question, although a different parameter was chosen, that of Kupffer cell clearance in the liver (Subramanian, McCleod, and Gans 1968). Rats that were subjected to 30–min surgeries that included cardiopulmonary bypass were compared with sham-operated animals that were subjected to all cannulation and other procedures except the actual bypass. In only those animals subjected to the bypass procedure were clearance values depressed, suggesting that the stress of the additional operative procedure had more to do with the decrements than the anesthetic. Although this study did not examine the type of injury these cells had incurred (cytokine immunology had not been invented yet), the approach was a good one that should now be repeated with modern immunologic technology.

In vitro techniques on human leukocytes may help answer these questions. When normal human leukocytes were subjected to incubation in media through which equipotent concentrations of vaporized anesthetic inhalants were bubbled, all but isoflurane caused significant drops in neutrophil and macrophage chemotactic migration (Moudgill et al. 1984). Of these, nitrous oxide was the most potent depressant. When human peripheral blood samples obtained after surgery were cultured in atmospheres containing surgical-use concentrations of common inhalant anesthetics, NK-cell function was temporarily depressed for 3–5 days (Tonnesen et al. 1984). Unfortunately, this study did not correct for changes in NK-cell number in that the assay system chosen used whole blood, but it did address the question of the role of endocrine stress on the depression. The patients were divided into two groups based on the anesthetic regimen each patient was subjected to. In one group, the regimen was designed to block the endocrine-mediated stress, but the patients in that group showed no differences from the other group. In other studies, samples from similar patients were examined for CD4/CD8 ratios, which were found to decline during cardiopulmonary bypass, cancer resection, and certain other general surgical procedures; although these values returned to normal within 24 hr in the latter two groups, they remained depressed for up to 6 days in the bypass patients (Pollock et al. 1987). The authors felt that this imbalance was caused by an increase in CD8$^+$ cells. Subjecting experimental animals to a variety of anesthetic inhalants alone or to anesthetic plus surgery resulted in the induction of stimulated NK-cell activity irrespective of the type of inhalant used (Markovic and Murasko 1990). Although the surgery further depressed base-line NK cell activity, it had no effect on the induced responses.

In conclusion, although a number of interesting approaches have already been used, answers to the question of the possibility of anesthetic immunosuppression suffer from the lack of a rigorous and critical examination. It is doubtful if the anesthesia associated with most surgical procedures puts the patient at immunologic risk, but long, technical operations like modern open heart surgery are now commonplace. As more complicated procedures are developed, the time under anesthesia increases as well. It is quite possible that such extended contact with these agents, together with the other stresses induced at the time of surgery, could temporarily alter host defenses sufficiently in the debilitated patient to predispose to infection. When such surgery takes place using the bypass apparatus, hemodilution can cause a 40–50% reduction in serum proteins, which might be a further complication (Finlayson 1989), and passing vigorously through the bubbling process affects cell membrane integrity severely. Even erythrocytes and platelets are affected adversely (Oeveren et al. 1985). Thus, how much of the temporary depression in immune function is caused by the inhalant anesthetics remains an open question.

Topical anesthetics have not received as much attention. However, of great interest to pulmonary immunologists is the finding that the use of lidocaine to increase cell yields in bronchoalveolar lavages results in impaired NK-cell function in the cells obtained (Renzi and Ginns 1990). Neither the cell number nor the viability was affected. Since lidocaine is used so frequently in this procedure in experimental animals as well as in human studies, the consequences on the findings may be widespread.

7. Medical Devices

New advances in medical technology allow the introduction of materials composed of new compounds as well as the use of invasive procedures that cause an interface between these substances and tissues ordinarily protected from the external environment. This technology has led to new problems involving the immune system. Some of these problems are inflammatory, some toxic, and some caused by contaminating antigens present in the device. The technology in this field is advancing so rapidly that immunotoxic evaluation cannot keep pace. Some of the problems stem from prosthetic or therapeutic devices, others from diagnostic agents given parenterally in a manner analogous to drugs.

Radiocontrast Media
During the radiologic evaluation of patients, various types of low-molecular-weight water-soluble radioiodinated materials are given patients, often intravenously. Some patients experience anaphylaxis-type reactions on administration of this type of agent. Rashes, urticaria, angioneurotic edema, smooth muscle spasm, hypotension, pulmonary edema, and even cardiac arrest may occur at unpredictable times and may result in a mortality of 1–5/100,000 (Moreau et al. 1988). In one sense, these reactions are among the most common produced by pharmaceutical preparations used in medical practice, e.g., in association with intravenous urography, computed tomography, and digital angiography.

A number of mechanisms have been postulated, but there does not seem to be any agreement on the exact chain of events leading to the reaction. Clinically, the reactions closely resemble true allergic reactions, yet premedication with antihistaminics or steroids does not seem to suppress the reactions, nor does histamine release occur in patients suffering from the reactions. There is scant evidence that the reactions are IgE mediated. Penetration of the low-molecular-weight agents past the blood–brain barrier with excitation of the hypothalamus has been proposed, as has nonspecific release of various mediator-related compounds, e.g., factor XII activation resulting in plasminogen conversion to plasmin and subsequent fibrinolysis, prekallikrein activation, nonspecific complement activation, basophil degranulation, leukotriene and/or PAF vasoactivity, and platelet aggregation (Lasser 1991; Moreau et al. 1988).

Hemodialyzers

Occasionally, some patients undergoing extracorporeal hemodialysis experience chest and back pain, dyspnea, hypotension, nausea, and vomiting as a result of dialysis with new units made with cuprophane dialysis membranes. There are at least four theories to explain the triggering events responsible for acute and chronic reactions associated with hemodialysis therapy: (1) endotoxin contamination of the dialyzer units; (2) nonspecific activation of the complement system by the membranes; (3) nonspecific activation of peripheral blood monocytes by dialyzer membranes, and (4) IgE-dependent reactions involving residual amounts of the sterilizing agent, ethylene oxide. Of these the first three are most relevant and may be interrelated.

Past evidence of endotoxin contamination had been obtained using the *Limulus* amoebocyte lysate test for the detection of bacterial endotoxin, but this reagent also reacted with the dialyzer membrane materials. When a newer, more endotoxin-specific *Limulus* test was used to test such patients being dialyzed with regenerated units, the only ones who still showed positive reactions were those with concurrent cirrhosis, malignancy, or infection. In the absence of such complications, the authors concluded that endotoxin contamination must be extremely rare and thus not a likely cause of most of the reactions (Taniguchi et al. 1990). Yet, bacterial endotoxin has been shown to be able to cross cuprophan and polysulfone membranes in vitro within the first 5 min of dialysis and be able to adsorb to these regenerated membranes (Laude-Sharp et al. 1990).

Patients experiencing dialyzer reactions have associated significant increases in certain complement cleavage fragments in their blood within minutes of beginning dialysis (Craddock et al. 1977; Hakim et al. 1984). During in vitro hemodialysis, such cleavage fragment values increased significantly, but not if the blood were treated with EDTA, a known inhibitor of complement activation. At the same time the alterations in complement components were taking place, peripheral blood monocytes could become activated in a number of ways: by direct contact with some biologically active material associated with the membranes, by microbial products such as bacterial lipopolysaccharide (LPS), or by activated complement fragments.

When whole blood was hemodialyzed in vitro for 2 hr, no stimulation of TNF-α or IL-1β was produced, although evidence was obtained that transcriptional coding of mRNA for these two cytokines had taken place (Schindler et al. 1990). This probably explains how these same cells were found to be primed to produce these factors if subsequently stimulated by LPS. In vivo measurements of TNF-α in patients undergoing hemodialysis also revealed that plasma levels of the cytokine were elevated, as was the cytokine production capacity of peripheral blood monocytes (Chollett-Martin et al. 1991). Further, this anomaly was only evident when cuprophane membranes were used and not with cellulose acetate or polysulfone membranes. Although LPS could stimulate TNF-α in cells obtained from these patients, it was not necessary, as the cells produced tenfold elevations of the factor spontaneously. Thus, not only does the use of an external immunotoxic material, i.e., dialyzer membrane, have the potential to alter immunologically important cells but, combined with other circumstances, may act synergistically with activated complement components and/or low levels of microbial products to induce biologically significant concentrations of potentially inflammatory cytokines.

In practice, some hemodialysis centers use new dialysis units (the disposable cartridge containing the dialysis membranes) for each use, whereas other centers reprocess the cartridges for reuse. Anaphylactic-like (anaphylactoid) reactions have been reported with "first-use" units, and it has been suggested that ethylene oxide reacting with the membrane somehow triggers an IgE-mediated response (Dolovich et al. 1984). Whether this is an antigen-specific or lectin-mediated reaction has not been determined. The use of reprocessed cartridges has been associated with a greater chance of outbreaks of infection and pyrogenic reactions. Cluster-case incidents of anaphylactoid reactions have been associated with reprocessed units, and to illustrate the complexity of trying to identify the causative agent, it has been pointed out that reprocessing involves different types of disinfectants, the reprocessing method (manual or automated), type of dialysate (e.g., bicarbonate, acetate, or both), and the use of heparin as an anticoagulant (Miller and Wilber 1991). One might also add contaminating materials of microbial origin. Although multivariate analysis indicated that heparin was the agent most associated with the reactions (more than threefold), followed by washing with bleach or H_2O_2 (2.5–fold), modification of reprocessing processes that included almost anything *except* removal of the heparin greatly reduced the incidence of clusters.

Latex Products

The use of latex products is widespread in the medical industry. Not only might there be prolonged, intimate patient contact with such materials (e.g., catheterization), but because of the threat of patient-acquired diseases (e.g., herpes, hepatitis, and AIDS), health care workers are also subject to long-term skin contact with latex gloves. Virtually the full range of allergic reactions have been reported from contact urticaria to increasing reports of anaphylaxis (Kelly, Setlock, and Davis 1991; Sussman, Tarlo, and Dolovich 1991). Some health care workers have developed inhalant asthma from nonskin contact. Water-soluble peptides in latex have been recognized as the offending allergens, and alternative products are being developed for use in those with problems.

8. Cigarette Smoking

Although the relevance of smoking to subsequent induction of lung cancer is beyond the scope of this text, undoubtedly immune factors are also involved. However, the present discussion is largely limited to direct immunotoxic effects. There is no doubt that tobacco smoking is associated with increased prevalence of infectious and inflammatory diseases of both the upper and lower airways. In addition to the human studies briefly summarized below, work has been done with experimental animal models, and in general the results parallel those obtained from humans (Johnson et al. 1990). Leukocyte responses are markedly changed in both the peripheral circulation and bronchoalveolar lavages. Neutrophils and monocytes are significantly increased in the circulation, although their function appears normal, but NK-cell function has been reported as depressed (Hughes et al. 1985). The total number of T lymphocytes is increased in all smokers, and although $CD4^+$ cells are increased in light and moderate smokers, that subpopulation is depressed in heavy smokers (reviewed in Holt 1987). In a subsequent study, total leukocytes, $CD4^+$ cells, and CD4/CD8 ratios were all reported to be statistically elevated in smokers compared to nonsmokers, although no attempt was made to analyze by degree of smoking (Tollerud et al. 1989). Results of proliferation assays of T lymphocytes from smokers have been mixed, some reporting normal and others reporting depressed responses. Holt points out several areas that need increased study: studies need to be done on age-stratified populations, since these values appear to change with age and length of smoking; functional suppressor and helper studies would be helpful; and in vitro responses to relevant antigens need to be done.

There are many reports that smokers have 10–20% lowered immunoglobulin (IgG, IgM, and IgA) levels in their sera, whereas IgE values are often higher than normal in light smokers (fewer than nine cigarettes per day) but below normal in heavy smokers. Secretory IgA concentrations are also lower than normal in the saliva of smokers but normal to high in bronchoalveolar lavage fluid.

Many cellular studies have been done on bronchoalveolar lavages. Both macrophages and neutrophils show significant increases, but the numerical lymphocyte population remains unchanged (Hunninghake et al. 1979). The macrophage population is clearly activated, as seen from both morphological and metabolic evidence. Thus, there is increased inflammatory potential of these cells, and they produce greater toxic oxygen radical releases. Their chemotactic functions are enhanced, but reports are mixed as to the efficiency of their opsonizing and killing ability (Holt 1987). The C3b receptor density is decreased, whereas reduction of Fc receptors appears to be limited to a subpopulation (Plowman 1982). Results of macrophage regulation of T-cell function have been mixed. Too often these studies are not comparable because they use different macrophage:lymphocyte ratios, which in itself produces different results. If the ratio is high, T-cell function will be suppressed (Holt 1986), and such ratios could indeed be achieved in vivo by the macrophage response seen in smokers. Studies on lymphocyte function have reported mixed results, partly because of nonuniformity of approaches and the varied presence of macrophages.

One lymphocyte study that offers a unique approach is that of determining chromosome damage in lymphocytes of smokers. Although there was a slightly increased (but statistically insignificant) rise in chromosome alteration frequency in smokers' lymphocytes, there was a significantly greater chromosome translocation frequency when the lymphocytes were subjected to X-irradiation (Au et al. 1991). What the significance of this finding of failure in DNA repair may mean in terms of subsequent immune function or health of the individual remains to be evaluated.

Various types of depressions in antigen-specific immune responses have been reported in smokers compared to nonsmokers, e.g., cytotoxic antibodies to fetal histocompatibility antigens in pregnant women, precipitating antibodies to numerous antigens, responses of workers to inhaled microbial antigens present in agricultural products, and influenza vaccine responses (reviewed in Holt 1987). Also, these workers exhibit more manifestations of IgE-mediated hypersensitivity. The suggestion has been made that smoking and excessive aeroallergen contact (i.e., such as that encountered by an agricultural product worker) lead to increased risk of IgE-mediated sensitization, but there is no such increase in smokers exposed to normal levels of aeroallergens, e.g., seasonal pollens. Unlike exposure to some immunotoxic substances, studies of cessation on the immune defects made in both experimental animals and humans suggest that all of these changes are reversible.

Thus, the immune effects on the lung most likely are attributable to the changes induced in the alveolar macrophage population. There is an increased inflammatory potential because of their heightened metabolic state as well as their marked relative increase in number to affect lymphocyte dysregulation. If the macrophage population is allowed to return to normal numbers and metabolic state, most evidence agrees that a state of immune normality returns, further attesting to the great resilience of the immune system.

The effect of environmental smoke on the health of others is currently the subject of much debate (see Chapter 10 for the effect of perinatal exposure). In a study of 9–year-old children of smoking parents, significantly higher eosinophil counts and serum IgE levels, particularly among boys, were encountered (Ronchetti et al. 1990). These changes are accompanied by an increased incidence of skin reactivity to environmental allergens, bronchial hyperresponsiveness (Weiss et al. 1985; Martinez et al. 1988), and increased prevalence of respiratory symptoms (Anonymous 1986). Thus, in this instance, the appearance of readily discernibie alterations in immune markers does seem to correlate with clinical disease. Few studies are available on subjects exposed to passive smoking that are similar in detail to those recounted above for active smokers (Johnson et al. 1990).

Although the incidence of precancerous conditions and other diseases of the oral cavity is known to be significantly elevated in chronic users of smokeless tobacco (Christen, McDonald, and Christen 1991), examination of the effects of smokeless tobacco on the immune system of humans is very rare. One approach used has been to study the effect of smokeless tobacco use on the incidence of dental caries, a subject complicated by the fact that most products have high concentrations of sucrose and glucose, substrates for caries-producing bacteria. Although salivary IgA and J-chain levels were higher in users than in controls, there were significantly lower levels in lactoferrin and lysozyme among users and only slight differences in the amount of *Streptococcus mutans* antibodies (Gregory et al. 1991). Although use of the product had a demonstrable effect of IgA synthesis, there was no clinical difference in the number of decayed, missing, or filled teeth between the study groups. The effects of smoking on gingival secretion and on calculus, plaque, and caries formation have been reviewed by Christen, McDonald, and Christen (1991).

9. Substances of Abuse

Many of the studies of immunotoxic effects of substances of abuse have been done in vitro by adding the test substance to normal cells, often in excessive doses in terms of the kinds of physiological tissue levels reached by these substances under realistic use. Although in vitro function studies done on leukocytes obtained from human drug users ought to be more relevant, they are complicated by many problems. Chronic, dependent users are often characterized by poor nutrition and personal hygiene. A problem associated with Δ^9-tetrahydrocannibinol (THC) use in particular is that its use may be limited to sporadic rather than consistent use (one joint/week versus twenty cigarettes/day), and little attempt has been made to correlate observed laboratory parameters with dose or usage. Further confounding studies of human users is the problem that many users are also cigarette smokers and/or are subject to a variety of substances (e.g., heroin, cocaine, and alcohol), and these may vary greatly in purity, being contaminated with other substances. Few studies have attempted to separate the effects of cigarette and marijuana smoking, but differences in phagocytic function in each group have been reported (Sherman et al. 1991). Although the possible additive immunosuppressive effect of substances of abuse in the induction of HIV infection is a worthy topic (Pillai and Watson 1990), the results of some studies are confusing because the HIV-seropositive and -seronegative populations of users were not segregated in the data analyses.

The effects of THC have been extensively reviewed by Friedman, Klein, and Specter (1991), who indicate that most work has been done either on rodents or on normal human lymphocytes treated in vitro. Although studies on leukocytes from users are rare, it is difficult to reconcile the laboratory treatment data with those obtained from users. For example, T-cell proliferation in response to PHA and Con A was inhibited in a dose-dependent fashion (5–10 μg/ml) if THC was present at the time of beginning incubation (Specter, Lancz, and Hazelden 1990), but no similar depressions were noted in lymphocytes from chronic users, i.e., those who smoked one cigarette per week for a year or longer (White, Brin, and Janicki 1975). Although there are other studies that report variable and transitory results, results obtained from hospitalized subjects given controlled doses of the substance showed a minimal effect on immmune parameters. It had no effect if added 24–48 hr after culture had commenced. The effect could not be reversed by the addition of IL-2 but could be if the time of THC contact was limited. Human B-cell numbers and function do not seem to be affected by THC use (Munson et al. 1976), but human NK-cell function was depressed when treated in vitro with THC and could be reversed by IL-2 (Specter et al. 1989).

Studies on lymphocytes from users of other substances are less precise, and the results are mixed. However, in one exceptional study that attempted to separate the effects of the various substances in multidrug users, lower levels of erythrocyte rosette-forming cell ($CD2^+$ T cells) populations in heroin users were reported than in those using both cocaine and heroin (Donahoe et al. 1986). Further, cocaine use alone (but not alcohol) was correlated with elevated levels of these populations such that the effect in multiusers was intermediate. This effect was not seen when the cells were analyzed cytofluorimetrically with monoclonal antibodies to the CD2 receptors, which suggests function rather than expression was being interfered with. Such a result would probably not be noticed today, since few laboratories now use the rosette technique. This effect could be dependent on morphine receptors that are known to occur on T cells in that the addition of morphine to human lymphocytes also inhibits T-cell rosette formation (Wybran et al. 1979).

Drugs of abuse may cause the formation of antibodies for cellular antigens. In one study, over 80% of sera tested from heroin addicts showed antibodies for MHC class I and II molecules, not directed to any specific allotype but toward either a single, nonpolymorphic antigen or a group of highly cross-reactive markers (Ameglio et al. 1988). This effect is without any known explanation but possibly reflects modulation of MHC allotype expression by heroin. What relevance this finding has to clinical resistance to infection is unknown, but it possibly could interfere with antigen presentation in infectious processes.

Both NK-cell number and function are reduced in heroin users but increased in cocaine users (Van Dyke et al. 1986). Cocaine added to NK cells in vitro was without this effect. The suggestion was made that cocaine exerts its effect via its known stimulation of catecholamine release and inhibition of norepinephrine reuptake by the sympathetic nervous system. Such findings throw considerable question on the relevance of in vitro studies that are separated from such important effects on the rest of the body.

In a related problem, the question arises what the potential immunosuppressive effect of long-term methadone maintenance therapy to reduce heroin dependency might be. This drug not only has been used in heroin aversion programs, it has itself also become a substance of abuse. The problem is confounded by the high incidence of AIDS and human T leukemia virus in intravenous drug users. To circumvent this problem, a study of seronegative intravenous drug users on methadone therapy was carried out. Significant reductions in T-cell responsiveness and NK-cell cytotoxicity function were found when compared with nonabusing controls (Klimas et al. 1991). This study is a good example of the paradoxical disparity of laboratory values; i.e., it showed significant *elevations* in certain lymphocyte subsets, notably CD4 helper cells as well as CD8 cytotoxic/suppressor cells, yet the proliferative responsiveness of these cells was reduced. The data alone do not explain the significance of the findings, however. Two significant inferences can be drawn from the study: (1) the widespread use of methadone programs for intravenous abusers may actually be immunosuppressive as well as (2) possibly enhancing the risk of HIV infectivity in intravenous abusers. Current opinion is that lymphocyte activation, e.g., by concurrent infection, enables the HIV agent to become infective. If similar activation is accomplished through methadone therapy, the user may be at additional risk. The study may also be an indication of what the effect of heroin alone might be.

Few studies are available on the effects of these substances on macrophages. Neutrophil and macrophage number and function have been reported depressed in mice and rabbits administered morphine (Tubaro et al. 1983). The functions included phagocytosis, killing, and superoxide anion production. In vivo, these effects were translated into decreased resistance to infection to *Candida* and *Klebsiella pneumoniae* in murine studies. Possibly this is brought about by morphine stimulation of PGE_2. Cocaine added to normal human macrophages also inhibits superoxide anion production in a dose-dependent manner (Chao et al. 1991). Bronchoalveolar macrophages from marijuana as well as tobacco smokers have been reported to have higher proliferative indices (eighteenfold and tenfold, respectively) than normal, which in part could explain the larger number of these cells found in these populations (Barbers et al. 1991).

Alcohol is another agent about which there is plenty of information consisting largely of anecdotal hearsay connecting it with immunosuppression. How much of the increased infections such as pneumonia or aspergillosis seen in chronic alcoholics are actually related to poor nutrition, cirrhosis, or immunotoxicity would be difficult to sort out. Most studies have been done on animals fed various regimens of alcohol and/or food or on normal leukocyte cultures to which alcohol has been added in vitro. It is difficult to attach much relevance to many of the in vitro studies that use ethanol at concentrations many thousandfold in excess (from 100 to 1,000 mg%) of the circulating levels that are considered in most states as presumed evidence of being under the influence of alcohol (0.1 mg%).

The better studies attempt to separate the effects of alcohol and undernutrition. For example, in one study mice were given either water or 20% ethanol ad libitum and divided into subgroups given either unrestricted, moderately restricted, or severely restricted food supplies (Blank, Duncan, and Meadows 1991). Splenic NK-cell function was significantly lower in those alcohol-consuming mice on unrestricted diet than those drinking water, whereas all groups on restricted diets had markedly depressed function regardless of liquid intake. The NK-cell function was also assessed after stimulation with recombinant IL-2. No significant difference was seen between the two groups on unrestricted diet, and although food-restriction depressed this parameter in all food restricted groups, the effect was curiously greater in the water-drinking groups. In a similar study proliferation of splenic lymphocytes to T-cell mitogens was diminished, but no change was seen in B-cell stimulation studies (Jerrells, Smith, and Eckardt 1990). These differences were also reflected in antibody responses; i.e., ethanol-fed mice showed a significant decrease in the primary antibody response to sheep red blood cells but not to a T-independent antigen.

The value of looking at normal leukocytes in vitro to which ethanol has been added is dubious in that such studies as the above have indicated that at the time of the killing, a detectable blood alcohol level was unnecessary for demonstration of depressed NK-cell function. Length of time of alcohol intake, amount consumed within a given time period, and the presence of alcohol metabolites (e.g., acetaldehyde) are all factors that seem to influence cell function and would be very difficult to duplicate in vitro. In addition to the reduced nutritional caloric intake characteristic of chronic alcoholics, alcohol doubtlessly interacts with other nutrients to alter enzyme induction and absorption of vitamins and to lower plasma levels of essential amino acids.

The selected examples of well-designed animal experiments above indicate that a better approach would be to examine lymphocyte and macrophage functions in chronic alcoholics. Unfortunately, few studies have looked at human subjects per se. A determination of basal and adenosine-stimulated cAMP levels was undertaken in a comparison study of lymphocytes obtained from chronic alcoholics, normal subjects, and patients with nonalcoholic liver disease (Diamond et al. 1987). Both parameters were considerably reduced in mixed lymphocytes and T cells from the alcoholics. How this interesting finding might relate to decreased resistance is problematic. On the one hand, increased cAMP accumulation in lymphocytes is inhibitory, and on this basis alone, one would not expect decreased basal levels to be connected with depression of immunity. Conversely, adenosine is an inhibitory immunomodulator of the central nervous system so that if the primary effect is here, then inhibition of key neurotransmitter production could adversely affect the immune system. Clearly, much more work needs to be done on human lymphocytes.

10. Heavy Metals

Various heavy metals have been studied from two points of view: their immunotoxicity (Koller 1980) and their ability to incite various forms of hypersensitivity diseases. The most serious of the latter is berylliosis, a chronic, severely disabling disease occurring in a minority of people exposed to the mineral that is characterized by cell-mediated-type hypersensitivity to the hapten and the production of granulomatous lesions. Human contact with this metal is limited to occupationally related exposures. Because nickel and chromium are found in coins, inexpensive jewelry, and metal clothing fasteners, they are major contact sensitins, particularly in women. In addition, chromium is often found in tanned leather products. Table 11-1 contains some of the well-known heavy metals that induce contact sensitivities.

Toxicologically, lead, cadmium, mercury in various chemical forms, arsenic, nickel, copper, magnesium, and zinc have all been studied. Lead has received much study, but there are problems of interpreting the results. Lead is often injected with infectious microorganisms, and the mortality is then measured. This does not necessarily mean that lead has interfered with the immune response. Its toxicity could simply have been a virulence enhancer of the microbes. Although the signs and symptoms of humans with elevated lead levels do not relate to increased rates of infections or tumors, many of these studies need to be reevaluated in light of current immunologic knowledge. This is especially critical with recent newspaper accounts of large numbers of American children who are exposed to lead from peeling paint and from various vaporized compounds.

Similar studies have been conducted with various inorganic and organic forms of mercury. The kinds of study that seem to be most relevant are those where long-term, low-level doses of the agent had been used. Data demonstrated that there were measurable depressions in such parameters as antibody responses with concomitant atrophic changes in the thymus and spleen (Blakley, Sisodia, and Mukkur 1980). If this exposure occurred to developing fetuses or infants, the result could well be serious. Even though we do not know of such serious human exposure, these kinds of data seem much more significant in predicting human toxicity for regulatory purposes. Although mercury compounds have not been used as pigments in paints for many years, a recent incident of toxicity in a child incriminated a mercuric compound in latex paint, but the material had been added as a fungicide, not as a pigment (Aronow et al. 1990). Again, this illustrates how a sudden introduction of a new commercial product or formulation may result in unanticipated toxicity.

There is a double association of nickel with increased tumor formation in mice challenged with a melanoma strain and with suppression of NK-cell activity (Smialowicz et al. 1985). Although NK cells are considered important in tumor recognition, it is not clear if the NK-cell repression led to tumor appearance or if the nickel acted as a direct carcinogen. The valence (and perhaps the presence of other ions in the compound) evidently contributes to the effects on the immune system. In a comparative study of Ni_3S_2, NiO, and $NiSO_4 \cdot H_2O$ inhalation, all compounds behave differently in inducing increases in nucleated cells in bronchopulmonary lavages, decrease in alveolar macrophage activity, and splenic NK-cell activity (Haley et al. 1990). To explain these diverse effects, more attention will have to be paid to the oxidation–reduction state of the metal ion (see gold, below), the oxidation potential of the ion, and their membrane interactions.

Some antiarthritic gold compounds (auranofin and gold sodium thiomalate) are able to inhibit in vitro activity of human IL-1 on lymphocytes at concentrations that correspond to levels found in the serum of patients receiving these drugs, possibly by interfering with another cytokine IFN-γ (Haynes et al. 1988; Harth, McCain, and Cousin 1990). Gold present in compounds in the Au(III) state is also a potent inducer of IgG autoantibodies to nucleolar antigens in mice (Schuhmann et al. 1990). It was hypothesized that T cells react with self proteins altered by the oxidized state of gold, Au(III), a metabolic state that can be induced in vivo.

Zinc and selenium are a special case—ordinarily the concern is about the *presence* of something as being unfavorable, but in the case of these metals, the *absence* is important. Zinc has been reported to be essential for maintaining normal immune response, and zinc deficiencies might be related to impaired function

(Fernandes et al. 1979). Zinc is necessary for proliferative responses of T cells and up-regulates these responses; it increases in vitro antibody responses and B-cell activation and restores some in vitro responses in lymphocytes from aged mice to competing toxins (reviewed by Malave et al. 1990; Pocino, Malave, and Baute 1990). The enhancement of T-cell proliferative responses is accompanied by increases in cells bearing IL-2 and transferrin receptors (Malave et al. 1990). The collective experience with selenium has been similar in that deficiency has been associated with a variety of depressed in vitro proliferative and phagocytic activities of both human and rodent leukocytes, whereas selenium supplementation is associated with restoration of these kinds of parameters (reviewed in Nair and Schwartz 1990). These effects are in part dose related in that microgram per milliliter amounts can be directly cytotoxic. Whatever the beneficial effects of selenium are on immune function, they appear to be independent of IL-1 or IL-2 concentration (Kiremidjian-Schumacher et al. 1990). Dietary levels of selenium at micronutrient concentrations have also been epidemiologically correlated with tumor morbidity.

11. Air Pollution

Of all possible immunotoxic agents, those with which the public is most concerned are air pollutants. Although there are anecdotal accounts about heavy air pollution and increased tumors and other diseases in certain areas like the Aral Sea region of Turkestan, there is little epidemiologic evidence that even the worst case scenarios result in widespread immunotoxicity. Epidemiologic studies on air pollutants are difficult because several pollutants occur together (e.g., ozone and oxides of sulfur or nitrogen), and it is impossible to ascribe a particular effect to a single substance (Koenig 1987). If compounds of lead, formerly used as fuel additives, were immunosuppressive, one would have expected epidemiologic evidence of increased infection/tumor incidence from large urban centers like Los Angeles; however, studies in areas such as this would have been complicated by the high levels of ozone occurring in such sunny areas. Ozone, sulfur dioxide, and nitrogen dioxide are the most commonly studied air pollutants, and all are certifiably toxic to respiratory tissues and functions (reviewed by Koenig 1987). Increased susceptibility to certain infections is seen in experimental animals exposed to these agents, but this enhancement is more likely caused by such things as direct epithelial toxicity, irritation of nerve endings, or decreased pulmonary function rather than immunotoxicity.

Another problem encountered in trying to assess the effects of air pollution on immune function is that the incidence of respiratory disease and its exacerbation are difficult to quantify. Asthmatics are extrasensitive to sulfur dioxide air pollution, but the effects result more as triggers of an existing state, not as antigenic or pathogenic inducers (McFadden 1984). In assessing air pollutants, one must consider that the entire respiratory apparatus is being affected, not just the immunologic cells that it contains. The mucociliary tissues of the airway linings are especially sensitive to environmental and infectious influences. Mucociliary clearance/transport, nasal mucus flow, and ciliary beat frequency are affected by a variety of indoor and outdoor air pollutants (reviewed in Pedersen 1990). If mucociliary clearance is compromised, increased opportunistic infection is a well-known result.

Air pollutants undoubtedly influence immune reactions against antigens to which individuals are already immunized. Dogs that had been exposed to ozone at 3 ppm showed increased respiratory resistance to acetylcholine or to aerosols of either antigen to which they had been immunized (Yanai et al. 1990). Although the sensitivity to acetylcholine was the same in immunized or nonimmunized dogs, no change in respiratory responsiveness was seen in unimmunized dogs at any antigen concentration. These data suggest that ozone evokes pharmacological changes in individuals with preexisting immune sensitivity who are also concomitantly being exposed to the relevant antigen. This study is one of the very few that have attempted to relate specific immune functions with defined exposure to air pollutants. In another controlled study of human exposure, healthy, nonsmoking volunteers were exposed for 2–hr periods on four separate days within a 6–day span to nitrogen dioxide, simulating what was considered a moderately heavy level of air pollution, 0.6 ppm (Rubinstein et al. 1991). These individuals were monitored for changes in pulmonary function and for changes in peripheral and bronchoalveolar leukocyte composition. No changes were found in any of the pulmonary function studies or in most of the lymphocyte subsets studied by FACS analysis. Only the percentage of NK cells ($CD16^+$) in the lavage fluids showed a significant rise (function was not tested).

Air pollution means more than just industrial or automotive emissions but includes indoor air quality as well. Not only is indoor air a significant source of allergens, it is also likely to contain significant concentrations of aldehydes, ammonia, radon, phenol, ozone, and other compounds with potentially inflammatory or immunotoxic effects. Emissions of these materials are derived from such sources as cigarette smoke, vapors from new synthetic carpets, wall board, and insulation (aldehydes), running of electric motors and office equipment (ozone), or ground water contamination in basements (radon). An overlooked air pollutant that leads to adverse respiratory effects, including high in vitro mutagenicity, is wood smoke from indoor wood-burning stoves (Keonig 1987), but its effect on specific immune functions has not yet been evaluated.

One aspect of indoor air pollution is "tight-" or "sick-building" syndrome. Inhabitants or workers complain of sinusitis, runny nose, eye irritation, headache, fatigue, and dizziness. As energy-efficient buildings have been designed to reduce heat loss, they have become more impervious to the introduction of outside air. The accumulation of vapors emanating from construction materials coupled with substances such as ozone from electric motor operations and possibly microbes being discharged from defective humidifying equipment combine to produce toxic effects. Other than for antigen-induced hypersensitivity pneumonitis or endotoxin-induced humidifier fever, no evidence is available to indicate that immunotoxicity is involved with regard to pollutants.

The microclimate within the home or building (chiefly temperature and humidity) coupled with availability of substrate combine to favor the growth of microbial agents that can be important agents in inducing allergic rhinitis and hypersensitivity pneumonitis, sources of microbially derived toxins, as well as infectious disease, e.g., Legionnaire's disease (Burge 1990; Dales, Burnett, and Zwanenberg 1991). Defective humidifiers have been incriminated in disseminating endotoxin-containing bacteria into the air and leading to a syndrome called humidifier fever (Rylander and Haglind 1984). Bacterial endotoxin is highly inflammatory and immunomodulatory. Microbes are an unlikely cause of sick-building syndrome in newly constructed buildings but may be involved in problems of older buildings in that dust has had more chance to accumulate, water leaks have contributed to enhancement of mold growth, etc.

12. Mycotoxins

Mycotoxins are secondary fungal metabolites with toxic and carcinogenic properties. They are stable to degradation and are commonly found in many agricultural products. When such products are stored under conditions that retain or promote moisture accumulation, favorable growth conditions are produced for the fungi. Specific fungi produce different kinds of these structurally diverse materials. Toxic effects are seen in livestock that have ingested contaminated feeds, and there is a potential that toxic effects could also occur following inhalation of mycotoxin-containing dusts. Dietary exposure to substances such as aflatoxin, ochratoxin, etc. has been shown to induce impairments in rodents of NK-cell function, antibody production, expression of delayed skin test hypersensitivity, and lymphocyte proliferative responses (reviewed in Pestka and Bondy 1990; Thurston, Richard, and Peden 1986). Although veterinary immunologists have not made the transition from experimental rodent data to livestock species yet, the relevance of these findings is significant in that dietary intake was also associated with increased susceptibility to *Salmonella* and *Listeria* infections, which are not only important in livestock productivity, but could represent a potential human health hazard as well. One particular toxin known as vomitoxin induces a disease when fed to mice strikingly similar to the human immunodeficiency disease of IgA nephropathy.

In a unique approach of assessing resistance to infection and immune responsiveness, a mycotoxin was administered either before or after to groups of mice that were also either immunized with sheep erythrocytes or challenged with a *Salmonella* infection (Bottex, Martin, and Fontanges 1990). Only when the mycotoxin was given after either the infection or immunization was an effect seen: increased mortality or depressed antibody production, respectively. These data recall the importance of timing in administering immunosuppressive therapeutics to inhibit induction of transplantation rejection and once again suggest that the temporal condition of the host at the time of xenobiotic contact greatly affects the outcome of exposure.

D. SELECTED DISEASES WITH IMMUNOTOXIC EFFECTS

Even by discussing immunotoxic/allergic reactions by organ system affected or by inducing agents, all of the important types of immunotoxicity disease are not really covered. There remain several important classes of human disease, many of which are difficult to study by experimental models, that must be discussed in a separate setting.

1. Occupational Asthma

A caution should be sounded against always trying to classify hypersensitivities separately from immunotoxicities because they can in fact occur together and even resemble each other. A good example is occupational asthma, a disease occurring idiosyncratically in workers exposed to a variety of chemicals and characterized by reversible airway obstruction. Clinically, patients suffering from occupational asthma may present with a spectrum of asthmatic responses following exposure or challenge; i.e., either early, late phase, dual, or even repetitive responses may be evoked (see Chapter 6). In addition, a hypersensitivity pneumonitis-like disease as well as a unique syndrome characterized by pneumonia and anemia may develop to the same chemicals (Zeiss 1989). Occupational asthma differs from IgE-mediated, atopic asthma in several respects. The disease may develop in people who are not necessarily hypersensitivity prone, and it often requires longer periods of exposure before sensitization leading to the development of signs and symptoms. There are numerous agents capable of inciting this disease (see Table 11–5 for a selected list of the most common types), and they can be divided generally into two groups. In one the offending materials are large-molecular-weight substances (usually 20–50 kDa), often protein, and the response induced is classical IgE-mediated asthma demonstrable by in vitro or in vivo testing (Novey et al. 1989). Exposure to vegetable products could include large- or small-molecular-weight substances. In these exposures, one must be careful to distinguish products of fungal contamination from those innate to the plant itself. Animal handlers and workers in enzyme production, fertilizer manufacture, printing, and soldering occupations are most at risk to the large-molecular-weight agents.

The other group consists of low-molecular-weight materials and more commonly induce the non-IgE-mediated, longer-lasting types of asthma. Genetic predisposition does not seem to be a factor in developing sensitivity to these stimulants as it is for that caused by the high-molecular-weight substances. More commonly this form is non-IgE-mediated, although the role of IgE antibodies to these haptens varies with the chemical. In the case of the acid anhydrides, the role is clear. Antigen-specific IgE antibodies to the anhydride hapten or to new antigenic determinants created by modification of host protein with the chemical are demonstrable and correlate well with immediate-onset disease (Zeiss et al.

TABLE 11–5.   Some Inciting Agents Causing Occupational Asthma

Large Molecular Weight	Low Molecular Weight
Enzymes	Chemicals
Subtilisin	Epoxy resins
Trypsin	Ethanolamines
Papain	Platinum salts
Antigens of animal origin	Several heavy metals
Urine, saliva, droppings	Isocyanates
Epithelial danders	Fabric finishers
Grain mits and weevils	Phthalic anhydrides
Ectoparasites	Dyes
(ova, pupae, feces, etc.)	Pyrethrum
Antigens of plant origin	Plicatic acid
Grain dust, flour	Drugs
Wood dusts	Piperazine
Castor beans	Synthetic penicillins
Coffee beans	Tetracycline
Gums acacia and tragacanth	Chloramine-T
Rosin	

1980). The role of such antibodies to toluene diisocyanates is less clear. Some of these smaller substances can induce IgE, but they are also irritative and can trigger airway responses in people with hyperreactive airways. Moreover, as in the case of toluene diisocyanate, the substance is pharmacologically active and capable of mimicking antigen-induced airway response. Workers in plastics, chemical synthesis, welding, and pharmaceutical processing industries are exposed to agents of this type.

Toluene Diisocyanate

Toluene diisocyanate (TDI) is widely used in polyurethane production and in the manufacture of plastics, foam insulation, and synthetic coatings. Since it has such widespread application, the number of workers exposed to the material is large. Inhalation of dilute amounts in sensitive individuals will trigger narrowing of the airways with a resultant decline in the forced expiratory volume in 1 sec (FEV_1). Although it is often thought of as an allergy, questions concerning an immunologic basis for TDI asthma were first prompted by observations that although TDI did not stimulate the release of histamine from peripheral human leukocytes in vitro, it did reduce the cAMP production produced by catecholamine stimulation (Van Ert and Batigelli 1975). At certain concentrations, bronchospastic responses could be evoked in all individuals challenged; i.e., there is a toxic, irritant effect at higher concentrations. Failure to produce sufficient quantities of cAMP from adenylate cyclase stimulation leads to the bronchial constriction and mucus hypersecretion characteristic of the disease. Thus, TDI appeared to act as a β-adrenergic blocker. Fewer than 15% of the symptomatic TDI asthmatics have TDI-specific IgE antibodies in their sera, and some may have positive skin tests to toluene isocyanate–albumin conjugates, but these reactions do not correlate with bronchial reactivity (Butcher, Jones, et al. 1977; Butcher et al. 1980; Butcher, Salvaggio, and O'Neil 1977).

In vitro testing of leukocytes from sensitive and nonsensitive individuals failed to show any histamine release when stimulated with TDI–albumin conjugates and confirmed the hypothesis that TDI was acting as a β-blocker. Significant TDI-induced inhibition of the rise of intracellular cAMP was noted following stimulation of human lymphocytes with isoproterenol and PGE_1 (Davies et al. 1977), but the dose level at which this happens must be critical. Most of the clinically sensitive persons demonstrated adverse bronchial responses when challenged by inhalation of TDI and, additionally, showed greater airways reactivity on mecholyl challenge than nonsensitive persons. Not only do sensitive people fail to exhibit a good correlation with circulating TDI-specific IgE, false-positive results may occur in asymptomatic workers (Butcher et al. 1983). These studies suggest that TDI might induce obstructive airways disease through pharmacological, not allergic, mechanisms and that TDI may be acting as a partial agonist. That antibodies develop at all in those with the disease is viewed by most as a result of the asthma, not the cause of it.

Animal models of TDI-induced asthma have been confined to the guinea pig. Karol (1983) reported induction of TDI-specific antibodies as measured by passive cutaneous anaphylaxis (PCA) in an apparent dose response to daily inhalations of TDI as low as 0.36 ppm. Higher doses were associated with a greater ease of antibody induction. Although skin testing was attempted, any positive reactions obtained were atypical for guinea pigs, being late-phase in nature and often reactive to the conjugate carrier itself, which was a guinea pig protein. In contrast, Cibulas et al. (1986), although able to induce airway hyperreactivity and pulmonary inflammation in guinea pigs with a similar protocol, were unable to demonstrate the induction of PCA antibodies at the time of these changes. The guinea pig can produce an increase in airway responsiveness that is associated with epithelial injury and acute airway inflammation including eosinophil infiltration of the tracheal mucosa as a result of a single exposure of 1 ppm TDI (Gordon et al. 1985). Such TDI exposure causes an acute increase in airway responsiveness to inhaled acetylcholine. That additional pharmacological mediators are also involved was shown by the ability of the substance P competitor capasaicin (as well as other substance P inhibitors) to prevent these TDI-induced altered responses (Sheppard et al. 1988). This TDI-induced increase in guinea pig bronchoconstriction to substance P is accomplished by inhibition of an endopeptidase that would normally degrade the neuropeptide, clearly not an immunologic mechanism.

The pattern of TDI-induced asthma includes sensitivity at very low doses, latency, and an anamnestic response in sensitized workers after reexposure, but neither the presence of IgE antibodies nor the β-blockade theory satisfactorily explains this pattern. Emerging evidence for the presence of antibodies of other classes, particularly IgG, needs to be evaluated for the possibility of cross-linking Fc receptors of mast cells and/or releasing mediators by other means (Zeiss et al. 1988).

Acid Anhydrides

Acid anhydrides (mostly phthalic and trimellitic) are industrial chemicals commonly used in a variety of applications, e.g., in paints, corrosion-resistant epoxy coatings, etc. The evidence with these chemicals suggests that inhalation can invoke quite a spectrum of types of immune injury. The evidence is good that these haptens must become attached to respiratory tract proteins to produce new antigenic determinants (Zeiss et al. 1980). Asthmatic reactions induced soon after inhalation correlate well with the presence of antigen-specific IgE antibodies, but other types of injury exist as well. A hypersensitivity pneumonitis-like reaction characterized by a delayed response (4–12 hr after exposure) with more systemic manifestations may also occur. This syndrome is accompanied by elevations in hapten–human serum albumin-specific circulating IgG, IgM, and IgA antibodies. An additional type of severe restrictive lung disease characterized by hemoptysis and anemia in addition to the lung pathology (pulmonary disease anemia or PDA syndrome) is also accompanied by high levels of circulating immunoglobulins to hapten proteins and hapten-coated erythrocytes (Turner et al. 1980). Studies of animal models of the late-onset type of disease show that the rising amount of hapten-specific antibody parallels the development of pulmonary lesions (Zeiss et al. 1988). Presumably immune complexes localized in situ activate complement, initiate macrophage or neutrophil influxes, and generate toxic oxygen radicals, but this remains to be proven with the acid anhydride model.

2. Anaphylaxis

One of the most alarming emergencies in medicine is the rapid development of systemic shock from anaphylaxis. The curious term means the opposite of prophylaxis and was originally applied to an antigen-induced sensitization that resulted in a serious systemic allergic reaction on subsequent challenge. Clinically the syndrome is characterized by severe upper or lower airway obstruction accompanied by secondary vascular collapse. Characteristic signs include laryngeal edema, hypotension, urticarial rash, angioedema, nausea and vomiting, hyperinflation of the lungs as a result of severe bronchoconstriction, and prominent eosinophil infiltration in the lungs and liver (Austen 1988). The attack may begin within seconds to minutes after exposure, which is usually via injection (includes administration of medicaments or venomous bites and stings). Less frequently, attacks may even be precipitated by ingestion of the offending agent, e.g., nuts, fish, egg white, or oral antibiotics. Fortunately, the reaction is uncommon; however, some agents such as heparin and protamine sulfate are used so frequently in cardiovascular surgery, cardiac catheterization, dialysis, and leukapheresis that the number of reactions encountered may be large (Weiler et al. 1990).

Most reactions have an IgE-mediated component that, when reacted with antigen, triggers widespread release of mediators from mast cells. What makes the reaction so generalized and life-threatening is unknown. Although anaphylaxis is a recognized risk in skin testing atopic individuals, there is no evidence that the atopic state is a requirement for its development, and it may develop in anyone, not necessarily the atopic (Terr 1985; Austen 1988). Major examples of drugs and diagnostic agents leading to IgE-mediated anaphylaxis are listed in Table 11–6. Were this the only mechanism of induction, predictability would be easily achieved through preskin testing with the intended therapeutic. But not only are there various IgE-independent mechanisms, some individuals are so sensitive that even application of the skin test has induced shock (Pinkowski and Leeson 1990). Additional well-known examples of anaphylaxis incitants are those related to venomous stings, especially honey bees, hornets, and fire ants.

Several examples of non-IgE-mediated anaphylaxis are also known. Transfusion reactions resulting from the intravascular reaction of recipient isoantibodies (e.g., anti-A or anti-B) for donor erythrocytes bearing either antigen resemble anaphylactic reactions duplicating some, but not all, of the same signs and symptoms. Damage is mediated by intravascular complement-dependent hemolytic reactions caused by naturally occurring antibodies. Systems primarily affected seem to be coronary artery constriction, hypotension, jaundice, and, in severe cases, disseminated intravascular coagulation and renal failure (Mollison, Engelfriet, and Contreras 1987). Transfusing plasma to IgA-deficient recipients carries the danger of inducing anti-IgA antibodies of the IgG class. Subsequent transfusion of IgA-containing blood into a pre-sensitized individual may trigger a similar reaction (Vyas, Perkins, and Fudenberg 1968). Formerly, intravenous administration of γ-globulin for treatment of B-cell immunodeficiency was often accompanied by anaphylactic reactions because of the presence of fine microprecipitates formed during the immunochemical manufacturing process. These precipitates, as well as the immune complexes formed in the anti-IgA recipients, most likely activated the complement cascade, which led to C3a, C4a, and C5a (anaphylatoxins) production and consequent widespread change in vascular permeability. It is important to recognize in γ-globulin infusions that there is no requirement for presensitization. This risk has been greatly reduced by treating the globulin by methods to prevent the formation of such precipitates.

There is considerable confusion concerning the immunologic mechanism of anaphylaxis owing to examples of agents that are capable of inducing the same clinical syndrome but that do not require specific immune sensitization. Such reactions are known as anaphylactoid or "anaphylaxis-like." A list of some of

TABLE 11–6.   Some Drugs, Diagnostic Agents, and Additives Causing Anaphylaxis and Anaphylactoid Reactions

Anaphylaxis-inducing Agents	Anaphylactoid-inducing Agents
Proteins and polypeptides	Nonsteroidal antiinflammatory drugs
Heterologous serum	Aspirin
Hormones	Aminopyrine
Insulin	Fenoprofen
Parathormone	Fluenamic acid
ACTH	Ibuprofen
Pitressin	Indomethacin
Estradiol	Mefenamic acid
Relaxin	Naproxen
Enzymes	Tolmetin
Trypsin	Zomepirac
Chymotrypsin	Sulfiting agents
Chymopapain	Sulfur dioxide
Penicillinase	Sodium sulfite
Asparaginase	Sodium bisulfite
Vaccines	Potassium bisulfite
Toxoids	Sodium metabisulfite
Allergy extracts	Potassium metabisulfite
Polysaccharides	Opiate narcotics
Dextran	Morphine
Iron dextran	Codeine
Acacia	Meperidine
Vitamins	Miscellaneous
Thiamine	Mannitol
Folic acid	Radiocontrast media
Antibiotics	Curare and d-tubocurarine
Penicillin	Dextrans
Streptomycin	IV immunoglobulins
Cephalosporin	
Tetracycline	
Amphotericin B	
Nitrofurantoin	
Diagnostic agents	
Sulfobromphthalein	
Sodium dehydrocholate	
Others	
Barbiturates	
Diazepam	
Phenytoin	
Protamine	
Aminopyrine	
Local and systemic anesthetics	
Some sulfas	
Latex peptides	

Source: Adapted from Terr (1985).

the most common medical products inducing antibody-independent responses in this category appears in Table 11-6. The mechanisms by which shock is induced are probably different depending on the nature of the inciting agent. Widespread complement activation most likely is responsible for that induced by infusion of high-molecular-weight dextran plasma volume expanders. Nonspecific mast cell release of histamine accounts for the reactions following administration of some agents such as opiates, and altered arachidonate metabolism may be an explanation for aspirin-induced reactions, but for many agents, the mechanism(s) remains obscure (see discussion concerning radiocontrast media above). Alternative explanations such as labile kinin-generating or unstable complement activating systems are attractive, but unproven. However, these theories point out the possibility of host predisposition. In some instances, repeated exposure combined with an anatomic defect that allows greater opportunity for antigen entry may enhance the chance of developing IgE-dependent reactions. In a retrospective study of anaphylactic reactions to water-soluble proteins present in latex materials (e.g., gloves, catheters) among pediatric patients, most (10/11) of the reacting patients were also afflicted with spina bifida, and one had a congenital genitourinary abnormality. Because these patients undergo multiple surgical procedures and require intermittent catheterizations, they are at increased exposure risk to this protein.

3. Hypersensitivity Pneumonitis and Organic Dust Toxic Syndrome

Inhalation of organic materials may activate a number of immunologic effectors and initiate a spectrum of inflammatory pulmonary diseases of complex pathogenesis. The clinical entities range from organic dust toxic syndrome (formerly called acute pulmonary mycotoxicosis) caused by the one-time inhalation of large amounts of mycelial/spore matter and various acute, chronic, and progressive forms of hypersensitivity pneumonitis (HP). Other than certain aspects of clinical presentation, the main difference between the toxic dust syndrome and the forms of HP is the requirement in the latter for prior immunologic sensitization. Several clinical forms of HP may occur and range from a short-term, classical acute form, a recurrent, subacute illness that is very difficult to distinguish from mild upper respiratory infections, and a serious, progressive form that does not resolve even when removed from agent exposure (Seaton and Morgan 1984).

A temporary acute respiratory illness known as organic dust toxic syndrome is often confused with hypersensitivity pneumonitis and can occur in individuals who have never been exposed to the agent previously (Von Essen et al. 1990). No radiologic chest infiltrates, severe hypoxemia, or physiological after effects occur in this form, and there are no demonstrable antigen-specific effectors present at the time of illness. It is caused by inhalation of high burdens of essentially the same types of contaminated products associated with HP. This short-term flu-like illness is much more common than HP, but its incidence could be reduced by dust curtailment methods.

The inhalants are most commonly but not always of microbial origin, and the responses can occur after a single inhalation of large doses or after chronic exposure to much lower amounts of offending material. The most common offending agents are agricultural wastes (spent sugar cane) or products (hay, feeds, etc.)

that have been microbially contaminated, especially by bacteria known as thermophilic actinomycetes or fungi (especially *Aspergillus*). Exposure to other industrial organic materials has also been incriminated in some outbreaks, and a list of many are presented in Table 11-7. Tracing the causes of case clusters is usually not difficult in an agricultural or industrial setting because of the obvious nature of the aerosols. However, HP may also arise in the home or in office buildings, where it is harder to identify because the source or nature of the aerosol is not so obvious, nor are large groups of affected individuals always involved. Moldy conditions about the home or in defective air conditioning systems and the dander or droppings of certain pets, e.g., parakeets or gerbils, are also known sources for this disease.

Cell walls of the representative microorganisms associated with these entities are known to incite inflammatory reactions (largely through enzymatic cascades like the alternative complement pathway), activate macrophages, initiate lymphocyte mitogenesis, and induce specific immune cytotoxic cells. The particular combination of any of these specific immunologic mechanisms together with undefined host factors may lead to one of these manifestations or, indeed, to no manifestation at all. Formerly, this disease was believed to be a pulmonary form of an Arthus reaction in which the presence of circulating precipitating antibodies reacted with inhaled protein antigens, leading to an immune-complex-mediated inflammation of the alveolar interstitium (Pepys, 1969). Although precipitins often accompany overt clinical disease, their presence is now considered only as evidence of antigenic contact rather than an indicator of pathogenesis (Burrell and Rylander 1981). Although toxic components are involved in HP induced by microbial aerosols, there are also ingredients capable of nonspecifically activating the complement system (Olenchock and Burrell 1976). Gram-negative bacteria are sources of highly inflammatory and immunomodulating endotoxin, and fungal spores and mycelia are rich in inflammatory glucans, immunomodulating mycotoxins, and proteolytic enzymes. This initial inflammatory event probably accounts for the toxic dust syndrome in the unsensitized. If the exposure is of suffient magnitude to allow aerosol-laden antigens to cross the air–blood bar-

TABLE 11-7.   Some Agents Causing Hypersensitivity Pneumonitis

Agent	Source
Fungi	
Aspergillus clavatus	Moldy malt, feeds, grains
A. fumigatus	
Cryptostroma corticale	Moldy maple bark
Aureobasidium pullulans	Moldy sequoia bark
Penicillium frequentans	Moldy cork dust
Penicillium casei	Cheese making
Bacteria	
Micropolyspora faeni and others	Moldy hay, compost, fodder, sugar cane; contaminated air conditioners
Flavobacterium	Contaminated humidifer water
Animal Sources	
Wheat weevils	Moldy flours and grains
Parakeets, chickens, pigeons; rodents	Proteins in droppings, urine
Pituitary snuff	Heterologous pituitary hormones
Amoebae	Contaminated humidifier water

rier, the host can be immunized. Subsequent antigen-specific effectors then leaving the vascular compartment could then inflict host injury (Burrell and Hill 1976; Burrell and Rylander 1981). Subsequent antigen-induced activation involves macrophage and T-cell-mediated pulmonary inflammation (Richerson 1983).

4. Multiple Chemical Sensitivity

It is necessary in any subject to know not only what properly belongs in that subject but also those matters that do not. With this guidepost, it is difficult to decide what to do with a controversial topic such as multiple chemical sensitivity (MCS). Basically, this is a syndrome characterized by various often vague symptoms (e.g., fatigue, irritability, anxiety, mood swings, memory lapses, and periods of confusion) but can affect almost any organ system. It is possibly brought on by stimulation of small quantities of many antigenically unrelated substances. Somehow, certain persons are adversely affected by synthetic chemicals in the environment at doses far lower than can be explained by accepted pathophysiological mechanisms. Although some illness may be triggered by foods or food additives, many patients (perhaps up to 80%) volunteer a history of acute or chronic exposure to a particular chemical, e.g., a pesticide or organic solvent, and some time later symptoms are triggered by inhalation or other contact with a wide variety of stimulants. The number of diverse chemical substances capable of stimulating a reaction in the sensitive patient often expands, and this feature is called the spreading phenomenon.

There are many difficulties encountered by anyone trying to understand MCS. Among them: there still does not exist any agreed-on working clinical definition of the disease; there are few objective, measurable signs that are diagnostic of the disease; and there are almost no molecular or cellular data or hypotheses that can be used by the laboratory scientist to evaluate it (Kahn and Letz 1990). Most clinical allergists believe that the vagueness and multiplicity of symptoms argue against their constituting a single disease process, especially in the absence of immunologic, biochemical, or histological abnormalities. Indeed, individuals suffering illnesses under the broad MCS umbrella consist of such diverse groups as chemical workers exposed to a variety of agents, particularly organic solvents; occupants of tight or sick buildings (discussed under Air Pollution above); people living near toxic waste sites or other areas receiving environmental contamination; consumers exposed to a wide variety of domestic materials; as well as those with legitimate psychosomatic disorders. The most difficult population to evaluate from the immunotoxicologic standpoint are people who have no known exposure to occupational materials, medical formulations, or cosmetics. Conceivably some patients in this mixed group may have such equally baffling disturbances as chronic fatigue syndrome or chronic Epstein-Barr infections.

Understanding of MCS is further complicated by the rather extreme polarity that exists among professional as well as lay groups concerned with this syndrome. Much of the confusion also stems from the superimposition of yet other controversies such that an objective evaluation of one of them (e.g., understanding MCS) soon gets involved in other arguments, e.g., the legitimacy of a field called clinical ecology. Clinical ecologists believe that certain forms of ill health are caused by exposure to food and extremely low levels of various synthetic chemicals in the environment. Since clinical ecologists have not yet put forward testable pathophysiological hypotheses to explain these diseases, and they use certain nonstandard diagnostic methods that have not been validated or accepted by allergists and others in classical medicine (Kahn and Letz 1990; Terr 1989), a discussion of MCS often gets clouded by disagreements on these points.

Two further complications serve to inflame objective understanding of this illness. One has been the involvement of legal suits seeking compensation and punitive damages against those accused of alleged negligence (Marshall 1986). Another unfortunate obstacle impeding understanding is that many of these unfortunate victims seem to belong to a group of people characterized by a psychological profile that might be dismissed as somatiform disorders. The role of depression and psychological stress on expression of symptoms is poorly understood, and many patients are probably dismissed with "It's all in your head," which does not solve anything.

No attempt is made to resolve or even explain these many confounding social matters that are germane to understanding MCS, nor is there any attempt to evaluate other theories offered to explain the disease, e.g., hyperreactivity of the olfactory, hypothalamus, and other parts of the limbic system. The reader is referred to the monograph by Ashford and Miller (1991) for details of the clinical ecology versus classical allergy argument and for clinical details about MCS, or to the more penetrable and balanced review of Hileman (1991). An older but worthwhile collection of reviews including the psychological aspects may be found in Cullen (1987), which also includes a critical assessment of the immune theories of MCS (Terr 1987).

Only the few immunologic reports available are assessed here, and unfortunately, most of these are even more anecdotal than many in the immunotoxicology field. Originally, ecological illness was defined as a type of allergy or even as an autoimmune disease, and this largely got the movement off to a bad start with classical allergists. Even today, precise words like "hypersensitivity" and "immunotoxicity" are used carelessly by those discussing MCS. The following discussion uses these words and evaluates the findings according to the same guidelines used elsewhere in this text.

The central thesis among those who invoke immunologic features in explaining MCS is that modern-day exposure to so many chemicals somehow damages the immune system in such a way that the individuals become hyperresponsive (or "sensitized") to many synthetic chemicals. The term "sensitized" is set off in quotes not in a derogatory way but rather to indicate it is not the way the word is used throughout this text. In clinical ecology usage, the term is used variously to denote immunologic as well as nonimmunologic sensitization.

In one fluorescent activated cell sorter (FACS) study comparing lymphocytes obtained from MCS patients and control subjects, no changes in $CD4^+$ T cells could be seen, but there were significant reductions in percentages of MCS $CD8^+$ lymphocytes, which caused significant increases in CD4/CD8 ratios in this population (Rea et al. 1986). To make their data more relevant to those from other laboratories, the authors compared their control data with data from several other studies on FACS analysis of human lymphocytes and found them consistent. Similarly, comparisons made of data from patients with chemically sensitive asthma or rheumatoid arthritis with data from other published sources were favorable. Such comparisons helped validate the effectiveness of the authors' use of the then new FACS technology. This is the best of several similar reports on lymphocyte ratios in MCS patients (others are reviewed by Levin and Byers

1987). But as in so many other studies of reputed immunotoxicity to specific agents, it is difficult to attach relevance to these findings in terms of using the data to explain the patients' disease. Do the abnormal CD4/CD8 ratios reflect a connection with causation, or is it simply another sign of the effects of the disease? If there is immune dysregulation, how does it affect the patient, and what, if anything, does it have to do with the manifestations of the patient's illness?

In other studies by several different groups on more highly selected but smaller sets of patients with environmentally triggered vascular disease, patient sera were measured for such things as immunoglobulins, immune complexes, C3, and C4. Although some patients in each group showed mild elevations, the response of any group was much less convincing than the lymphocyte data and not statistically analyzed. A suggestion was made that the illness was caused by vascular depositions of immune complexes and complement-mediated damage, but no in situ proof of localization was offered, nor was any attempt made to identify the offending antigen.

In conclusion, there is no evidence available to suggest that there is an immune etiopathogenesis of MCS. Rather, it is one of many disturbances that can be shown to have an effect on certain immunologic parameters, the significance of which remains unknown. A possible example of how immunologists may contribute to the understanding of MCS is shown by a study in which mice were given graded doses of benzene or toluene in drinking water for 28 days and monitored for hypothalamic norepinephrine, circulating corticosterone, ACTH, and lymphocyte-derived IL-2 activity (Hsieh, Sharma, and Parker 1991). Norepinephrine and steroid levels were elevated only in animals given the higher doses of solvents, and at these same levels, IL-2 activity was depressed. The implication was that the solvent certainly stimulated hypothalamic–pituitary–adrenocortical activity, which would be immunosuppressive. Could inhalation/olfaction of such solvents accomplish the same thing, and if it could, how would this relate to the other target organ systems and MCS symptoms? We are a long way from an answer, but carefully controlled and designed experiments such as this are a start.

5. Pneumoconiosis

A better example of a disease where a definitive pathogenic xenobiotic is known and that is accompanied by immunologic changes that contribute to the development of the disease would be any of the mineral pneumoconioses. Obviously, these well-characterized diseases are caused by the chronic inhalation of mineral dusts and not strictly by immunologic causes. Yet, both molecular and cellular aspects of the immune system are affected and are manifested in several different ways. Since these immunologic features contribute to the pathology of the process, the diseases quite properly could be considered to have immunotoxic components and may serve as examples for those wishing to make similar connections with other diseases. The literature on the immunologic aspects of the mineral pneumoconioses is extensive, and several reviews are available (Burrell 1981; Davis 1986; Scheule and Holian 1991; Burrell and Lapp 1992).

There are four major, occupational minerals that have an immunologic impact on the lung: asbestos (particularly chrysotile), silica or quartz, beryllium, and coal mine dust. Each has an immunotoxic potential to induce either hypersensitivity (as in the case of beryllium) or other types of immune injury. These agents have many things in common, yet each is distinctive. Both silicon dioxide (silica) and asbestos occur in nature in different crystallographic forms, which influences their biological properties. Moreover, freshly fractured silica appears more toxic than aged dusts because the former are more highly charged in such a way that the particles react with aqueous media. The result is production of hydroxyl ions, which initiate an oxidative chain reaction leading to macrophage membrane damage through peroxidation (Vallyathan et al. 1988). Additional confounders occur in coal mine dust, which is a very heterogeneous material mineralogically as well as organically and contains many contaminating materials such as silica. Much of the cellular reactivity, and consequently some of the immune responses, are additionally determined by site of deposition, which in turn is dependent on such physical properties as particle size and fiber length (Scheule and Holian 1991). Immunologic data have been obtained from occupationally exposed workers, experimental animals exposed to relevant concentrations of material, and to some extent from in vitro studies. Concern is not only for the immunologic effects but also for how cytokine networks are stimulated to induce the fibrosis that is so characteristic of many clinical forms of the pneumoconioses (see Davis 1986; Scheule and Holian 1991 for these aspects).

Beryllium exists in nature as an element or as ions of very insoluble salts and functions as a hapten to combine with carrier proteins in vivo to become complete antigens. Beryllium induces in some exposed workers and experimental animals all of the signs of classical delayed-type hypersensitivity, i.e., positive skin test sensitivity as well as in vitro correlates of cell-mediated immunity, e.g., macrophage migration inhibition or lymphocyte transformation. Antigen-specific reactivity can be passively transferred by lymphoid cells, but not serum, and the antigen can induce specific tolerance by the oral route. In vitro lymphocyte transformation tests using subcytotoxic doses of antigen have proven valuable in detecting sensitized workers with undetectable clinical disease without exposing them to the potentially harmful metal, even at the low dilutions used in skin testing. The test can be used on peripheral blood leukocytes as well as on bronchoalveolar lavage (BAL) suspensions (Newman et al. 1989). In addition to its haptenic role, beryllium can function as an immunologic adjuvant. The inflammation in some immunologically sensitized individuals is so great as to result in severe and often progressive systemic disease.

Polyclonal immunoglobulin levels, particularly IgA and IgG, are often elevated in miners with disease, and although these changes tend to occur in the more clinically complicated types of disease, there is a poor correlation in amount with radiologic severity. These levels as well as other immune parameters are confounded by smoking.

Alveolar macrophages respond initially to inhaled particles and do so dramatically. Silica is a well-known macrophage toxin (Vigliani and Pernis 1959), but in addition to lysis, in vivo evidence suggests that macrophages become highly activated as evidenced by several parameters (Driscoll et al. 1990). Not only are activated macrophages important in generating toxic radicals and inflammatory cytokines, they influence other cells such as neutrophil chemotaxis, lymphocyte regulation, and fibroblast stimulation (Davis 1986).

Results from studies on lymphocytes obtained from dust-exposed humans are conflicting but in general show depressed responsiveness. It is not clear whether these effects are caused by a direct action of particles on the lymphocytes or the result of indirect regulation from affected macrophages because there is evidence for both. Some studies have reported increases in CD8[+] cells, thus making the

CD4/CD8 ratios reduced (Tsang et al. 1988). Also, some evidence exists that the $CD8^+$ cell activity is enhanced, suggesting that immunosuppression could be a result (Kinugawa et al. 1990). Results from studies with human NK cells have been exceedingly variable, reporting enhanced, depressed, and no effects that no doubt reflect differences in protocols (Burrell and Lapp 1992).

The result of this immune modulation has been seen in two ways: by the effect on resistance to infectious agents or incidence of cancer and by the association with autoimmunity. The synergistic relationship between tuberculous infection and silicosis has long been recognized. Both the bacteria and the silica particles are profound immunomodulating agents, and both are very inflammatory, albeit by different pathways. In an interesting study of the relationship with other infectious disease, silica suspensions were intratracheally injected into specific pathogen-free (SPF) and SPF-maintained rats and studied histologically (Campbell et al. 1980). Results of these animals were compared with those from rats maintained under ordinary conditions, subject to the usual endemic bacterial infections found in any animal care facility. Even after 12 months, the lungs from the SPF-maintained animals mainly showed granulomata with little tendency to form hyaline deposits. Silicosis developed much more rapidly and became more severe in the ordinary infection-prone controls.

Although certain mineral forms of asbestos are known human carcinogens, the epidemiologic evidence suggests that the mortality from lung cancer among coal miners is less than expected (Costello, Ortmeyer, and Morgan 1974). Whether this reflects immune modulation (e.g., macrophage activation) or the fact that the pattern of smoking in coal miners is affected by prohibition of smoking during working hours is uncertain.

The possible connection between autoimmunity and the various pneumoconioses originates with the suggestion that macrophages are stimulated to initiate immune responses to altered serum proteins adsorbed to quartz particles (Scheel et al. 1954). Quite apart from its pathogenic properties, silica has been studied for its adjuvant effects on the immune system. The demonstration of circulating autoantibodies in the sera of workers with pneumoconiosis or in experimental animals has often focused on the presence of antiimmunoglobulins (rheumatoid factor, RF) or antinuclear antibodies (ANA). The general experience has been that although such autoantibodies are found in varying frequencies in workers with coal workers pneumoconiosis (CWP), coal miners with rheumatoid arthritis, asbestos workers, and silicotics, other than for the tendency of ANA frequency to be higher and that of RF to be associated in those with rheumatoid arthritis, there are conflicting reports concerning correlation between their presence and the state of clinical disease or extent of exposure.

Autoantibodies to organ antigens have also received some attention, but many of the studies used nonspecific simple tissue homogenates as in vitro antigens that only demonstrate antibodies against serum globulins, in other words, RF (Esber and Burrell 1967). When globulin-free tissue extracts are carefully prepared, one can identify collagenous components to which sera from a variety of workers with CWP (Burrell 1972) as well as animals with experimental silicosis or CWP have been shown to react. When such antibody is passively administered over a long period of time to experimental animals unexposed to the dusts, focal localization may be seen on the alveolar septa as well as monocytic infiltration, an increase in alveolar interstitial tissue, distention of the distal airways, and increased localization of inhaled bacteria (Burrell, Flaherty, and DeNee 1974).

Pronounced immunoglobulin localization has been demonstrated in the hyaline cores and on the fibroblast cells forming layers around human silicotic nodules, although the antigens to which these react are different. Localization in the hyaline core was shown to be antibodies reacting with other human globulins (Vigliani and Pernis 1959), whereas that in the fibroblast layer is directed against collagenous products of the fibroblasts (Burrell 1972).

6. Splenectomy

Although it may be regarded as an unusual topic in immunotoxicology, splenectomy is included here because it represents a well-defined event that leads directly to profound immunodeficiency in some subjects, and it might serve as instructive material for studies regarding the effects of xenobiotics. Although splenectomy is a valuable therapeutic strategy for treating certain diseases such as idiopathic thrombocytopenic purpura, splenic malignancies, thalassemia, etc., and is often necessary following trauma, it is now considered dangerous to remove the total organ. Where possible, it is much preferable to leave a small part of the spleen in place. Splenectomy may lead to severe infection or sepsis of two types: that appearing in the immediate 10–day postoperative period and that occurring years later. It is the latter type that is of concern from the immunologic point of view.

Statistically, patients who have undergone total splenectomy suffer a greater incidence of infections from certain encapsulated bacteria (e.g., penumococci, meningococci, and *Haemophilus influenzae*). The capsule has a polysaccharide coating that inhibits phagocytosis. These people tend to suffer more from fulminating (overwhelming) infections, especially septicemic infections; however, this septicemia differs in several clinically important details from that occurring in normal individuals (Sherman 1984). The appearance of such an infection seems to be unpredictable and may happen years later (as long as 41 years in one case), and these subjects are considered to be at hazardous risk for the rest of their lives. The individuals are also at risk of activating latent viral infections or reactivating malaria from previous infections. The consequences of overwhelming postsplenectomy infection are extremely serious and often fatal (reviewed in Stryker and Orton 1988).

The rate of overwhelming sepsis in asplenic individuals has ranged mostly in the 2.5–2.8% range (reviewed by Sherman 1984). An enormous number of splenectomies are performed annually and why the long-term mortality rate is not higher must be considered carefully. Do these people who suffer this complication represent some abnormal subset with predisposing conditions? In addition to these types of infections, should these people in later years acquire a malignancy or an immunodeficiency unrelated to the splenectomy or become intravenous drug abusers, they are at a greater disadvantage against these kinds of infections as well as opportunists.

Among its many functions, the spleen is a blood filter, which explains its strategic importance in septicemias. Also, it seems to be the site of opsonizing IgM antibody production, an essential means of defense against encapsulated bacteria. Although these antibodies may be made elsewhere, for unknown reasons the spleen seems to be a preferred site. Asplenic individuals can make enough opsonins eventually, but the lag could play a significant role in dealing with a septicemia or some other kind of overwhelming infection.

There are a number of strategies that can be used prophylactically to insure that the person either devoid of a spleen or who is scheduled to undergo elective splenectomy can avail himself. The risk of pneumococcal infection can be substantially reduced by administration of polyvalent pneumococcal vaccine for most of the common strains of pneumococci, ideally before surgery or within 12 hr of removal. The spleen has good regenerative powers and can often reconstitute near normal immune function if a small part is left behind, although there are reports of overwhelming postsplenectomy sepsis in patients with such partial spleens. remaining (Sass et al. 1983). Patients with splenectomies should be carefully instructed about precautions to follow at the first sign of any febrile illness because prompt action is essential. Antibiotic prophylaxis has also been used for children with good results, although the practice in general is controversial.

References

Abelson, P. H. 1991. Excessive fear of PCBs. *Science* 253:361.

Ameglio, F., A. Benedetto, P. Marotta, et al. 1988. A high proportion of sera of heroin addicts possess anti-HLA class I and class II reactivity. *Clin. Immunol. Immunopathol.* 46:328–34.

Anonymous. 1986. The health consequences of involuntary smoking: A report of the Surgeon General. USPHS, DHHS Publication No. (CDC) 87–8398. Washington: U.S. Government Printing Office.

Aronow, R., C. Cubbage, R. Wiener, et al. 1990. Mercury exposure from interior latex paint—Michigan. *Morbid. Mortal. Weekly Rep.* 39:125–26.

Ashford, N. A., and C. S. Miller. 1991. *Chemical Exposures: Low Levels and High Stakes.* New York: Van Nostrand Reinhold.

Au, W. W., D. M. Walker, J. B. Ward, et al. 1991. Factors contributing to chromosome damage in lymphocytes of cigarette smokers. *Mutat. Res.* 260:137–44.

Austen, K. F. 1988. The anaphylactic syndrome. In *Immunological Diseases*, 4th ed., ed. M. Samter, D. W. Talmage, M. M. Frank, et al., pp. 1119–33. Boston: Little, Brown.

Baldo, B. A., and D. G. Harle. 1990. Drug allergenic determinants. In *Mongographs in Allergy,* Vol. 28: *Molecular Approaches to the Study of Allergens*, ed. B. A. Baldo, pp. 11–51. Basel: Karger.

Barbers, R. G., M. J. Evans, H. Gong, and D. P. Tashkin. 1991. Enhanced alveolar monocytic phagocyte (macrophage) proliferation in tobacco and marijuana smokers. *Am. Rev. Respir. Dis.* 143:1092–95.

Bekesi, J. G., J. Roboz, A. Fischbein, et al. 1985. Immunological, biochemical, and clinical consequences of exposure to polybrominated biphenyls. In *Immunotoxicology and Immunopharmacology*, ed. J. H. Dean, M. I. Luster, A. E. Munson, and H. Amos., pp. 393–406. New York: Raven Press.

Bekesi, J. G., J. P. Roboz, S. Solomon, et al. 1983. Altered immune function in Michigan residents exposed to polybrominated biphenyls. In *Immunotoxicology*, ed. G. C. Gibson, R. Hubbard, and D. V. Parke, pp. 182–92. New York: Academic Press.

Bernstein, D. I., J. S. Gallagher, M. Grad, and I. L. Bernstein. 1984. Local ocular anaphylaxis to papain enzyme contained in a contact lens cleansing solution. *J. Allergy Clin. Immunol.* 74:258–60.

Blakley, B. R., C. S. Sisodia, and T. K. Mukkur. 1980. The effect of methylmercury, tetraethyl lead, and sodium arsenite on the humoral immune response in mice. *Toxicol. Appl. Pharmacol.* 52:245–54.

Blank, S. E., D. A. Duncan, and G. G. Meadows. 1991. Suppression of natural killer cell activity by ethanol consumption and food restriction. *Alcohol Clin. Exp. Res.* 15:16–22.

Bock, S. A., H. A. Sampson, F. M. Atkins, et al. 1988. Double-blind placebo-controlled food challenge as an office procedure: A manual. *J. Allergy Clin. Immunol.* 82:986–97.

Bottex, C., A. Martin, and R. Fontanges. 1990. Action of a mycotoxin (diacetoxyscirpenol) on the immune response of the mouse—interaction with an immunomodulator (OM-89). *Immunopharmacol. Immunotoxicol.* 12:311–25.

Brown, D. P., and M. Jones. 1981. Mortality and industrial hygiene study of workers exposed to polybrominated biphenyls. *Arch. Environ. Health* 36:120–29.

Burchiel, S. W., W. M. Hadley, S. L. Barton, et al. 1988. Persistent suppression of humoral immunity by 7,12–dimethylbenz[a]anthracene in B6C3F1 mice: Correlations with changes in spleen cell surface markers detected by flow cytometry. *Int. J. Immunopharmacol.* 10:369–76.

Burge, H. 1990. Bioaerosols: Prevalence and health effects in the indoor environment. *J. Allergy Clin. Immunol.* 86:687–701.

Burrell, R. 1972. Immunological aspects of coal workers' pneumoconiosis. *Ann. N.Y. Acad. Sci.* 200:94–105.

Burrell, R. 1981. Immunological aspects of silica. In *Health Effects of Synthetic Silica Particulates*, ed. D. D. Dunnom, pp. 82–93. Phildelphia: American Society for Testing Materials.

Burrell, R., D. K. Flaherty, and P. B. DeNee. 1974. Effect of lung antibody on normal lung structure and function. *Am. Rev. Respir. Dis.* 109:106–13.

Burrell, R., and J. O. Hill. 1976. The effect of respiratory immunization on cell-mediated immune effector cells of the lung. *Clin. Exp. Immunol.* 24:116–24.

Burrell, R., and Lapp, N. L. 1992. The immunology of the mineral pneumoconioses. In *Immunology and Allergy Clinics of North America*, ed. D. Banks, pp. 379–400. Philadelphia: W. B. Saunders.

Burrell, R., and R. Rylander. 1981. A critical review of the role of precipitins in hypersensitivity pneumonitis. *Eur. J. Respir. Dis.* 62:332–43.

Butcher, B. T., R. N. Jones, C. E. O'Neil, et al. 1977. Longitudinal study of workers employed in the manufacture of toluene-diisocyanate. *Am. Rev. Respir. Dis.* 116: 411–21.

Butcher, B. T., C. E. O'Neil, M. A. Reed, and J. E. Salvaggio. 1980. Radioallergosorbent testing of toluene diisocyante-reactive individuals using *p*-tolyl isocyanate antigen. *J. Allergy Clin. Immunol.* 66:213–16.

Butcher, B. T., C. E. O'Neil, M. A. Reed, and J. E. Salvaggio. 1983. Radioallergosorbent testing with *p*-tolyl monoisocyanate in toluene diisocyanate workers. *Clin. Allergy* 13:31–34.

Butcher, B. T., J. E. Salvaggio, and C. E. O'Neil. 1977. Toluene diisocyanate pulmonary disease: Immunopharmacologic and mecholyl challenge studies. *J. Allergy Clin. Immunol.* 59: 223–27.

Campbell, M. J., M. M. Wagner, M. P. Scott, et al. 1980. Sequential immunological studies in an asbestos-exposed population. II. Factors affecting lymphocyte function. *Clin. Exp. Immunol.* 39:176–82.

Chao, C. C., T. W. Molitor, G. Gekker, et al. 1991. Cocaine-mediated suppression of superoxide production by human peripheral blood mononuclear cells. *J. Pharmacol. Exp. Ther.* 256:255–58.

Chollett-Martin, S., G. Stamatakis, S. Bailly, et al. 1991. Induction of tumor necrosis factor-alpha during haemodialysis. Influence of the membrane type. *Clin. Exp. Immunol.* 83:329–32.

Christen, A. G., J. L. McDonald, Jr., and J. A. Christen. 1991. *The Impact of Tobacco Use and Cessation on Nonmalignant and Precancerous Oral and Dental Disease and Conditions.* Indiana School of Dentistry Teaching Monograph. Indianapolis: Indiana University School of Dentistry.

Cibulas, W., Jr., C. G. Murlas, M. L. Miller, et al. 1986. Toluene diisocyanate-induced airway hyperreactivity and pathology in the guinea pig. *J. Allergy Clin. Immunol.* 77: 828–34.

Corbett, J. A. 1974. *The Biochemical Mode of Action of Pesticides*, pp. 107–64. New York: Academic Press.

Costello, J., C. E. Ortmeyer, and W. K. C. Morgan. 1974. Mortality from lung cancer in U.S. coal miners. *Am. J. Publ. Health* 64:222–24.

Craddock, P. R., J. Fehr, K.L Brigham, et al. 1977. Complement and leukocyte-mediated dysfunction in hemodialysis. *N. Engl. J. Med.* 296:769–74.

Crispe, I. N., M. J. Bevan, and U. D. Staerz. 1985. Selective activation of Lyt 2^+ precursor T cells by ligation of the antigen receptor. *Nature* 317:627–29.

Crofford, L. J., J. I. Rader, M. C. Dalakas, et al. 1990. L-Tryptophan implicated in human eosinophilia-myalgia syndrome causes fasciitis and periomyositis in the Lewis rat. *J. Clin. Invest.* 86:1757–63.

Cullen, M. 1987. Workers with multiple chemical sensitivities. *Occup. Med. State Art Rev.* 2:655–804.

Dales, R. E., R. Burnett, and H. Zwanenburg. 1991. Adverse health effects among adults exposed to home dampness and molds. *Am. Rev. Respir. Dis.* 143:505–9.

Davies, R. J., B. T. Butcher, C. E. O'Neil, and J. E. Salvaggio. 1977. The in vivo effect of toluene diisocyanate on lymphocyte cyclic adenosine monophosphate production by isoproterenol, prostaglandin, and histamine. *J. Allergy Clin. Immunol.* 60:223–29.

Davis, G. S. 1986. Pathogenesis of silicosis: Current concepts and hypotheses. *Lung* 164:139–54.

de Weck, A. L. 1990. Drug allergy, immunotherapy, immune complexes and anaphylaxis. *Curr. Opin. Immunol.* 2:548–57.

Diamond, I., B. Wrubel, W. Estrin, and A. Gordon. 1987. Basal and adenosine receptor-stimulated levels of cAMP are reduced in lymphocytes from alcoholic patients. *Proc. Natl. Acad. Sci. U.S.A.* 84:1413–16.

Dolovich, J., C. Marshall, E. K. M. Smith, et al. 1984. Allergy to ethylene oxide in chronic hemodialysis patients. *Artif. Organs* 8:334–37.

Donahoe, R. M., J. Nicholson, J. Madden, et al. 1986. Coordinate and independent effects of heroin, cocaine, and alcohol abuse on T cell E rosette formation and antigenic marker expression. *Clin. Immunol. Immunopathol.* 41:254–64.

Driscoll, K. E., R. C. Lindenschmidt, J. K. Maurer, et al. 1990. Pulmonary response to silica or titanium dioxide: Inflammatory cells, alveolar macrophage-derived cytokines, and histopathology. *Am. J. Respir. Cell. Mol. Biol.* 2:381–90.

Emslie-Smith, A. M., A. G. Engel, J. Duffy, et al. 1991. Eosinophilia myalgia syndrome. I. Immunocytochemical evidence for a T-cell mediated immune effector response. *Ann. Neurol.* 29:524–28.

Esber, H. J., and R. Burrell. 1967. An immunologic study of experimental silicosis. *Environ. Res.* 1:171–77.

Fernandes, G., M. Nair, K. Onoe, et al. 1979. Impairment of cell-mediated immune function by dietary zinc deficiency in mice. *Proc. Natl. Acad. Sci. U.S.A.* 76:456–61.

Fine, J. S., T. A. Gasiewicz, and A. E. Silverstone. 1989. Lymphocyte stem cell alterations following perinatal exposure to 2,3,7,8-tetrachlorodibenzo-*p*-dioxin. *Mol. Pharmacol.* 35:18–25.

Fingerhut, M. A., W. E. Halperin, D. A. Marlow, et al. 1991. Cancer mortality in workers exposed to 2,3,7,8-tetrachlorodibenzo-*p*-dioxin. *N. Engl. J. Med.* 324:212–18.

Finlayson, D. C. 1989. Immunologic changes in critically ill patients after anesthesia and surgery. *Anesthesiol. Clin. North Am.* 7:883–95.

Fiore, M. C., H. A. Anderson, R. Hong, et al. 1986. Chronic exposure to aldicarb-contaminated groundwater and human immune function. *Environ. Res.* 41:633–45.

Fleming, L. E., A. M. Ducatman, and S. L. Shalat. 1991. Disease clusters: A central and ongoing role in occupational health. *J. Occup. Med.* 33:818–25.

Fraser, D. W., T. R. Tsai, W. Orenstein, et al. 1977. Legionnaire's disease. Description of an epidemic of pneumonia. *N. Engl. J. Med.* 297:1189–97.

Friedman, H., T. Klein, and S. Specter. 1991. Immunosuppression by marijuana and its components. In *Psychoneuroimmunology*, 2nd ed., ed. R. Ader, D. L. Felten, and N. Cohen, pp. 931–53. San Diego: Academic Press.

Fries, G. F. 1986. The PBB episode in Michigan: An overall appraisal. *CRC Crit. Rev. Toxicol.* 16:105–56.

Garattini, S. 1977. TCDD poisoning at Seveso. *Biomedicine* 26:28–29.

Gordon, T., D. Sheppard, D. M. McDonald, et al. 1985. Airway hyperresponsiveness and inflammation induced by toluene diisocyanate in guinea pigs. *Am. Rev. Respir. Dis.* 132:1106–12.

Gregory, R. L., J. C. Kindle, L. C. Hobbs, and H. S. Malmstrom. 1991. Effect of smokeless tobacco use in humans on mucosal immune factors. *Arch. Oral Biol.* 36:25–31.

Greiner, J. V., R. N. Ross, and M. R. Allansmith. 1988. Ocular allergy. In *Immunological Diseases*, 4th ed., ed. M. Samter, D. W. Talmage, M. M. Frank, et al., pp. 1917–44. Boston: Little, Brown.

Hakim, R. M., J. Breillatt, J. M. Lazarus, and F. K. Port. 1984. Complement activation and hypersensitivity reactions to dialysis membranes. *N. Engl. J. Med.* 311:878–82.

Haley, P. J., G. M. Shopp, J. M. Benson, et al. 1990. The immunotoxicity of three nickel compounds following 13–week inhalation exposure in the mouse. *Fund. Appl. Toxicol.* 15:476–87.

Hamilton, H. E., D. P. Morgan, and A. Simmons. 1978. A pesticide (dieldrin)-induced immunohemolytic anemia. *Environ. Res.* 17:155–64.

Harth, M., G. A. McCain, and K. Cousin. 1990. The modulation of interleukin-1 production by interferon-gamma, and the inhibitory effects of gold compounds. *Immunopharmacology* 20:125–34.

Haynes, D. R., I. R. Garrett, M. W. Whitehouse, et al. 1988. Do gold drugs inhibit interleukin-1? Evidence from an in vitro lymphocyte activating factor assay. *J. Rheumatol.* 15:775–78.

Hermanowicz, A., and S. Kossman. 1984. Neutrophil function and infectious disease in workers occupationally exposed to phosphorganic pesticides: Role of mononuclear-derived chemotactic factor for neutrophils. *Clin. Immunol. Immunopathol.* 33:13–22.

Hileman, B. 1991. Multiple chemical sensitivity. *Chem. Eng. News.* 69(29):26–42.

Hoffman, R. E., P. A. Stehr-Green, K. B. Webb, et al. 1986. Health effects of long-term exposure to 2,3,7,8-tetrachlorodibenzo-*p*-dioxin. *J.A.M.A* 255:2031–38.

Holt, P. G. 1986. Down-regulation of immune responses in the lower respiratory tract: The role of alveolar macrophages. *Clin. Exp. Immunol.* 63:261–70.

Holt, P. G. 1987. Immune and inflammatory function in cigarette smokers. *Thorax* 42:241–49.

House, R. V., L. D. Lauer, M. J. Murray, et al. 1987. Suppression of T-helper cell function in mice following exposure to the carcinogen 7,12–dimethylbenz[a]anthracene and its restoration by interleukin-2. *Int. J. Immunopharmacol.* 9:89–97.

Howard, S. K., P. R. Werner, and S. D. Sleight. 1980. Polybrominated biphenyl toxicosis in swine: Effects on some aspects of the immune system in lactating sows and their offspring. *Toxicol. Appl. Pharmacol.* 55:146–53.

Hsieh, G. C., R. P. Sharma, and R. D. R. Parker. 1991. Hypothalamic-pituitary-adrenocortical axis activity and immune function after oral exposure to benzene and toluene. *Immunopharmacology* 21:23–32.

Hughes, D. A., P. L. Haslam, P. J. Townshend, et al. 1985. Numerical and functional alterations in circulatory lymphocytes in cigarette smokers. *Clin. Exp. Immunol.* 61:459–66.

Hunninghake, G. W., J. E. Gadek, O. Kawanami, et al. 1979. Inflammatory and immune processes in the human lung in health and disease: Evaluation by bronchoalveolar lavage. *Am. J. Pathol.* 97:149–78.

Jerrells, T. R., W. Smith, and M. J. Eckardt. 1990. Murine model of ethanol-induced immunosuppression. *Alcohol Clin. Exp. Res.* 14:546–50.

Johnson, J. D., D. P. Houchens, W. M. Kluwe, et al. 1990. Effects of mainstream and environmental tobacco smoke on the immune system in animals and humans: A review. *CRC Crit. Rev. Toxicol.* 20:369–95.

Kahn, E., and G. Letz. 1990. Clinical ecology: Environmental medicine or unsubstantiated theory? *J. Allergy Clin. Immunol.* 85:437–39.

Karol, M. H. 1983. Concentration dependent immunologic response to toluene diisocyanate (TDI) following inhalation exposure. *Toxicol. Appl. Pharmacol.* 68:229–41.

Kawabata, T. T., and K. L. White. 1989. Metabolism of 7,12–dimethylbenz[a]anthracene by splenic microsomes. *FASEB J.* 3:A604.

Kelly, K., M. Sctlock, and J. P. Davis. 1991. Anaphylactic reactions during general anesthesia among pediatric patients. *Morbid. Mortal. Weekly Rep.* 40:437–43.

Kerkvliet, N. I., L. Baecher-Steppan, B. B. Smith, et al. 1990. Role of the Ah locus in suppression of cytotoxic T lymphocyte activity in halogenated aromatic hydrocarbons (PCBs and TCDD): Structure–activity relationships and effects in C57Bl/6 mice congenic at the Ah locus. *Fund. Appl. Toxicol.* 14:532–41.

Kerkvliet, N. I., L. Baecher-Steppan, and J. A. Schmitz. 1982. Immunotoxicity of pentachlorophenol (PCP): Increased susceptibility to tumor growth in adult mice fed technical PCP-contaminated diets. *Toxicol. Appl. Pharmacol.* 62:55–64.

Kilbourne, E. M., J. T. Bernhert, Jr., M. Posada de la Paz, et al. 1988. Chemical corelates of pathogenicity of oils related to the toxic oil syndrome epidemic in Spain. *Am. J. Epidemiol.* 127:1210–27.

Kilbourne, E. M., J. G. Rigau-Perez, C. W. Heath, Jr., et al. 1983. Clinical epidemiology of toxic-oil syndrome. *N. Engl. J. Med.* 309:1408–14.

Kinugawa, K., F. Hyodoh, A. Andoh, et al. 1990. Elevated binding activity of $CD8^+$ cells with phytohaemagglutinin by asbestos fibers in vitro. *Clin. Exp. Immunol.* 80:89–93.

Kiremidjian-Schumacher, L., M. Roy, H. I. Wishe, et al. 1990. Selenium and immune cell functions. I. Effect on lymphocyte proliferation and production of interleukin 1 and interleukin 2. *Proc. Soc. Exp. Biol. Med.* 193:136–48.

Kirtland, H. H. III, D. N. Mohler, and D. A. Horwitz. 1980. Methyldopa inhibition of suppressor-lymphocyte function. *N. Engl. J. Med.* 302:825–32.

Klimas, N. G., N. T. Blaney, R. O. Morgan, et al. 1991. Immune function and anti-HTLV-I/II status in anti-HIV-1–negative intravenous drug abusers. *Am. J. Med.* 90:163–70.

Koenig, J. Q. 1987. Pulmonary reaction to environmental pollutants. *J. Allergy Clin. Immunol.* 79:833–43.

Koller, L. D. 1980. Immunotoxicology of heavy metals. *Int. J. Immunopharmacol.* 2:269–79.

Kumar, A., M. R. Weatherly, and D. C. Beaman. 1991. Sweeteners, flavorings, and dyes in antibiotic preparations. *Pediatrics* 87:352–60.

Labro, M. T. 1990. Cefodizime as a biological response modifier—a review of its in vivo, ex vivo and in vitro immunomodulatory properties. *J. Antimicrob. Chemother.* 26:37–47.

Ladics, G. S., T. T. Kawabata, and K. L. White. 1991. Suppression of the in vitro immune response of mouse splenocytes by 7,12–dimethylbenz[a]anthracene metabolites and inhibition of immunosuppresion by alpha-naphthoflavone. *Toxicol. Appl. Pharmacol.* 110:31–44.

Landrigan, P. J., K. R. Wilcox, Jr., J. Silva, Jr., et al. 1979. Cohort study of Michigan residents exposed to polybrominated biphenyls: Epidemiologic and immunologic findings. *Ann. N.Y. Acad. Sci.* 320:284–94.

Lasser, E. C. 1991. Pseudoallergic drug reactions: Radiographic contrast media. *Immunol. Allergy Clin. North Am.* 11:645–58.

Laude-Sharp, M., M. Caroff, L. Simard, et al. 1990. Induction of IL-1 during hemodialysis: Transmembrane passage of intact endotoxins (LPS). *Kidney Int.* 38:1089–94.

Leung, D. Y. M., A. R. Rhodes, and R. S. Geha. 1987. Atopic dermatitis. In *Dermatology in General Medicine*, ed. T. B. Fitzpatrick, A. Z. Eisen, K. Wolff, et al., pp. 1385–1408. New York: McGraw-Hill.

Levin, A. S., and V. S. Byers. 1987. Environmental illness: A disorder of immune regulation. *Occup. Med. State Art Rev.* 2:669–82.

Lü, Y.-C., and Y.-C. Wu. 1985. Clinical findings and immunologic abnormalities in yu-cheng patients. *Environ. Health Perspect.* 59:17–29.

Malave, I., J. Rodriguez, Z. Araujo, and I. Rojas. 1990. Effect of zinc on the proliferative response of human lymphocytes—mechanism of its mitogenic action. *Immunopharmacology* 20:1–10.

Markovic, S. N., and D. M. Murasko. 1990. Anesthesia inhibits poly-I:C induced stimulation of natural killer cell cytotoxicity in mice. *Clin. Immunol. Immunopathol.* 56:202–9.

Marshall, E. 1986. Immune system theories on trial. *Science* 234:1490–92.

Martinez, F. D., G. Antognoni, F. Macri, et al. 1988. Parental smoking enhances bronchial responsiveness in nine-year-old children. *Am. Rev. Respir. Dis.* 138:518–23.

Mathews, K. P. 1984. Clinical spectrum of allergic and pseudoallergic reactions. *J. Allergy Clin. Immunol.* 74(Suppl.):558–66.

McFadden, E. R., Jr. 1984. Pathogenesis of asthma. *J. Allergy Clin. Immunol.* 73:413–24.

Miller, G. B., Jr., and J. Wilber. 1991. Update: Acute allergic reactions associated with reprocessed hemodialyzers. *Morbid. Mortal. Weekly Rep.* 40:147–53.

Mollison, P. L., C. P. Engelfriet, and M. Contreras. 1987. Haemolytic transfusion reactions. In *Blood Transfusions in Clinical Medicine*, 8th ed., pp. 587–636. Oxford: Blackwell.

Moreau, J.-F., P. LeSavre, H. de Luca, et al. 1988. General toxicity of water-soluble iodinated contrast media. Pathogenic concepts. *Invest. Radiol.* 23(Suppl. 1):S75–S78.

Moudgill, G. C., J. Gordon, and J. B. Forest, et al. 1984. Comparative effects of volatile anesthetic agents and nitrous oxide on human leukocyte chemotaxis in vitro. *Can. Anesth. Soc. J.* 31:631–37.

Munson, A. E., J. A. Levy, L. S. Harris, et al. 1976. Effects of Δ 9 tetrahydrocannabinol of the immmune system. In *Pharmacology of Marijuana*, ed. M. C. Braudas and S. Szaras, pp. 187–99. New York: Raven Press.

Nair, M. P. N., and S. A. Schwartz. 1990. Immunoregulation of natural and lymphokine-activated killer cells by selenium. *Immunopharmacology* 19:177–83.

Newman, L. S., K. Kreiss, T. E. King, et al. 1989. Pathologic and immunologic alterations in early stages of beryllium disease. Reexamination of disease definition and natural history. *Am. Rev. Respir. Dis.* 139:1479–86.

Nikolaidis, E., B. Brunstrom, L. Dencker, and T. Veromaa. 1990. TCDD inhibits the support of B-cell development by the bursa of Fabricius. *Pharmacol. Toxicol.* 67:22–26.

Novey, H. S., I. L. Bernstein, L. S. Mihalas, et al. 1989. Guidelines for the clinical evaluation of occupational asthma due to high molecular weight (HMW) allergens. Report of the Subcommittee on the Clinical Evaluation of Occupational Asthma due to HMW Allergens. *J. Allergy Clin. Immunol.* 84:829–33.

Oeveren, W., M. D. Kazatchkine, B. Descamps-Latscha, et al. 1985. Deleterious effects of cardiopulmonary bypass. *J. Thorac. Cardiovasc. Surg.* 88:888–99.

Olenchock, S. A., and R. Burrell. 1976. The role of precipitins and complement activation in the etiology of allergic lung disease. *J. Allergy Clin. Immunol.* 58:76–88.

Pedersen, M. 1990. Ciliary activity and pollution. *Lung* 168:368–76.

Pepys, J. 1969. Hypersensitivity diseases of the lungs due to fungi and organic dusts. *Monogr. Allergy* 4:1–147.

Pestka, J. J., and G. S. Bondy. 1990. Alteration of immune function following dietary mycotoxin exposure. *Can. J. Physiol. Pharmacol.* 68:1009–16.

Pillai, R. M., and R. R. Watson. 1990. In vitro immunotoxicology and immunopharmacology—studies on drugs of abuse. *Toxicol. Lett.* 53:269–83.

Pinkowski, J. L., and M. C. Leeson. 1990. Anaphylactic shock associated with chymopapain skin test. *Clin. Orthoped. Rel. Res.* 260:186–90.

Plowman, P. N. 1982. The pulmonary macrophages of human smokers: Fc receptor concentrations on heavily particle-laden cells. *Hum. Toxicol.* 1:433–42.

Pocino, M., I. Malave, and L. Baute. 1990. Zinc administration restores the impaired immune response observed in mice receiving excess copper by oral route. *Immunopharmacol. Immunotoxicol.* 12:697–713.

Pollock, R., F. Ames, P. Rubio, et al. 1987. Protracted severe immune dysregulation induced by cardiopulmonary bypass: A predisposing etiologic factor in blood transfusion-related AIDS? *J. Clin. Lab. Immunol.* 22:1–5.

Rajka, G. 1960. Prurigo Besnier (atopic dermatitis) with special reference to the role of allergic factors. I. The influence of atopic hereditary factors. *Acta Dermatol. Venereol.* 40:285–306.

Raphals, P. 1990. Does medical mystery threaten biotech? *Science* 250:619.

Rea, W. J., A. R. Johnson, S. Youdim, et al. 1986. T and B lymphocyte parameters measured in chemically sensitive patients and controls. *Clin. Ecol.* 4:11–14.

Reggiani, G. 1980. Acute human exposure to TCDD in Seveso, Italy. *J. Toxicol. Environ. Health* 6:27–43.

Renzi, P. M., and L. C. Ginns. 1990. Natural killer activity is present in rat lung lavage and inhibited by lidocaine. *Immunopharmacol. Immunotoxicol.* 12:389–415.

Richerson, H. B. 1983. Hypersensitivity pneumonitis—pathology and pathogenesis. *Clin. Rev. Allergy* 1:469–83.

Ronchetti, R., F. Macri, G. Ciofetta, et al. 1990. Increased serum IgE and increased prevalence of eosiophilia in 9–year-old children of smoking parents. *J. Allergy Clin. Immunol.* 86:400–7.

Rubin, R. L., and R. W. Burlingame. 1991. Drug-induced autoimmunity—a disorder at the interface between metabolism and immunity. *Biochem. Soc. Trans.* 19:153–59.

Rubinstein, I., T. F. Reiss, B. G. Bigby, et al. 1991. Effects of 0.60 PPM nitrogen dioxide on circulating and bronchoalveolar lavage lymphocyte phenotypes in healthy subjects. *Environ. Res.* 55:18–30.

Rylander, R., and P. Haglind. 1984. Airborne endotoxins and humidifier fever. *Clin. Allergy* 14:109–12.

Sampson, H. A. 1988. IgE-mediated food intolerance. *J. Allergy Clin. Immunol.* 81:495–504.

Sass, W., M. Bergholz, A. Kehl, et al. 1983. Overwhelming infection after splenectomy in spite of some spleen remaining and splenosis. *Klin. Wochenschr.* 61:1075–79.

Scheel, L. D., B. Smith, J. Van Riper, and E. Fleisher. 1954. Toxicity of silica. II. Characteristics of protein films adsorbed to quartz. *Arch. Ind. Hyg. Occup. Med.* 9:29–36.

Scheule, R. K., and A. Holian. 1991. Immunologic aspects of pneumoconiosis. *Exp. Lung Res.* 17:661–85.

Schindler, R., G. Lonnemann, S. Shaldon, et al. 1990. Transcription, not synthesis, of interleukin-1 and tumor necrosis factor by complement. *Kidney Int.* 37:85–93.

Schneeberger, E. E., M. DeFerrari, M. J. Skosskiewicz, et al. 1986. Induction of MHC-determined antigens in the lung by interferon-γ. *Lab. Invest.* 55:138–43.

Schuhmann, D., M. Kubickamuranyi, J. Mirtschewa, et al. 1990. Adverse immune reactions to gold. 1. Chronic treatment with an Au(I) drug sensitizes mouse T cells not to Au(I) but to Au(III) and induces autoantibody formation. *J. Immunol.* 145:2132–39.

Seaton, A. 1984. Asbestos-related diseases. In *Occupational Lung Diseases*, 2nd ed., ed. W. K. C. Morgan and A. Seaton, pp. 323–76. Philadelphia: W. B. Saunders.

Seaton, A., and W. K. C. Morgan. 1984. Hypersensitivity pneumonitis. In *Occupational Lung Diseases*, 2nd ed., ed. W. K. C. Morgan and A. Seaton, pp. 564–608. Philadelphia: W. B. Saunders.

Selman, J., M. Rissenberg, and J. Melius. 1991. Eosinophilia–myalgia syndrome: Follow-up survey of patients. New York, 1990–1991. *Morbid. Mortal. Weekly Rep.* 40:401–3.

Sheppard, D., J. E. Thompson, L. Scypinski, et al. 1988. Toluene diisocyanate increases airway responsiveness to substance P and decreases airway neutral endopeptidase. *J. Clin. Invest.* 81:1111–15.

Sherman, M. P., L. A. Campbell, H. Gong, Jr., et al. 1991. Antimicrobial and respiratory burst characteristics of pulmonary alveolar macrophages recovered from smokers of marijuana alone, smokers of tobacco alone, smokers of marijuana and tobacco, and nonsmokers. *Am. Rev. Respir. Dis.* 144:1351-56.

Sherman, R. 1984. Management of trauma to the spleen. *Adv. Surg.* 17:37-71.

Slade, M. S., R. L. Simmons, and E. Yunis. 1975. Immunodepression after major surgery in normal patients. *Surgery* 78:363-72.

Smialowicz, R. J., R. R. Rogers, M. M. Riddle, et al. 1985. Immunologic effects of nickel. II. Suppression of natural killer cell activity. *Environ. Res.* 36:56-66.

Specter, S., G. Lancz, and J. Hazelden. 1990. Marijuana and immunity—tetrahydrocannabinol mediated inhibition of lymphocyte blastogenesis. *Int. J. Immunopharmacol.* 12:261-67.

Specter, S., M. Rivenbark, C. Newton, et al. 1989. Prevention and reversal of delta-9-tetrahydrocannibinol induced depression of natural killer cell activity by interleukin-2. *Int. J. Immunopharmacol.* 11:63-69.

Spreafico, F., A. Vecchi, M. Sironi, and S. Filippsechi. 1983. Problems in immunotoxicological assessment: Examples with different classes of xenobiotics. In *Immunotoxicology*, ed. G. G. Gibson, R. Hubbard, and D. V. Parke, pp. 343-57. New York: Academic Press.

Stehr-Green, P. A., P. H. Naylor, and R. E. Hoffman. 1989. Diminished thymosin$_{\alpha\text{-}1}$ levels in persons exposed to 2,3,7,8-tetrachlorodibenzo-*p*-dioxin. *J. Toxicol. Environ. Health* 28:285-95.

Street, J. C. 1981. Pesticides and the immune system. In *Immunologic Considerations in Toxicology*, ed. R. P. Sharma, pp. 46-66. Boca Raton: CRC Press.

Stross, J. K., I. A. Smokler, J. Isbister, and K. R. Wilcox. 1981. The human health effects of exposure to polybrominated biphenyls. *Toxicol. Appl. Pharmacol.* 58:145-50.

Stryker, R. M., and D. W. Orton. 1988. Overwhelming postsplenectomy infection. *Ann. Emerg. Med.* 17:161-64.

Subramanian, V., J. McCleod, and H. Gans. 1968. Effect of extracorporeal circulation on reticuloendothelial cell function. *Surgery* 64:775-84.

Sussman, J. L., S. Tarlo, and J. Dolovich. 1991. The spectrum of IgE-mediated responses to latex. *J.A.M.A.* 265:2844-47.

Taniguchi, T., S. Katsushima, K. Lee, et al. 1990. Endotoxemia in patients in hemodialysis. *Nephron* 56:44-49.

Ten, R. M., G. M. Kephart, M. Posada, et al. 1990. Participation of eosinophils in the toxic oil syndrome. *Clin. Exp. Immunol.* 82:313-17.

Terr, A. I. 1985. Anaphylaxis. *Clin. Rev. Allergy* 3:3-25.

Terr, A. I. 1986. The atopic worker. *Clin. Rev. Allergy* 4:267-88.

Terr, A. I. 1987. "Multiple chemical sensitivities": Immunologic critique of clinical ecology theories and practice. *Occup. Med. State Art Rev.* 2:683-94.

Terr, A. I. 1989. Clinical ecology. *Ann. Intern. Med.* 111:168-78.

Thomas, P., H. Ratajczak, D. Demetral, et al. 1990. Aldicarb immunotoxicity: Functional analysis of cell-mediated immunity and quantitation of lymphocyte subpopulations. *Fund. Appl. Toxicol.* 15:221-30.

Thomas, P., H. Ratajczak, H. Eisenberg, et al. 1987. Evaluation of host resistance and immunity in mice exposed to the carbamate pesticide aldicarb. *Fund. Appl. Toxicol.* 9:82-89.

Thomas, P. T., W. W. Busse, N. I. Kerkvliet, et al. 1988. Immunologic effects of pesticides. In *The Effects of Pesticides on Human Health*, eds. S. R. Baker and C. F. Wilkinson, pp. 262-95. New York: Princeton Scientific Publishers.

Thomas, P. T., and R. E. Faith. 1985. In *Immunotoxicology and Immunopharmacology*, ed. J. H. Dean, M. I. Luster, A. E. Munson, and H. Amos, pp. 305-13. New York: Raven Press.

Thurston, J. R., J. L. Richard, and W. M. Peden. 1986. Immunomodulation in immunotoxicoses other than aflatoxicosis. In *Diagnosis of Mycotoxicoses*, ed. J. L. Richard and J. R. Thurston, pp. 149-61. Boston: Martinus Nijhoff.

Tollerud, D. J., J. W. Clark, L. M. Brown, et al. 1989. The effects of cigarette smoking on T cell subsets. A population-based survey of healthy Caucasians. *Am. Rev. Respir. Dis.* 139:1446–51.

Tonnesen, E., M. S. Huttel, N. J. Christensen, et al. 1984. Natural killer cell activity in patients undergoing upper abdominal surgery: Relationship to the endocrine stress response. *Acta Anesthesiol. Scand.* 28:654–60.

Tryphonas, H., M. I. Luster, G. Schiffman, et al. 1991. Effect of chronic exposure of PCB (Aroclor-1254) on specific and nonspecific immune parameters in the rhesus (*Macaca mulatta*) monkey. *Fund. Appl. Toxicol.* 16:773–86.

Tsang, P. H., F. N. Chu, A. Fischbein, et al. 1988. Impairments in functional subsets of T-suppressor (CD8) lymphocytes, monocytes, and natural killer cells among asbestos-exposed workers. *Clin. Immunol. Immunopathol.* 47:323–32.

Tubaro, E., G. Borelli, C. Croce, et al. 1983. Effect of morphine on resistance to infection. *J. Infect. Dis.* 148:656–66.

Turner, E. S., J. J. Pruzansky, R. Patterson, et al. 1980. Detection of antibodies in human serum using trimellityl-erythrocytes: Direct and indirect hemagglutination and hemolysis. *Clin. Exp. Immunol.* 39:470–76.

Vallyathan, V., X. Shi, N. S. Dalal, et al. 1988. Generation of free radicals from freshly fractured silica dust. *Am. Rev. Respir. Dis.* 138:1213–19.

Van Dyke, C., A. Stesin, R. Jones, et al. 1986. Cocaine increases natural killer cell activity. *J. Clin. Invest.* 77:1387–90.

Van Ert, M., and Battigelli, M. C. 1975. Mechanism of respiratory injury by TDI (toluene diisocyanate). *Clin. Allergy* 35:142–47.

Vigliani, E., and B. Pernis. 1959. An immunological approach to silicosis. In *Proceedings of the Pneumoconiosis Conference*, ed. A. J. Orenstein, pp. 395–407. London: J.& A. Churchill.

Von Essen, S., R. A. Robbins, A. B. Thompson, and S. I. Rennard. 1990. Organic dust toxic syndrome—an acute febrile reaction to organic dust exposure distinct from hypersensitivity pneumonitis. *J. Toxicol. Clin. Toxicol.* 28:389–420.

Vos, J. G. 1977. Immune suppression as related to toxicology. *CRC Crit. Rev. Toxicol.* 5:67–97.

Vyas, G. N., H. A. Perkins, and H. H. Fudenberg. 1968. Anaphylactoid transfusion reactions associated with anti-IgA. *Lancet* 2:312–15.

Ward, E. C., M. J. Murray, L. D. Lauer, et al. 1986. Persistent suppression of humoral and cell-mediated immunity in mice following exposure to the polycyclic aromatic hydrocarbon 7,12-dimethylbenz[a]anthracene. *Int. J. Immunopharmacol.* 8:13–22.

Webster, R. C., and H. I. Maibach. 1985. Dermatotoxicology. In *Environmental Pathology*, ed. N. K. Mottet, pp. 181–94. New York: Oxford University Press.

Weiler, J. M., M. A. Gellhaus, J. G. Carter, et al. 1990. A prospective study of the risk of an immediate adverse reaction to protamine sulfate during cardiopulmonary bypass surgery. *J. Allergy Clin. Immunol.* 85:713–19.

Weiss, S. T., I. B. Tager, A. Munoz, et al. 1985. The relationship of respiratory infections in early childhood to the occurrence of increased levels of bronchial responsiveness and atopy. *Am. Rev. Respir. Dis.* 131:573–78.

White, S. C., S. C. Brin, and B. W. Janicki. 1975. Mitogen-induced blastogenic responses of lymphocytes from marijuana smokers. *Science* 188:71–72.

Wilhemsson, A., S. Cuthill, M. Denis, et al. 1990. The specific DNA binding activity of the dioxin receptor is modulated by the 90 kd heat shock protein. *EMBO J.* 9:69–76.

Worlledge, S. M. 1973. Immune drug-induced hemolytic anemias. *Semin. Hematol.* 10:327–44.

Wybran, J., T. Appelboom, J. P. Famey, and A. Govaerts. 1979. Suggestive evidence for receptors for morphine and methionine enkephalin on normal human blood lymphocytes. *J. Immunol.* 123:1068–72.

Wysocki, J., Z. Kalina, and I. Owczarzy. 1985. Serum levels of immunoglobulins and C-3 component of complement in persons occupationally exposed to chlorinated pesticides. *Med. Pract.* 36:111–17.

Yamashita, U., and T. Hamaoka. 1982. Selective suppression of host T-cell and macrophage activities during 7,12–dimethylbenz[a]anthracene-induced carcinogenesis. *Gann* 73:773–82.

Yanai, M., T. Ohrui, T. Aikawa, et al. 1990. Ozone increases susceptibility to antigen inhalation in allergic dogs. *J. Appl. Physiol.* 68:2267–73.

Yokoyama, A., N. Yamashita, Y. Mizushima, and S. Yano. 1990. Inhibition of natural killer cell activity by oral administration of theophylline. *Chest* 98:924–27.

Zeiss, C. R. 1989. Reactive chemicals as inhalant allergens. *Immunol. Allergy Clin. N. Am.* 9(2):235–44.

Zeiss, C. R., C. L. Leach, L. J. Smith, et al. 1988. A serial immunologic and histopathologic study of lung injury induced by trimellitic anhydride. *Am. Rev. Respir. Dis.* 137:191–96.

Zeiss, C. R., D. Levitz, R. Chacon, et al. 1980. Quantitation and new antigenic determinant specificity of antibodies induced by inhalation of trimellitic anhydride in man. *Int. Arch. Allergy Appl. Immunol.* 61:380–88.

Zwetchkenbaum, J. 1990. *Insights in Allergy*, Vol. 5, No. 2, *Food Allergy.* St. Louis: C.V. Mosby.

12

Regulatory Immunotoxicology

A. INTRODUCTION

During the last 20 years, the United States has been moving toward requiring the performance of immunotoxicity testing of chemicals prior to their introduction into the marketplace. Among the forces driving the process are an increased perception that immune defects might have life-threatening effects and may lead to litigation. The awareness has been heightened by the dissemination of chemicals into the environment, the accidental exposure of humans to putatively immunotoxic chemicals, and the AIDS epidemic. Interest in immunotoxicity was stimulated by such events as the dioxin controversy of the 1970s. At the same time, military personnel in Viet Nam were exposed to a defoliant called Agent Orange, which contained small concentrations of dioxin. It was alleged that dioxin induced health-related effects, including immunotoxicity, in exposed subjects. Although recent data have suggested that guinea pigs used in the animal studies were extremely sensitive to the effects of dioxin, the human health-related effects are still being debated (Roberts 1991).

Another notorious incident at that time was the accidental human exposure to polybrominated biphenyls in Michigan. Although there are conflicting data on decrements in immune function in exposed subjects as measured in laboratory tests, there has been no evidence of increased infections, tumors, or other adverse health-related effects (see Chapter 7). The AIDS epidemic of the 1980s has shown dramatically how severe immunosuppression can lead to a slow and painful death and raises the question of whether exposure to chemical substances can trigger similar consequences. Recently, much media attention has been given to the multiple chemical hypersensitivity syndrome. Although the syndrome may not be mediated by immune reactions, the misuse of the term "hypersensitivity" has connoted a detrimental chemical-induced effect on the immune system.

Concomitant with this rise in public awareness, increased litigation claiming chemical-induced damage to the immune system first appeared in 1980. The number of suits has increased dramatically in the last 10 years following successful litigation by the plaintiffs. Two of the more celebrated were the Woburn and Alcolac legal decisions. In the former suit, community members claimed immune system dysfunction after drinking water from a well contaminated with small concentrations of carbon tetrachloride and chloroform. Moreover, the plaintiffs claimed that the extent of immune system dysfunction was sufficient to increase the future risk of developing diseases such as cancer. The only evidence of immune dysregulation was alterations in lymphocyte subsets in peripheral blood (Byers et al. 1988). The plaintiff's medical experts testified that the changes in lymphocyte subsets were consistent with chemical-induced immune dysregulation. The court awarded damages ranging from $75,000 to $500,000 to five plaintiffs. In the Alcolac case, the plaintiffs alleged that exposure to toxic waste from a chemical plant damaged their immune systems and caused "chemically induced AIDS." Moreover, the immunosuppression was responsible for adverse health-related effects. Flow cytometry measurements of lymphocyte subsets were used to document the immunosuppression. Although there was little evidence of increased infections or malignancies, medical experts employed by the plaintiffs suggested that each of the 31 plaintiffs was immunosuppressed. The court awarded the plaintiffs $49 million (Cornfeld and Schlossman 1989).

In response to public pressures, the Environmental Protection Agency (EPA) has issued immunotoxicity testing guidelines for biochemical pesticides, and the agency is considering issuing testing guidelines for chemical pesticides. Similarly, the Food and Drug Administration (FDA) is revising its "Redbook" of acceptable testing protocols to include immunotoxicity testing. The following is a description of the scientific concerns and testing protocols of both the FDA and the EPA.

B. FOOD AND DRUG ADMINISTRATION

The food, Drug, and Cosmetic act (FDCA) of 1938 grants the FDA the authority to regulate chemicals in food, drugs, and cosmetics. Other laws have expanded the FDA responsibility for regulating food additives, food dyes, and drugs used in the treatment of animal diseases. New drugs used in animals or humans are regulated by the FDCA and the Public Health Service Act. The regulation of biologicals, vaccines, cytokines, and growth factors is mandated by the latter legislation.

Only four centers at the FDA are involved in basic immunotoxicity research and development. Included in this group are the Center for Food Safety and Applied Nutrition (CFSAN), the Center for Drug Evaluation and Research (CDER), the Center for Biologics Evaluation and Research (CBER), and the National Center for Toxicology Research (NCTR). The CFSAN has been active in immunotoxicology research for the last 15 years and has developed in vitro techniques to screen for immunotoxic food constituents, direct additives, and contaminants. The efforts of the CBER are confined to the understanding of clinical immunosuppression. This center also evaluates the safety of products produced by recombinant DNA technology, including monoclonal antibodies, cytokines, and growth factors. Most classical pharmaceuticals are evaluated by the CDER. The NCTR has no direct involvement in safety evaluation of drugs or biologics, but it has played an indirect role by development of in vivo testing protocols.

1. Immunotoxic Concerns within the FDA

Generally, all of the centers have the same concerns about immunotoxicity. Hypersensitivity, autoimmunity, immunomodulation, and antigenicity are scientific areas receiving a great deal of attention within the FDA. Specific concerns follow.

Autoimmune Reactions
Many pharmaceuticals have been associated with the induction of autoimmune responses in humans. These include such commonly used substances as penicillin, procainamide, phenytoin, and lithium. These responses differ from typical au-

toimmune disease in that the response abates after the offending agent is removed from the host. The FDA has concerns in two specific areas: (1) autoimmunity or autoimmune responses caused by exposure to pharmaceuticals and (2) the role of drugs in the aggravation of preexisting autoimmune disease in humans.

Laboratory studies can be implemented to ascertain whether the biopharmaceutical agent induces the formation of autoantibodies or, in the case of monoclonal antibodies used to treat disease, cross-reactivity with other host tissues. Immunohistology studies using fresh frozen tissue from unrelated adults and fetuses can define both the presence and pattern of cross-reactive antibodies. Since multiple tissues (e.g., kidney, thyroid, intestine) from several donors are usually used in such studies, phenotype variability and intensity of reactivity can be determined. Simple ELISAs or RIAs can be used to determine the presence of antibodies directed toward endogenous proteins such as tissue plasminogen activator.

Sensitization

Sensitization may be produced following repeated exposure to a foreign material. This results in an alteration of the host immune system so that the sensitized host responds to extremely low concentrations of antigen with the elicitation of immediate and/or delayed hypersensitivity reactions. Hypersensitivity is the most common drug-induced reaction in humans (deWeck 1983), accounting for approximately 15% of all reactions. Classic examples of sensitizers are the penicillins, and the β-lactam family of antibiotics (Alanis and Weinstein 1983).

In the pharmaceutical industry, sensitization is rarely considered in preclinical testing since experience and a historical data base have suggested that sensitization data derived from animals do not readily predict human responses (Parke 1983). Thus, the extent of sensitization is usually considered only in human clinical trials of the pharmaceutical. Although hypersensitivity testing of nonpharmaceuticals is not mandated by the FDA, some manufacturers of cosmetics and fragrances voluntarily test ingredients for their potential to induce skin sensitization.

Antigenicity

In humans, some drugs or chemicals are antigenic. The immune response differs from sensitization and autoimmune responses in that the antibodies are of the IgG and IgM isotypes and the serological reactivity is directed toward the drug or chemical rather than host tissue. The antigenicity may result from the fact that some small-molecular-weight chemicals or their metabolites bind to host protein, creating a conjugate capable of eliciting an immune response. It is also conceivable that endogenous human proteins produced by recombinant DNA technology have small differences in structure or stereochemistry when compared to natural molecules. Antigenicity may be a consequence of these small changes in the recombinant protein. This effect is most pronounced in products produced in eukaryotic or prokaryotic cells. Conversely, biopharmaceuticals produced by human cells or transformed human cell lines usually are not antigenic because the glycosylation pattern and stereochemistry are identical to that produced in the body. However, minor additional structural changes induced by the manufacturing or formulation process may render such molecules antigenic. The antigenicity of biopharmaceuticals can be determined in simple laboratory tests such as the enzyme-linked immunosorbent assay (ELISA). This assay has replaced the radioimmunoassay in many laboratories and is cost effective, rapid, sensitive, and adaptable to large sample volumes.

Depending on the xenobiotic, the presence of specific antibodies may have either a beneficial or a detrimental effect. For example, antibodies may react with toxicants in the serum, thus preventing the chemical from reaching target or metabolizing organs. On the other hand, antibodies directed toward pharmaceuticals or recombinant-technology-derived proteins may cause a loss of biological efficacy.

The loss of biological efficacy is a concern for the FDA, especially with regard to recombinant proteins or monoclonal antibodies for human use. Data from animal studies suggest that antibody neutralization of heterologous proteins is a common event. Humans seem to be unique in that a segment of the population given the same homologous protein will develop high levels of protein-specific antibodies; however, product neutralization is not commonly reported.

Another concern of the FDA is immune complex disease induced by biopharmaceuticals, i.e., where chemical or biopharmaceutical substances form such complexes and induce damage to the glomeruli of the kidney or the intima of the small capillaries.

Inadvertent Reactions

Immunotherapeutic agents can cross-react with nontarget tissue sites. For example, monoclonal antibodies directed toward T-cell determinants may react with the same site present on other tissues. It is also conceivable that therapeutics designed to augment or inhibit the function of specific immunocompetent cells may have indirect or nonspecific effects on other cells. Indirect activation of T cells is achieved by the administration of murine anti-CD3 antibody, which cross-links receptors on the cell initiating cellular activation. The activated cells then release TNF, IFN-γ, and perhaps IL-2 (Waldman 1991), which can then induce a variety of responses in other tissues and cells.

The administration of superphysiological concentrations of a biopharmaceutical may also cause immune responses. For example, high doses of tissue plasminogen activator may evoke an immune response to the endogenous protein. Normally, the molecule is only present in small quantities that fail to stimulate the immune system. When the cross-reactivity of the biopharmaceutical has been determined in prospective or retrospective studies, the in vivo sequelae of the interaction should be determined in animal models or isolated human organ perfusion studies. If test systems are not available, clinical studies should be undertaken to ascertain, using radiolabeled product, the biodistribution of the material in the body (Anonymous 1987).

Immunomodulation

Two types of immunomodulation have been described. The most common form is immunosuppression, which predisposes subjects to infections or neoplastic conditions. Of major concern to the FDA are immunosuppressive therapeutic agents used to treat subjects with preexisting immunodeficiency and chronic disease such as systemic lupus erythematosus or organ graft rejection.

Immunoenhancement is also a concern to the FDA, since some pharmaceuticals (e.g., levamisole) are likely to cause enhanced activity of the immune system. There are new areas of drug development (e.g., cytokines, growth factors) that have wide-ranging effects on the immune system. These biopharmaceuticals may enhance one facet of the immune response while inhibiting other mechanisms. Reactions involving the production of biologically active cytokines may be difficult to discern in whole-animal studies. Therefore, in vitro assays for the detection of cytokines have been developed in humans and mice (Chapter 9). Other assays used to measure cytokines may include colony-forming assays, microtoxicity testing, or autoradiography.

Indirect Immunotoxicity

Many of the new pharmaceuticals are produced by normal or transformed human cells. Other bioproducts are synthesized by bacteria, yeast, or fungi. The vector used to synthesize the pharmaceutical may produce additional products or supply contaminants that influence or cause immunotoxicity in humans. Human pathogens such as *Mycoplasma* species, Epstein–Barr virus (EBV), cytomegalovirus, hepatitis B virus, or retroviruses can infect cell lines. Tissue culture safety tests using virus-susceptible cell lines derived from humans, simians, and other species can be used to identify the presence of viral contamination. In addition, assays available for the detection of EBV and retrovirus DNA have been recommended by the FDA for safety assessment of cell lines used to produce monoclonal antibodies or pharmaceuticals. Emphasis has been placed on testing procedures with a sensitivity of 10 pg DNA per dose.

Mouse viruses (e.g., Hantaan and K viruses) present in murine cell lines can also cause human infection. Since the K virus is rarely found in mouse colonies, current interest is focused on contamination with the Hantaan virus. Methods similar to those described for detection of human viruses are used to ascertain murine viral particles in susceptible cell lines (Anonymous 1987).

Other viruses can be present in ascitic fluids used to produce monoclonal antibodies. A murine antibody production test can be used to detect polyoma, Hantaan, pneumonia, adenoma, hepatitis, Sendai, and LCM virus infections. Because of the possibility of nonspecific reactions, all positive reactions must be confirmed by alternate methods, which may include complement fixation, immunofluorescence, or hemagglutinin assays (Anonymous 1987).

Many of the recombinant DNA vectors are Gram-negative bacteria, and the cell walls of these bacteria contain endotoxins that have both potent pharmacological and immunologic effects. The pyrogenicity potential of a product can be best determined by the in vivo rabbit pyrogenicity test. A fever in test rabbits injected with the test material indicates that the product contains substances that may cause a fever in humans. Because a derived product of the blood of the horseshoe crab gels in the presence of minute amounts of endotoxins, the *Limulus* amebocyte (LAL) assay is a good in vitro method to detect endotoxins in test material.

Negative pyrogen or LAL tests do not exclude the possibility of adverse reactions in humans. Some biological agents or pharmaceuticals are pyrogenic only in humans. These materials can be detected by incubating the biological with human monocytes and testing for production of the pyrogen IL-1 (Anonymous 1985).

2. FDA Drug Licensing

For a drug to be sold, the FDA must grant marketing approval. The manufacturer must fulfill technical requirements for two petitionary applications. In the initial Investigative New Drug (IND) application, the manufacturer requests approval to pursue additional studies. In addition to a plan for clinical studies, the manufacturer supplies information on the toxicology, pharmacology, synthesis, and manufacture of the compound. After completion of the clinical studies, a New Drug Application (NDA) is usually filed with the agency. The application includes the results of all clinical and toxicology studies that demonstrate both the biological efficacy and safety of the product. Additional information on post-marketing surveillance may also be included in the package.

3. Immunotoxicity Testing

Most centers within the FDA do not require immunotoxicity testing on pharmaceuticals. Rather, testing is performed on a case-by-case basis depending on the concern of the agency. The concern level for a particular compound is a function of several variables including structure-activity relationships to known immunotoxicants, therapeutic use at superphysiological levels, the population at risk, and projected population exposure estimates.

Data from standard toxicity studies may also raise the concern level of the agency. In standard studies, any aberrations in blood cells, serum proteins, lymphoid organ weights, or histopathology of immunocompetent organs may suggest the need for immunotoxicity testing. Also suggestive of immunosuppressive effects would be an increased incidence of opportunistic infections or cancers in chronic or carcinogenicity studies. An abnormal incidence of maternal infections or abnormalities in fetal immunocompetent organs gleaned from in utero toxicity studies would also suggest the necessity for immunotoxicity testing.

The FDA requires that toxicity or safety assessment studies be performed in both rodent and nonrodent species because it is widely believed within the agency that tests in a single species will not be predictive of effects in humans. Moreover, the use of two species in the test protocols may demonstrate the existence of metabolic differences or receptor specificity in animals and man for a given material. This increases the possibility of detecting adverse effects when both rodent and nonrodent species are used as test animals.

In the design of immunotoxicology studies, the nature of the drug, dose regimen, the route of administration, the target population, and the animal model must be taken into consideration (Graham 1987). Also, the data may be influenced by the purity of the product and the tissue half-life. When the bioproduct is used in high concentrations or over extended periods of time, careful consideration should be given to the level of antigenic contaminants in the preparation relative to the active material. Finally, the immune response is dependent on prolonged contact with the antigen in the host system. Thus, products that persist in the host system are more antigenic than products with a tissue half-life of 10 min. These factors need to be taken into consideration in designing or evaluating immunotoxicity. If possible, the route of administration and the drug regimen should be similar to that used in man.

The major criteria for the proper species selection are pharmacological activity similar to man and the lack of an immune response to the test molecule. Since cytokines and other endogenous human proteins react only in species closely related to humans, primates may be the animal of choice. However, human stem cells can be placed in SCID-hu mice to generate a functional human hematopoietic system (Namikawa et al. 1990; Kamel-Reid and Dick 1988). These mice have normal human CD4/CD8 ratios in peripheral blood and respond to mitogens, alloantigens, and antibodies to CD3 (Kaneshima et al. 1990). Hence, these mice or other transgenic mice may be used to test the effects of endogenous proteins on the human immune system (Galbraith 1987; Graham 1987). To increase the possibility of detecting a toxic effect in humans, additional studies are performed in rodents. Data from rodent studies are often difficult to interpret. Within 2–3 weeks following exposure to the protein, rodents often form neutralizing antibodies that cause a loss of biological efficacy or immune complex disease (Graham 1987).

Although the range of doses used in toxicity studies is not usually specified, the Center for Drugs and Biologics has recommended specific doses for testing of monoclonal antibodies. One dose should be equivalent to the highest anticipated clinical use, with two others being multiples of that dosage. Animals should be sacrificed at a time when there is a maximum toxic effect (Anonymous 1987).

Most centers of the FDA use a flexible approach in the choice of ex vivo tests used in immunotoxicity testing. The panel of tests is directed at determining, in mechanistic terms, the nature of possible immunologic lesions. In practice, the protocols are defined after discussions between the agency and the manufacturer.

The CFSAN is the only arm of the FDA having defined protocols for the study of immunotoxicity. The center assigns concern levels from I to III, with III being the highest level of concern. Compounds assigned the lowest concern level (level I) would be tested in short-term acute exposure studies. Usually, these studies would be less than 30 days in duration. Ninety-day studies would be used when compounds are assigned a level II concern status. At the highest level of concern, long-term studies of immunotoxicity may be required. In addition, the agency may recommend long-term chronic and in utero exposure, evaluation of carcinogenicity potential, the collection of absorption, distribution, and metabolism data, and short-term mutagenicity studies (Hinton 1991).

The animal of choice for CFSAN immunotoxicity studies is the rat because it is most often used for toxicological safety evaluations. Several strains have been used, including the Sprague–Dawley, Spartan, and Osborne–Mendel strains (Hinton et al. 1987). Most of these strains are not inbred but colony bred using a standard genetic pool. Hence, the data are more representative of the general population (Hinton 1991). Studies on the inbred Fischer 344 rats could result in increased defects with a genetic component.

Historically, CFSAN has required, in all studies, the inclusion of select endpoints that may suggest immunotoxicity. Among the endpoints are hematology measurements, serum chemistries, histopathology, and organ and body weights. Alterations in total white blood cell or differential counts are common hematology measurements. Reduced serum protein levels and/or altered albumin/globulin ratios may indicate immunotoxic effects.

In the CFSAN guidelines proposed by Hinton, more extensive histopathological analyses are required (Hinton 1991). Routine gross and histological evaluations of spleen, lymph nodes, thymus, Peyer's patches, and bone marrow are required. In unfixed tissue, the determination of cellularity and viability of some immunocompetent organs (e.g., spleen, lymph node, bone marrow) is mandated. In essence, the numbers and viability of total nucleated cells and lymphocytes per gram of wet weight of tissue is determined. Since the weight of some tissues (e.g., spleen) is influenced by exogenous factors unrelated to immunotoxicity (Chapter 9), this measurement may yield data of questionable value. Moreover, there may be changes in subpopulations of nucleated cells (e.g., lymphocytes) that would not be detected in the assay. In addition, evaluation of stained lymphoid organs includes a description of the distribution of lymphocytes in T- and B-cell-dependent areas, indications of cellular proliferation or activation in any area, the density of cell populations, and the presence or absence of activated macrophages.

When there is a high concern level about the immunotoxicity of the test material, an enhanced testing protocol is undertaken. All of the testing can be performed on the core group of animals used in standard, required studies. Enhanced testing has both prospective and retrospective components. In this approach there is a need to divide tissue and blood for immediate and future analyses. For example, one-half of the spleen is processed for cellular analyses; the other half is fixed in Bouin's fixative and stored in alcohol for histological evaluation. The blood is also divided so that cellular analyses can be immediately performed. Serum is recovered from the blood samples, filter-sterilized, and refrigerated for future use.

The testing approach is flexible in that the testing addresses specific endpoints, and numerous tests can be used in the prospective portion of the study. The rationale for the use of some tests is unclear. For instance, lymphocyte transformation assays have been evaluated by other governmental agencies and rejected for use in most testing because of the large inter- and intraassay variation (Luster et al. 1988). If immunotoxic effects are observed in the prospective study, additional studies using stored tissues and blood from the animals in the prospective study would be undertaken. The minimum assays required in the retrospective study are shown in Table 12-1. If the retrospective study does not confirm the data from the prospective study, no further studies would be undertaken. Additional testing would be mandated if the data are inconclusive or confirm the original data (Hinton 1991).

The additional studies are usually invasive and require a separate group of animals. Since most of the additional studies have been validated in the mouse,

TABLE 12-1.   FDA Suggested Expanded Testing on Core Animals for Immunotoxicity of Food Additives[a]

Prospective Study	Retrospective Study
Hematology	Hematology
T- and B-cell determinations in blood or spleen	None
Absolute numbers per microliter, T cell/B cell, and T_h/T_s	None
Histopathology	Histopathology
None	B cells in spleen and lymph nodes
T cells in the spleen	None
None	Micrometric analyses of spleen and lymph node
None	Morphometric analysis of thymus
Electrophoresis	Electrophoresis
None	Immunoglobulins
Cellularity and viability	None
None	Autoantibodies
NK-cell function	None
Mitogenic stimulation	None
Macrophage phagocytic index	None

[a]Other tests include complement function, cytokines (IL-2 and IFN-γ), and hematopoietic stem cell assays.

that is the animal of choice. The studies can be performed on a "satellite" group of animals during standard subchronic studies or on another set of animals at a different time. To allow proper evaluation of effects on the primary or secondary immune responses and recovery from effects, testing is performed from 3 to 6 weeks. The basic testing protocol is shown in Table 12–2.

Additional testing may also be required on a case-by-case basis when a protocol, study design, or execution is faulty. Some examples of a faulty study design are use of animals that are unusually sensitive or resistant to the test molecule, use of barrier facilities that preclude the possibility of infection, failure to measure endpoints specified in basic testing protocols, and small animal numbers unsuitable for proper statistical analyses (Hinton 1991).

4. Risk Assessment

The FDA has no unified method of assessing risk based on preclinical testing, but pharmacokinetics, tissue distribution, and persistence in tissues are major considerations in such determination. Immunotoxic effects would be considered in the context of the target population and intended usage of the material.

C. ENVIRONMENTAL PROTECTION AGENCY

The EPA has the mandate to regulate chemicals under two Congressional Acts. the Federal Insecticide, Fungicide and Rodenticide Act (FIFRA) makes it illegal to manufacture, sell, or distribute pesticides without the written approval of the EPA. The Office of Pesticide Programs (OPP) administers FIFRA. Other chemicals are regulated under the Toxic Substances Control Act (TSCA). This act also authorizes the EPA to regulate chemicals before and after they reach the marketplace.

TABLE 12–2.   FDA Suggested Additional Invasive Tests for Immunotoxicity of Food Additives

Evaluation of the antibody-mediated response
   T-cell-dependent antigen:
      measurements of serum antibody titers of primary (e.g., IgM) and secondary (e.g., IgG) responses
   T-cell-independent antigen:
      measurement of serum antibody titers of primary (e.g., IgM) response
Evaluation of the T-cell-mediated response
   Contact sensitization protocol
   Mixed lymphocyte response (MLR)
Host defense models
   Validated mouse models
      Humoral immunity
      Influenza
      Delayed hypersensitivity to infection
      Listeria
      Plasmodium
   Tumor resistance
      PYB6 sarcoma

1. EPA Approval for the Use of a Chemical under FIFRA

In the development of a chemical under FIFRA guidelines, the manufacturer can conduct limited field studies using a total of 10 acres nationwide. If the data from the field studies foster commercialization of the product, an Experimental Use Permit (EUP) is filed with the EPA. Along with a plan to conduct additional field studies in approximately 4,000 acres at different sites across the country, the manufacturer may provide limited toxicology data, plant residue analyses, and weed tolerance patterns. In addition, the manufacturer must undertake additional toxicology and environmental studies.

Extensive laboratory testing is required for the registration of pesticides. These studies include acute toxicity studies using various routes of exposure, 90–day subchronic toxicity studies, 2–year chronic oncogenicity and toxicity studies, developmental and reproduction studies, in vitro mutagenicity testing, and a metabolism study. In cases where there is the possibility of repeated skin exposure, a dermal sensitivity study may also be required.

2. EPA Approval of a Chemical under TSCA

In 1978–1979, under the administration of the EPA, TSCA inventoried all chemicals manufactured or imported into the United States. Excluded from the inventory were chemicals already regulated by the EPA or FDA and chemicals manufactured solely for export, research, or test marketing. In order to place new chemicals on the TSCA inventory, manufacturers must submit a Premanufacturing Notice (PMN) to the EPA prior to the introduction of the chemical into commerce. The PMN presents data on chemical structure, manufacturing process, potential impurities in the product, the proposed usage, and projected annual production volume. Within 90 days of receipt of PMN, the EPA must grant approval or disallow the usage of the chemical.

The volume of a chemical partially determines the level of testing. Chemicals manufactured or imported at low volumes (e.g., less than 1,000 kg/year) may be exempt from PMN review. Chemicals produced or imported in higher quantities trigger performance of a core battery of tests. These tests include in vitro mutagenicity testing; acute oral toxicity tests in rats and rabbits, and a 28–day repeat dose oral study in rats.

In certain circumstances the EPA would consider additional testing. Certainly, a structure–activity relationship to a known toxicant would likely require additional testing. Near-total release of high production volumes (e.g., 1,000,000 kg/year) of chemical into the environment during the course of normal or intended use would trigger additional testing. Alternatively, testing is mandated when the chemical persists in the environment or exposure of large populations (e.g., 100,000 workers) is possible.

3. Immunotoxicology Concerns of the EPA

The EPA is interested in immunosuppression induced by chemicals, and it has also voiced concern about hypersensitivity reactions. However, the guinea pig hypersensitivity test is the only test mandated. The status of current and proposed immunotoxicity testing guidelines is discussed below.

Biochemical Pesticides

When there is the possibility of significant human exposure from the air or foodstuffs, OPP has issued guidelines for the required immunotoxicity testing of biochemical pesticides including enzymes, plant and insect growth regulators, pheromones, and plant hormones. A screening panel known as the tier approach to testing, shown in Table 12–3, was designed to identify compounds with potential immunotoxic activity. Compounds testing positive can then be tested further in a second panel or tier. The studies can be performed in either rats or mice in 30–day subchronic testing protocols. In addition to the immunotoxicity studies, a study of delayed hypersensitivity reactions in guinea pigs is required (Anonymous 1991). In the immunotoxicology studies, material is administered by the oral, inhalation, or dermal exposure routes. The highest dose should produce some signs of overt toxicity such as body weight depression, whereas the lowest dose should not produce any evidence of immunotoxicity. All animals should be observed for a 30–day observation period.

The immunotoxicology protocol is unique in its requirement for several control groups each containing ten animals in each dose group. Also, there is a concurrent vehicle control group. If the immunotoxicity of the vehicle in undefined, a separate untreated control group is suggested. Finally, a positive immunosuppressed control group of animals ($n = 5$) is required for each ex vivo assay to verify sensitivity of the species.

The progression from tier I to tier II (Table 12–3) becomes automatic when statistically significant dose-related immunotoxic effects are observed in tier I tests, data from other sources suggest immunotoxicity for the material, or tier I data cannot be definitively interpreted (Anonymous 1991). The tier II tests selectively probe recovery from effects, the biological relevance of the dysfunction, and the nature of the cellular defect. Risk assessment is determined using data and information from the tier II tests.

Microbial Pesticides

There is no required immunotoxicity testing for microbial (e.g., bacteria, fungi, and viruses) pesticides. When viruses known to affect human health are used as microbial pesticides, the agency can request a standard immunotoxicity study

TABLE 12–3.   Immunotoxicity Testing for Biochemical Pesticides

Tier I
  Cellularity and viability
    Spleen
    Thymus
    Bone marrow
  Humoral immunity (either of the following)
    Primary or secondary response to antigen
    Plaque-forming culture
  Cell-mediated immunity (any of the following)
    Mixed lymphocyte response
    Delayed hypersensitivity response
    Cytotoxic T-cell functional assay
  Nonspecific immunity
    Natural killer cells
    Macrophage function
Tier II
  Recovery from effects
  Host defense and tumor challenge models
  Additional ex vivo assays

(Sjoblad 1988). In most circumstances, the ability of animals to clear the agent, following administration by several routes, is used as an index of normal immune function.

Chemical Pesticides

Immunotoxicity testing of chemical pesticides, herbicides, and fungicides is not designed as a tiered approach. The EPA believes that extensive toxicity testing is already required for registration (Sjoblad 1988). Nevertheless, the agency has requested that additional immunologic endpoints be included in standard 90–day subchronic studies (Table 12–4). It is also possible that the measurement of immunologic endpoints will be required in other studies. To ascertain effects on the developing immune system in standard reproduction studies, the cellularity, viability, and weights of lymphoid organs (e.g., spleen, lymph node, and thymus) must be measured in both mother and offspring. In addition, the determination of natural killer cell function might be required in chronic or oncogenicity studies. These latter points are still undergoing discussion within the EPA.

TSCA-Regulated Chemicals

The TSCA does not require immunotoxicity testing for chemicals under their regulation. This applies to both immunomodulation and hypersensitivity. This may reflect the fact that the chemical industry has a large data base on chemicals that have been in the marketplace for many years. If immunotoxic effects induced by exposure to chemicals were prevalent, they should have already been described.

Recently, the EPA has attempted to harmonize guidelines for testing of chemicals. Because TSCA has not initiated any activity to require immunotoxicity test-

---

TABLE 12–4.   Panel for Immunotoxicity Testing of Chemical Pesticides

Screen
    Serum immunoglobulin isotype levels (IgG, IgA, IgM)
    Organ weights
      Spleen
      Thymus
      Lymph node
    Cellularity and viability
      Spleen
      Thymus
      Bone marrow
Special immunocytochemistry–histochemistry
Evaluation of "premature" deaths of dosed animals
Risk evaluation
    Host resistance to infectious agents or tumors
Specific cell-mediated immunity
    Mixed lymphocyte reaction
    Delayed-type sensitivity (skin test)
    Cytotoxic lymphocyte reaction
Nonspecific cell-mediated immunity
    NK-cell activity
    Macrophage function
Time course for recovery from effects

Source: Modified from Sjoblad (1988).

ing, and OPP has already proposed guidelines, it is likely that the OPP guidelines will be adopted by both FIFRA and TSCA.

4. Unreasonable Risk

The EPA has proposed several definitions for an immunotoxic effect. The following are current definitions: functional impairments in ex vivo or in vivo parameters resulting in pathological lesions influencing performance; reversible or compensatory effects on the immune system; reversible or irreversible decreases in responses to additional biological challenges and induction of immune dysfunction or inappropriate suppressive or stimulatory responses in components of the immune system (Anonymous 1991).

In the assessment of human risk, the EPA can decide that immunotoxic effects have a threshold effect level, and thus, conventional safety or uncertainty factors (tenfold multiples) can be used to ascertain safe levels of exposure. In the determination of "unreasonable risk to human health" the EPA considers a number of factors concerned with the relationship of adverse animal data to human health, the effects on the environment, the benefits of the proposed chemical compared to other products, and, finally, the economic consequences of the introduction of the compound into the market.

5. Regulation of Compounds on the Basis of Immune System Effects

Neither the FDA nor the EPA has banned a commercial product on the basis of immunotoxicity. Some compounds have been regulated by the FDA on the basis of an association with hypersensitivity reactions. Yellow dye No. 5 and sulfites were regulated by the FDA on the basis of their potential to enhance allergic reactions. However, it is clear that sulfites induce "asthma-like" reactions by nonimmunologic mechanisms. Cosmetic ingredients have been regulated for the presence of some eighteen to twenty sensitizers including lead, mercury, and vinyl chloride. Both agencies regulate sensitizers in a similar manner. If the benefits of the molecule outweigh the sensitization potential, a warning label is required on the product. Neither agency usually bans a product solely on the basis of sensitization potential.

Other governmental agencies have also regulated compounds on the basis of hypersensitivity. By Supreme Court mandate, OSHA is required to enact the most protective permissible exposure limits to eliminate health risks. The prospect of sensitization has moved OSHA to regulate exposure to eight classes of chemicals. Included in this group are isocyanates, picric acid, subtilisins, and captafol.

Recently, the EPA has regulated exposure limits for tributyltin oxide on the basis of immunotoxicity (Kranjc et al. 1987), and regulation is also pending for 2,4–dichlorophenol.

D. CONCERNS ABOUT CURRENT IMMUNOTOXICITY TESTING

Many of the ex vivo host defense and tumor challenge assays used in the standard immunotoxicity assays were developed over the last 15 years by the National Toxicology Program (NTP). There were four objectives of the NTP: (1) to evaluate the effects of a toxic chemical on the immune system; (2) to determine the relationship between alterations in immune function and general or specific organ toxicity; (3) to establish correlations between decrements in host resistance and immune function; and (4) to define a battery of ex vivo tests to study immunotoxicity (Table 12-5). The program has successfully met or exceeded all of its goals. The success of the program is more significant when one considers that the program is composed of intraagency groups from the National Cancer Institute (NCI), the National Institute of Environmental Health Sciences (NIEHS), the National Center of Toxicology Research (NCTR), and the National Institute of Occupational Safety and Health (NIOSH). Because of its unique expertise in immunotoxicology, the NIEHS has assumed leadership in the program.

1. Choice of Test Animal

A major concern of toxicologists is the development and validation of assays in the B6C3F1 mouse. Most standard immunotoxicity studies performed for EPA or FDA registration require the use of the rat and/or dog. At this time, none of the ex vivo assays have been validated for use in these species. Moreover, there are no validated tumor models in the rat or dog, and some host defense studies developed for the mouse cannot be adapted to the rat. Recently, the EPA has undertaken studies to validate the assays in the rat and primate but not the dog.

2. Validation of Ex Vivo Parameters

Several of the ex vivo parameters required for immunotoxicity testing of chemicals have not been validated adequately in the rat. These parameters include bone marrow cellularity, determination of immunoglobulin subclasses, and histological evaluation of Peyer's patches and lymph nodes.

3. Sensitivity of Ex Vivo Assays

It is unclear whether the assays developed and validated by the NTP can detect all immunotoxic events. Certainly, tier I studies can detect the most potent immunotoxicants (Luster et al. 1988). Less potent immunotoxicants may not be detected in the assays, especially if the effect is on a specific subpopulation of lymphocytes or interferes with the more subtle effects of cytokine interaction. This may be because there is an over reliance on histopathology to define lesions in the immune system. Moreover, some biopharmaceuticals (e.g., cytokines) may have no overt effect on the histology of immunocompetent organs, yet they exert immunomodulatory effects.

4. Predictive Nature of Rodent Ex Vivo Assays

There has been a tendency to ascribe biological significance to data gleaned from rodent ex vivo assays. At the present time there are no published data suggesting that decrements in such assays correlate with decrements in human immune function. Such correlations are not possible for the following reasons. First, there may be differences in metabolism of the test material when rodent and man are compared. Hence, the material may be nontoxic in man. Second, there may be significant differences in the function of immunocompetent cells in vivo versus

TABLE 12–5.   NTP Tier Testing for Immune Alterations after Chemical Exposure

Tier I
  Hematology
    White blood cell count and differential
  Organ weights
    Body
    Spleen
    Thymus
    Kidney
    Liver
  Histology
    Spleen
    Thymus
    Lymph node
  Humoral immunity
    PFC to T-cell-dependent and -independent antigens
  Cell-mediated immunity
    Lymphocyte transformation with concanavalin A
  NonSpecific immunity
    Natural killer cell function
Tier II
  T- and B-cell enumeration in the spleen
  Humoral immunity
    Quantitation of IgG response to sheep RBCs
  Cellular immunity
    T-cell cytolysis of tumors
    Delayed hypersensitivity response
  NonSpecific immunity
    Macrophage function
  Host resistance
    Syngeneic tumors
      PYB6 sarcoma
      B16F10 melanoma
    Bacterial models
      Listeria
      Streptococci
    Viral
      Influenza
    Parasitic
      Plasmodium yoelii

in vitro assays (Hou and Zheng 1988). Third, chemicals administered by one route of exposure may not be toxic when given by a second route (e.g., testing performed by oral route but humans exposed by inhalation route). Fourth, data derived from acute studies in animals may not be reproduced in longer-term exposures of humans to a given material. Because of these and other problems associated with immunotoxicity testing, it is difficult to extrapolate animal data to humans (see Chapter 10 for further discussion).

E. CONCLUSIONS

In summary, immunotoxicology is undergoing a paradigm shift from academic research to application in the safety assessment of chemicals and select biologicals. It must be recognized that data from immunotoxicity testing in standard studies have several limitations. It is clear that the ex vivo and in vivo assays can detect severe immunotoxic events in the mouse. Whether immunotoxicants of less potency can be detected in the assays is open to question. Moreover, it is unclear whether the same assays can detect immunotoxic effects in the rats; however, data from current studies, over the next 2 years, will resolve this question. Finally, the extrapolation of animal data to the human condition is open to question.

Despite these criticisms of the assay systems and the scientific approach, both the EPA and the FDA have developed immunotoxicity testing protocols. Because of the nature of the agencies and their scientific interest, the approaches are different. The EPA utilizes a screening approach, whereas the FDA has opted for a problem-solving approach. The major disadvantage of the screening approach proposed by the EPA is that the immunotoxicity determinations are added to 90–day subchronic studies, which are usually feeding studies. No attempt is made to study the inhalation effects of chemicals, and only minimal effort is directed toward studying the immunotoxic effects on skin. The FDA problem-solving approach seems more rational, since it addresses, in mechanistic terms, the nature and biological relevance of the defect.

Why undertake the studies if there are such reservations concerning the value of the testing approach? Perhaps the answer to the question is that this is the first step in an evolving testing scenario. Naturally, the ex vivo and in vivo assays used in the testing protocols are the most familiar to the regulators and immunotoxicologists. In fact, the assays may yield some meaningful information. Clearly, there are more advanced technologies (e.g., flow cytometry) that may give more meaningful mechanistic information in a more efficient manner. Building on data from these initial studies, one may be able to develop more efficient biologically relevant protocols within the next 10 years.

References

Alanis, A., and A. J. Weinstein. 1983. Adverse reactions associated with the oral use of penicillins and cephalosporins. *Med. Clin. North Am.* 67:113–29.

Anonymous. 1985. *Points to Consider in the Production and Testing of New Drugs and Biologicals Produced by Recombinant DNA Technology.* Washington: FDA Office of Biologics Research and Review, Center for Drugs and Biologics.

Anonymous. 1987. *Points to Consider in the Manufacture and Testing of Monoclonal Antibody Products for Human Use.* Washington: FDA Office of Biologics Research and Review, Center for Drugs and Biologics.

Anonymous. 1991. *Identifying and Controlling Immunotoxic Substances. Background Paper. U.S. Congress, Office of Technology Assessment, Publication No. OTA-BP-BA-75*, pp. 3–63. Washington: U.S. Government Printing Office.

Byers, V. S., A. S. Levin, D. M. Ozonoff, and R. W. Baldwin. 1988. Association between clinical symptoms and lymphocyte abnormalities in a population with chronic domestic exposure to industrial solvent-contaminated domestic water supply and a high incidence of leukemia. *Cancer Immunol. Immunother.* 27:77–81.

Cornfeld, R. S., and S. F. Schlossman. 1989. Immunologic laboratory tests: A critique of the Alcolac decision. *Toxics Law Reporter* Sept. 6, pp. 381–90.

deWeck, A. L. 1983. Immunopathological mechanisms and clinical aspects of allergic reactions to drugs. In *Handbook of Experimental Pharmacology*, Vol. 63. Allergic Reactions to Drugs. eds. A. L. deWeck and H. Bundgaard, pp. 75–133. New York: Springer-Verlag.

Galbraith, W. M. 1987. *Safety Evaluation of Biotechnology Derived Products*, pp. 3–14. New York: Alan R. Liss.

Graham, C. E. 1987. *Safety Evaluation of Biotechnology Derived Products*, pp. 183–87. New York: Alan R. Liss.

Hinton, D. M. 1991. Testing guidelines for evaluation of the immunotoxic potential of direct food additives. *(Personal Communication)*.

Hinton, D. M., J. J. Jessop, A. Arnold, R. H. Albert. 1987. Evaluation of immunotoxicity in a subchronic feeding study of triphenyl phosphate. *Toxicol. and Indus. Hlth.* 3:71–89.

Hou, J., and W. F. Zheng. 1988. Effect of sex hormones on NK and ADCC activity in mice. *Int. J. Immunopharmacol.* 10:15–22.

Kamel-Reid, S., and J. E. Dick. 1988. Engraftment of immune-deficient mice with human hematopoietic stem cells. *Science.* 242:1706–9.

Kaneshima, H. C., B. Chen, C. Baum, et al. 1990. Today's SCID-Hu mouse. *Science.* 348:561–2.

Kranjc, E. I., J. G. Vos, P. W. Wester, et al. 1987. *Toxicity of Bis(tri-n-butyltin) Oxide (TBTO) in Rats.* Washington: USEPA, FYI-OTS-0687–0550 Seq. A. 84–870000132.

Luster, M. I., A. E. Munson, P. T. Thomas, et al. 1988. Development of a testing battery to assess chemical-induced immunotoxicity: National Toxicology Program guidelines for immunotoxicity evaluation in mice. *Fund. Appl. Toxicol.* 10:2–19.

Namikawa, R., K. N. Weilbaecher, H. Kaneshima, et al. 1990. Long term hematopoiesis in the SCID-hu mouse. *J. Exp. Med.* 172:1055–63.

Parke, A. L. 1983. Clinical manifestations of drug induced syndromes. In *Immunotoxicology*, ed. G. G. Gibson, R. Jubbard, and D. O. Parke, pp. 27–40. New York: Academic Press.

Roberts, L. 1991. Dioxin risks revisited. *Science* 251:624–26.

Sjoblad, R. D. 1988. Potential future requirements for immunotoxicity testing of pesticides. *Toxicol. Ind. Health* 4:391–94.

Waldman, T. A. 1991. Monoclonal antibodies in diagnosis and therapy. *Science* 252:1657–62.

Index

Acetylation polymorphism 222
Acetylcholine 198, 272
Acetylcholinesterase, inhibition 128
Achlorhydria 241
Acid anhydrides 270, 272
ACTH 56, 274
Actinomycin D 197
Activation, cellular 49–54
Activation, receptor-mediated 54
Acute oral toxicity test 302
Acute phase proteins 64–65, 190, 219
Adaptive responses 36–38, 245
ADCC 13, 80, 81, 92, 95, 99, 106, 114, 149,
 193
Additives, food and drug 252–253, 300
Addressins 12
Adenoma 297
Adenosine deaminase 138
Adenoviruses 128, 192
Adenylate cyclase 95, 110, 127
Adhesins 97, 141, 195
Adjuvant 32, 158, 159
Adrenalectomized animals 198
α-Adrenergic stimulation 111, 128
β-Adrenergic blockade 111, 128, 271–272
β-Adrenergic function, viral interference 224
Adrenoreceptors 38
Adult respiratory distress syndrome 95
Adverse responses 37–38
Aeroallergens 223
Aflatoxin 144, 269
Agammaglobulinemia 138, 139
Agent Orange 2, 250, 293
Agranulocytosis 114, 151, 152, 255
AIDS 3, 137, 147, 164, 168, 181, 191, 216,
 217, 227, 241, 293
Air pollution 154, 267–268
Albumin:globulin ratio 200, 299
Alcolac, litigation 293
Aldehdye dehydrogenase, atypical 222
Aldehydes 268
Aldicarb 248
Allergenicity, predicting 214
Allergic encephalomyelitis 129
Allergic responses 38
Allergic respiratory disease 115
Allergic rhinitis 219, 239
Allergoid 165–166
Allergy 2, 37
Allergy of infection 120–121
Allergy, defined 104
Allergy, genetic factors 219–220
Allergy, in vitro assays 124, 125

Allergy, risk factors 214, 219–220
Allopurinol 253
Alum 159–160
p-Aminophenol derivatives 115
Aminophyllin 150
Aminopyrine 151, 274
p-Aminosalicylic acid 115
Amitriptyline 151
Ammonium groups 254
Amphetamine 38
Amphotericin B 274
Anamnestic response 9
Anaphylactoid reactions 119, 128, 260,
 273–274
Anaphylatoxins 84, 85, 87, 128
Anaphylaxis 37, 241, 253, 260, 272–275
Anemia, hemolytic 114, 116, 131
Anesthetics 256–258
Angioedema, hereditary 138, 139
Angioedema 236
Angioneurotic edema 258
Aniline 246–247
Animal data, extrapolating to humans
 228–232
Animal models, adequacy 41
Animal models, choice of 41, 306
Animal models of predicting immune injury
 125
Animal-derived allergens 239, 270
Anti-idiotypic antibodies 115, 169
Antibiotics 241
Antibody-dependent cellular cytotoxicity *See*
 ADCC
Antibody neutralization 296
Antibody production, inhibition 117
Anticholinesterase effects 248
Antigen, definition 4
Antigen, molecular recognition 31
Antigen, presentation 13–14, 31, 90
Antigen, processing 28, 29, 140, 144
Antigen-presenting cells 13, 14, 28, 29, 109,
 140, 149
Antigenic mimicry 129
Antigenicity 294–295
Antilymphocyte globulin 177
Antinuclear antibodies 256, 281
Antithyroid drugs 152
α_1-Antitrypsin inhibitor 219
Aplastic anemia 142, 151, 152, 193, 222
Arachidonic acid 59–60, 106, 172
Aral Sea 267
Aroclor 1260 246
Arsenic 265

Arsphenamines 151
Arthus reaction 116, 276
Arylsulfatase 95
Asbestos 37, 119, 144, 223, 245, 279, 281
Ascaris 112
Ascites tumors 218
Ash, fly 144
Ash, volcanic 119
Asparaginase 253, 274
Aspergillosis 184, 265
Aspirin 61, 115, 119, 183, 253, 274
Assay validation 306
Assessment, accessory functions 194–197
Assessment, antibody-mediated system
  184–188
Assessment, cell mediated immunity 188–194
Assessment, complement 196
Assessment, human cytokines 197–198
Assessment, immune function in animals
  197–207
  Antibody mediated immunity 201–202
  Cell mediated immunity 202–205
Assessment, monocyte function 193–194
Assessment, neutrophils 194–195
Assessment, NK cells 192–193
Assessment, T cells 188–192
Assessment, Tc function 191–192
Asthma 4, 95, 110–113, 127, 128, 150, 219,
  254, 267
Asthma, animal models 112–113
Asthma, occupational 111–112, 128
Asthma, perinatal predisposition 223, 224
Ataxia telangiectasia 138
Atopic dermatitis 237–238
Atopy 106, 111, 219, 273
Autoimmune hepatitis 255
Autoimmunity 114, 117, 128–131, 139, 149,
  158, 172, 174, 175, 248, 281, 294
Azathioprine 172–173, 183

B cell dysfunction 217
B cell maturation 187
B cells 186–187
B cells, IgE production 105
B lymphocytes 162, 164, 165, 168, 171, 174
B lymphocytes, antigen-presentation 14
B lymphocytes, origin and development 11–12
B lymphocytes, xenobiotic effects on 142,
  143, 145–147
Bacteriophage ΦX 174 186
Barbiturates 199, 274
Basement membrane, alveolar 115
Basement membrane, glomerular 115, 117
Basenji-Greyhound dog, asthma model 112
Basic-staining granules 94
Basophil degranulation 125, 126
Basophil histamine release 108
Basophils 93–94, 106, 108, 122, 126, 127
BCG 159
Benz(a)pyrenes 218
Benzene 38, 142–143
Benzocaine 237
Benzodiazepines 151
Beryllium 122, 160, 237, 279, 280
Betastatin 163
Biochemical pesticides 294, 303
Biodistribution 296
Biopharmaceuticals 290
Bis(tris-n butyltin) 200
Blocking antibody 166

Bone marrow 107, 142, 171, 199, 200, 299,
  306
Bordetella exotoxin 161
Boyden chamber 195
Bradykinin 94, 106
Bronchial smooth muscle 106
Bronchoalveolar lavage 145, 150, 229, 258,
  261, 264, 268, 280
Bronchoconstriction 106, 109, 110, 112, 113
Bronchoprovocation testing 109
Buehler test 123
Bursa of Fabricius 11
Bursin 164
Byssinosis 120, 215

C1 82, 86
C1 esterase, inhibitor 139, 196
C1-INH 84, 86
C1q 117, 118
C3 85, 86, 118, 182, 196
C3, antibodies 118
C3 convertase 81, 83, 87
C3, deficiency 139
C3a 86, 87
C3b 83, 84, 86, 95
C3b 117
C3 NeF 84
C4 196
C4 binding protein 84
C5a 86, 87, 95
C5-C9, deficiency 139
C6 83, 86
C7 83, 84, 85
C8 83, 84, 86
C9 83, 84, 86
C-reactive protein 98
Cadmium 131, 237, 265
Caffeine 241
Calcium concentration 202
Calmodulin 52
cAMP 53, 110, 128, 141, 172, 265
Candidiasis 168, 217
Captafol 305
Captopril 151
Carbamazepine 145, 151
Carbaryl 247
Carbimazole 151
Carbon monoxide 38, 144
Carbon tetrachloride 40, 293
Carcinogenesis 44, 46, 215, 251
Cardiomyopathy 193
Castor beans 270
Catechol 142, 143
Catecholamines 56–57, 170, 198
Cats, allergy to 224
CD2 12, 187, 263
CD3 27, 177, 187
CD3, antibodies 192
CD3/TCR 191
CD3/Ti-expressing Tc lymphocytes 193
CD3:TCR complex 92
CD4 26, 29, 31, 181, 187, 201
CD4+ cells 37, 91, 99, 148, 149
CD4+ cells, in DTH 121
CD4/CD8 ratios 148, 227
CD5 187, 201
CD6 187
CD8 26, 29, 31, 187, 201, 204
CD8+ cells in DTH 121
CD11/CD18 97

CD11b   187, 201
CD16   92, 187, 189, 201
CD19   187
CD21   187
CD23   106, 187
CD25   187, 201
CDw29   187
CD35   187
CD45   187, 189
CD56/CD57   187
CD59   84
CD markers, defined   10–11, 189
Cefodizime   256
Cell cycle   49–50
Cell-mediated responses, defects   138
Cellularity analyses   299, 300, 304, 306
Center for Biologics Evaluation and Research (CBER)   294
Center for Drug Evaluation and Research (CDER)   294
Center for Food Safety and Applied Nutrition (CFSAN)   294
Cephalosporin   274
Cephalothin   115
CH$_{50}$ 196
Charcoal   45
Charcot-Leyden crystals   95
Chediak-Higashi disease   193
"Chemical AIDS"   148, 294
Chemical approval, EPA   302
Chemical pesticides   294, 304
Chemiluminesence   145, 195
Chemotaxis   85, 88, 96, 172, 182, 191, 193, 195
Chloramine-T   270
Chloramphenicol   114, 115, 151, 152, 228
Chlordane   37
Chlorhexidine   254
Chlorinated hydrocarbons   237, 248
Chloroform   293
Chloroquine   151
Chlorpromazine   43, 115, 131, 152
Chlorpropamide   151
Chlorthalidone   36, 131, 151
Chlordane   37
Cholinergic stimulation   110, 111, 128
Chromates   237, 265
Chronic atrophic gastritis   241
Chronic granulomatous disease   138, 139
Chymase   94, 106
Chymopapain   228, 274
Chymotrypsin   274
Cigarette smoking   144, 154, 218, 223, 260–262, 264
Cimetidine   152, 183
Clinical effects, immunotoxicity   236–242
Clinical ecology   277, 278
Clinical immunosuppression   294
Cluster-case incidents   235
Co-culture experiments   188
Cobra venom factor   118
Cocaine   263, 264
Codeine   107, 274
Coffee beans   270
Colchicine   43
Collagen-generating factors   145
Collagenase   109
Colony-forming assay   297
Colony stimulating factors   10, 70–71, 142
Complement   196, 201

Complement activation, biologic consequences   85, 86
Complement activation, overview   80, 81–83
Complement, activation mechanisms   80
Complement, alternative and classical pathways   81, 82, 86, 196
Complement, amplification loop   82
Complement, component deficiencies   86, 138, 139
Complement, lytic pathway   82, 83
Complement, regulation   83, 84
Complement system   81–87
Complement, alternative pathways   118, 119, 196, 206
Complement, glomerulonephritis   116
Complement, component deficiency   130
Complement, non-specific activation   118–120, 128, 259, 273, 276
Complement, alternative pathway   139
Complement, guinea pig   229
Compound 48/80   107, 128
Concanavalin A   190, 203
Conglutinin   84
Connective tissue mast cells   93
Connective tissue antibodies   127
Contact allergen   204
Contact dermatitis   121, 122, 123, 172, 254
Contact lenses   240
Contrasuppressor cells   170
Coombs and Gell system   105, 113, 115, 116, 120
Copper   266
Corticosteroids   146, 153, 170, 171–172, 183, 198, 222, 228, 279
Corticotropin-releasing factor   56
Cosmetics   238, 295, 305
Coumarin resistance   222
Crohn's disease   241
Cromolyn   112
Cross-reactivity   295–296
Cryptococcosis   217
Cryptosporidiosis   217, 241
Cuprophan   259
Curare   274
Cutaneous basophil reactions   126
Cutting oils   237
Cyclooxygenase pathway   59–60, 109, 253
Cyclophilin   175
Cyclophosphamide   173–174, 184
Cyclosporin   174–175
Cystic fibrosis   222
Cytokines   30, 62–71, 87, 99, 191, 196
Cytokines, concerns about research   62
Cytokines, evaluation   294, 297, 298
Cytokines, hematopoiesis regulators   69–71
Cytokines, immune respone enhancement   27–28, 29
Cytokines, inflammation activators   69
Cytokines, innate immunity mediators   63–67
Cytokines, Lymphocyte regulators   67–68
Cytokines, rodent   205–206
Cytolytic Lymphocyte reaction (CLR)   203, 207
Cytomegalovirus   158, 181, 217, 241, 297
Cytotoxic antibodies   113–116
Cytotoxic cell assays   203
Cytotoxic lymphocytes (CTLs)   91, 92, 99, 100, 120, 122, 149, 165
Cytotoxic T cells   13, 31, 227
Cytoxan   191

Danders, epithelial   270
Dapsone   151
DDT   37, 230, 247
Debrisoquine 4–hydroxylase deficiency   222
Decay-accelerating factor   84
Delayed toxicological response   38
Delayed type hypersensitivity   91, 120–126, 159, 160, 165, 229
Delayed-in-time reactions   126–127
Delayed-type hypersensitivity, assessment   123–126
Delayed-type hypersensitivity, predicting   226
Delayed-type hypersensitivity reaction   194, 204, 206
Delayed-type hypersensitivity, reactions in lung   123
Dermatitis herpetiformis   120
Dermatoses, occupational   236–237
Desensitization, in toxicity   37
Desipramine   151
Detergent enzymes   108
Dextran plasma volume expanders   274
Diabetes   182
Diabetes, Type B insulin-resistant   115, 129
Diabetes, type 1   175
Diacylglycerol   51–52
Diapedesis   88
Diazepam   274
Dichloroethane   228
2,4–Dichlorophenol   305
Diclofenac   115
Dieldrin   248
Diethyl fumarate   247
Diethylstibestesterols   228
DiGeorge syndrome   16, 138, 139
7,12–Dimethylbenz[a]anthracene   249
Dimethylnitrosamine   227
Dinitrochlorobenzene   194, 237
Dinitrofluorobenzene   123, 126, 237
Dioxins   200, 247, 249–252, 293
Diphtheria toxoid   185
Disseminated intravascular coagulation   114
Diuretics   182
Diurnal variation   183, 231
Dose regimen   298, 299, 303
Dose-response relationships   34–36
Double signalling   225
Doxepin   151
Drug efficacy   36
Drug idiosyncrasies   221
Drug licensing   297–298
Drug metabolism   40–41
Drug-induced lupus   131
Drug-induced reactions   222–223
Drug-induced allergy/immunotoxicity   252–256
DTH   See Delayed-type hypersensitivity
Dust, coal mine   144, 223, 279, 281
Dust, cotton   223
Dust, organic   154, 239
Dust, wood   270
Dyes   270

Ectoparasites   270
Eczema   138
ED$_{50}$ 35
Edema, pulmonary   97, 109, 168, 258
EDTA   45
Efficacy, definition   36

Elastase   109, 204
Electron spin resonance   195
ELISA   184, 196, 295–296
Encapsulated bacteria   282
Endocrine stress   257
Endogenous protein   299
Endopeptidase   272
β-Endorphin   56, 170
Endothelial cells   88, 91, 96–97, 107, 117, 163, 171, 195
Endothelial cells, antigen presenting   10, 14
Endothelium, high   18
Endotoxin   79, 97, 118, 119, 161, 163, 188, 190, 202, 225, 226, 259, 268
Enkephalins   56
Enterotoxin, E. coli   161
Environmental Protection Agency (EPA)   294, 301–305
Eosinophil chemotactic factor of anaphylaxis   57–59, 94, 107
Eosinophils   81, 87, 94–95, 106, 107, 109, 115, 120, 127, 193
Eosinophil-derivedneurotoxin   95
Eosinophilia-myalgia syndrome   241–242
Eosinophilia   246, 262
Epidemiology   1, 217, 218, 235
Epitopes   1, 200
Epithelial cells   109, 115, 238
Epoxy resins   237, 270
Epstein-Barr virus   181, 297
Erythema multiforme   254
Erythropoiesis   199
Estradiol   274
Ethacrynic acid   151
Ethanol   37, 41, 45, 264–265
Ethanolamines   270
Ethosuximide   131
Ethylenediamine   237
Exotoxins   99, 161
Experimental Use Permit (EUP)   302
Exposure, duration and frequency   40

Fab fragment   21
Fabric finishers   270
Factor B   83, 86, 182, 196
Factor D   84
Factor H   83, 84
Factor I   83, 84, 87
Factor V   96
Factor VIII   96, 97
Factor VIII antibodies   255
Factor XII   94
Factor XII activation   258
Fc region, interaction with xenobiotic   153
Fc, immunoglobulin   14, 21, 120, 128
Federal Insecticide, Fungicide and Rodenticide Act (FIFRA)   301–302
Fenoprofen   274
Fibrin   88, 122, 126
Fibrinogen   96
Fibroblasts   14, 122
Fibronectin   88, 96, 145
Fibrosis   90, 127
Fibroblast-stimulating factors   145
FK-506   175–176
Flow cytome try (FACS)   186, 189, 193, 200, 294
Fluenamic acid   274
Folic acid   274
Follicular dendritic cells   14

Food allergy   236, 240–241
Food and Drug Administration (FDA)
    294–301
Food constituents   294
Food intolerance   127–128, 241
Food, Drug, and Cosmetic Act (FDCA)   294
Formaldehyde   144
Fragrances   295
Free radicals   183
Freund's adjuvant   123, 126, 159, 160
Functional impairment   305
Fungi as allergens   119, 223, 239
Furosemide   36, 37

Gastroenteropathy   241
Gastrointestinal manifestations, immunotoxi-
    city   240–242
Gaucher's disease   182
Genetic basis, for immunotoxicity   137, 139,
    140, 238
Genetic risk factors   221, 222, 224
Gentamycin   151
Gerbils   275
Germinal centers   199
Giant Cells   90, 122
Giant papillar conjunctivitis   240
Gliadin   128
Glomerulonephritis   3, 116, 117, 129, 130, 196
Glucans   276
Glucocorticoids   56–57, 231
Glucose-6–phosphate dehydrogenase defi-
    ciency   222
Gluten   120
GM-CSF   94
Gold salts   115, 131, 266
Goodpasture's nephritis   129
Gp120   148, 149
Graft vs. host reaction   173
Grain dust, flour   270
Grain mites and weevils   270
Gram-negative bacteria   297
Granulocyte dysfunction   217
Granulocytes   10, 114, 163
Granulocytes, antibodies to   152
Granuloma   122, 139
Granulocytopenia   217
Graves disease   115, 127, 129
Griseofulvin   131
Growth factors   294
Growth hormone   56, 198
Guillain-Barre Syndrome   3
Guinea pig maximization test   123, 248
Gums   270, 274

H-2 or Mls loci   203
Haemophilus   181
Halothane-induced hepatitis   222
Hantaan virus   297
Haptens   113, 114, 126
Heat shock proteins   129–130
Heavy metals   265, 270
Helper:suppressor (T4:T8) ratio   189
Hematology   299
Hematopoiesis   10, 11, 14, 141, 298
Hemodialysis membranes   119, 259–260
Hemoglobin   38
Hemolysin   196
Hemolytic anemia   248, 255–256
Heparin   115, 260, 273
Hepatitis B virus   297

Hepatotoxins   198
Heroin   115, 263
Herpes   192
Herpes simplex   217
Herpes zoster   182
Hexachlorobenzene   228
Hexachlorophene   34
Histamine   57–59, 94, 95, 97, 106, 109, 112,
    113, 126
Histamine, decarboxylation toxicity   241
Histamine, non-specific release   128
Histamine, release   141
Histamine-releasing factors   109, 220
Histopathology   299
Histoplasmosis   122
HIV infection   147, 148, 181, 245, 263, 264
HLA-Dr   187
HLA-Dr marker   197
Hodgkin's disease   182, 190
Homograft   2
Horseradish peroxidase   195
Host defense models   206
Human encephalomyocarditis virus   197
Human maximization test   248
Human repeat patch test   125
Humidifier fever   268
Hydantoin   253
Hydralazine   131
Hydrogen peroxide   88, 109, 145, 195
Hydroquinone   142, 143
Hydroxyl radicals   88, 145, 195, 204–205, 279
5–Hydroxytryptamine   See serotonin
Hyper-IgE syndrome   184
Hyperbilirubinemia   222
Hyperplasia   127
Hyperresponsiveness   111, 112, 114, 248, 268,
    270
Hypersensitivity   293, 294, 295, 302, 304, 305
Hypersensitivity, defined   104
Hypersensitivity, different from toxicity   104
Hypersensitivity-like reactions   127–128
Hypersensitivity, mediators   58
Hypersensitivity pneumonitis   95, 104, 119,
    122, 172, 222, 268, 272, 275–276
Hypertrophy, smooth muscle   127
Hypogammaglobulinemia   138, 145, 146, 181,
    190
Hypophosphatemia   182
Hypothalamus   56

Iatrogenic disease   119, 171, 224, 253
Ibuprofen   274
Idiopathic pulmonary fibrosis   95
Idiosyncratic reactions   105, 125, 127, 131,
    220, 226, 253
Idiotype   24, 169
IFN-α 56, 167, 197
IFN-β 66, 99, 197
IFN-Γ 29, 30, 31, 44, 66, 88, 90, 91, 93, 97,
    99, 159, 162, 165, 174, 197
IFN-Γ, inhibition   149
IFN-Γ, stimulation   142
IgA   22, 25, 120, 184
IgA, deficiency   273
IgA, depressions   146
IgA, in airways   238
IgA, in food intolerance   241
IgA, nephropathy   269
IgA, secretory piece   25
IgA, selective deficiency   138

IgA, synthesis   21
IgD   22, 25
IgE   22, 25, 105–106, 160, 165, 184, 223, 224
IgE vs. non-IgE mediation   270
IgE+   109, 220
IgE, ADCC   95
IgE, allergen-specific   106, 113
IgE, depressions   146
IgE, function in normal health   106
IgE, gene regulation   219–220
IgE, hyperglobulinemia   138
IgE, in airways   238
IgE, in atopic dermatitis   237
IgE, in DTH   121, 126
IgE, in food allergy   241
IgE, lectin cross-linking   153
IgE, regulation   125, 170, 219–220
IgE, T cell modulation   120
IgE-dependent responses   105, 109, 111, 127
IgE-mediated   95, 100, 127, 128, 253
IgG   22, 24, 184
IgG, elevated   37
IgG, subclasses   24, 186, 200
IgM   22, 24–25
IgM deficiency   138, 139
IL-1   29, 55–56, 63–64, 97, 99, 193, 194, 196,
   205, 297
IL-1, depression   142, 143, 149
IL-1, stimulation   145
IL-2   30–31, 55–56, 67–68, 91, 92, 122, 159,
   163, 167, 168, 170, 172, 174, 175, 177, 192,
   196, 203, 205, 225
IL-2, homology with *Gp120*   142
IL-2, therapy   93
IL-3   70, 94, 142, 176
IL-4   30–31, 68, 94, 142, 160, 168, 175, 196,
   205
IL-5   69, 91, 94, 160, 175, 197
IL-6   56, 64–65, 142, 160, 165, 172, 197
IL-7   70, 197
IL-8   65
IL-9   68
IL-10   68
Immediate-type hypersensitivity   105–109
Immune adherence   85
Immune competence, restoration   16
Immune complex disease   116–118, 129, 296
Immune dysfunction, consequences   215–219
Immune enhancement, non-antigen specific
   224–226
Immune function, nervous system effects
   54–57
Immune function, stress effects   55
Immune response   298
Immune response, antigen-specific   9, 79, 98
Immune response, cellular interactions   10,
   27–32
Immune response, induction   29
Immune response, non-antigen specific   9, 79,
   98
Immune response, primary   158
Immune response, secondary   9
Immune response, types of   4
Immune system, reserve   98, 227
Immune system, vulnerable points   140–141
Immunity, antigen-specific vs. non antigen-
   specific   4,5
Immunity, definition   1
Immunity, degrees of protection   1
Immunodeficiency diseases   2, 3, 137

Immunodeficiency, reconstituting   158, 167
Immunodeficiencies, primary   181
Immunodeficiencies, secondary to other dis-
   eases   181–183
Immunodeficiencies, secondary, diagnosis
   183–197
Immunoenhancement   296
Immunoglobulin   21–25
Immunoglobulin, allotypes   24
Immunoglobulin, depressions   132, 146
Immunoglobulin, deficiencies   99
Immunoglobulin, domains   24
Immunoglobulin, enyzme digestion   21–22
Immunoglobulin, elevation   138, 149
Immunoglobulin, gene superfamily   21, 26–27
Immunoglobulin, heavy chains   21, 23
Immunoglobulin, idiotypes   24
Immunoglobulin, light chains   21, 23
Immunoglobulin, mechanism of action   80
Immunoglobulin, non-specific reactions with
   128
Immunoglobulin, cytoplasmic   187
Immunoglobulin, degradation rate   186
Immunoglobulin, half-life (T/2)   186
Immunoglobulin, isotype catabolism   186
Immunohistochemistry   200
Immunohistology   295
Immunologic enhancement   159
Immunologic tolerance   129
Immunomodulation, by endocrines   153
Immunomodulation, by microbial substances
   153, 160–161, 225
Immunomodulators, peptides   163–164
Immunomodulators, synthetic polymers
   165–166
Immunomodulation   158, 161, 294, 296, 304
Immunopharmacology   49, 170
Immunopotentiation   2, 3
Immunoproliferative disease, X-linked   138
Immunoregulation   32
Immunosuppressants   5, 32, 168–177, 245,
   269, 296, 302
Immunosuppression, natural   169–170
Immunosuppression, PGE₂   170
Immunosuppression, therapeutic   158, 170–
   177, 218
Immunotoxicity, genetic component   8
Immunotoxicity, problems predicting   226
Immunotoxicity, indirect effects   198
Immunotoxicity testing with drugs   298–301
Immunotoxicity testing, concerns   302–307
Immunotoxicology   7, 11
Immuntoxicology, problems studying   214–215
Immunotoxicology, regulatory   Chap 12
In utero exposure   299
Inadvertent reactions   296
Indirect immunotoxicity   297
Indomethacin   61, 115, 151, 274
Infectious disease   98, 114, 120, 137, 139, 142
Infectious disease, associated with defects   138
Infectious disease, decreased resistance
   215–219
Infectious disease, enhancing immunotoxicity
   154
Inflammation   97, 172
Inflammation, acute   87
Inflammation, chronic   90, 99
Inflammation, mediators   58
Inflammatory factor of anaphylaxis (INF-α)
   107

Influenza virus   181, 202, 206
Inhalation exposure   142, 145
Innate immunity   9
Inosiplex   167
Inositol triphosphate   51–52, 54
Insulin   170, 183, 274
Insulin receptor antibodies   115
Integrins   97
Interdigitating cells   14, 18
Interferons   66–67, 192, 196, 197, 205–206, See
   IFN sub-types
Intratracheal challenge test   108
Intravenous gamma globulin   273, 274
Intrinsic factor-Vitamin B$_{12}$ complex   241
Investigative New Drug (IND) application   297
Ionomycin   203
Iron-dextran   43, 274
Irritants, non-specific   111, 122
ISCOMS   166
Isocyanates   305
Isoflurane   257
Isohemagglutinins   185
Isoniazid   41, 115, 131, 151, 222

J-chains   24, 25
Jones-Mote reactions   126

K virus   297
Kallikreins   94, 139
Kaposi's sarcoma   217
Keyhole limpet hemocyanin   186
Kinins   128
Kuppfer cells   79, 257

Laboratory data, relating to humans disease
   215
Lactase deficiency   127
Lactoferrin   90
LAK cells   13, 92, 100, 115, 150, 168, 203
Langerhans cells   14, 122, 124
Laser nephelometry   184
Late phase reactions   96, 109–110, 117, 120,
   127, 224
Latex peptides   260, 274, 275
LATS   127
LCM virus   297
LD$_{10}$ 206
LD$_{30}$ 206
LD$_{50}$ 34, 35, 39, 42
Lead   38, 45, 265–266
Lectins   128
Legionella   239
Legionnaire's disease   268
Lethality, as an endpoint   35
Leukemia   142, 182
Leukopenia   256
Leukotrienes   61, 113
Levamisole   151, 166–167, 296
Lewis lung carcinoma   218
Lidocaine   150, 258
Limbic system   278
Limulus amebocyte (LAL) assay   259, 297
Lipid A   160–161, 163, 165
Lipopeptides   164
Lipopolysaccharide, bacterial   See Endotoxin
Liposomes   162, 164–165
Lipoteichoic acid   161
Lipoxygenase pathway   59–60, 109
Listeria   143, 203, 206, 227, 249
Lithium   131, 294

Litigation   293
Long term effects   139
Love Canal   2, 235
Low density lipoproteins   90, 245
Low molecular weight stimulants   113, 122
LTB$_4$ 88, 95, 109
LTC$_4$ 58, 61, 94, 95, 96
LTD$_4$ 58, 61, 95
LTE$_4$ 58, 61
Lung reactions   109, 122
Lupus erythamatosus, drug-induced   222
Lupus erythamatosus, systemic   129, 130
Lymph nodes   18–21, 199, 299
Lymphatic system   17–18
Lymphoblasts   12
Lymphocytes, activation   50–54
Lymphocytes, allogeneic   191, 203
Lymphocytes, mitogenesis   126, 143, 145, 244,
   246, 249, 280
Lymphocytes, seeding   10
Lymphocyte subsets   200
Lymphocyte (CTL) assays   191
Lymphocyte transformation test   190–191,
   203, 300
Lymphocytes   193
Lymphocytes, rodent phenotypes   201
Lymphoid cells, lineage   10
Lymphoid interstitial pneumonia   217
Lymphoid tissue atrophy   198
Lymphokine-activated cells   See LAK cells
Lymphoma   142, 182, 217
Lymphotoxin   See TNF-β
Lysophospholipase   95
Lysosomes   89, 172

Macrophage   204–205, 207
Macrophages/monocytes   10, 14, 81, 87, 90–
   91, 93, 99, 163, 172, 182, 191, 193
Macrophages/monocytes, xenobiotic effects
   on   142, 143–145, 149
Macrophages, activated   204, 205
Macrophages, defensive functions   14
Macrophages, glomerulonephritis   116
Macrophages, in DTH   121, 127
Macrophage-derived growth factor   145
Magnesium   266
Major basic protein   95, 100, 247
Malnutrition   183
Manganese dioxide   144
Mannitol   274
Marijuana   262
Mast cells   10, 58, 88, 93–94, 107, 108, 111,
   121, 128, 236
Measles   182
Mediators, hypersensitivity and inflamma-
   tion   57–62
Medical devices   258
Mefenamic acid   274
Melanoma   218
Melanoma cells   204, 207
Membrane attack complex   84
Membrane signalling   52–51
Menetrie's disease   182
Meningoencephalitis   206
Meperidine   274
Meprobamate   151
Mercapatans   237
Mercaptopurine   40
Mercury   40, 131, 265–266, 305
Metabolic effects, alteration of   33, 37, 40, 41

Metabolic defects   138, 152
Metabolic differences   298, 299, 306
Metallothionein   35
Metamizole, sodium   222
Methacholine   221
Methadone   264
Methanol   45
Methicillin   255
Methimazole   151
Methisoprinol   *See Inosiplex*
Methotrexate   173
Methyl piperonylate   107, 128
Methylchlorthiazide   36
Methylcholine   112
Methylcholanthrene   131
α-Methyldopa   114, 115, 131, 151, 228, 252, 255
Methylhydrazine   39
Metiamide   151, 152
Metroprolol   224
MHC Class I   26, 31, 92, 97, 101, 191, 203, 227
MHC Class II   26, 28, 29, 30, 91, 97, 99, 159, 163, 170, 173, 183, 191, 197, 202, 203
MHC Class II, expression   109
MHC Class II, xenobiotic effects on   144, 149, 263
MHC gene complex   26, 125
MHC markers   11
Microbial inhalants   275
Microbial pesticides   303
Microclimate   268
Microenvironment   10, 12, 28, 30, 32
Microflora, as modifiers of toxicity   41
Micronutrients as immunotoxicants   149
Microtoxicity testing   297
Migration inhibition factor   69
Mipafox   38
Mites   223, 224
Mitogenic stimulation   187–188, 298
Mitomycin-C   203
Mixed lymphocyte reaction (MLR)   191, 194, 203
Moloney sarcoma virus   218
Monoclonal antibody   176, 294, 296
Monosodium glutamate   241
Morphine   107, 254, 274
Mouse ear swelling test   124
Mucosal mast cells   93
Mucous cell metaplasia   127
Mucous secretion   106, 108, 109, 110
Multiple chemical sensitivity   2, 104, 276–279, 293
Multiple sclerosis   129, 190
Mumps   194
Muramyl dipeptide (MDP)   99, 161–162, 165
Murine local lymph node assay   124
Murine viruses   201
Mutagenicity   299, 302
Mutagenesis   44
Myasthenia gravis   115, 129
Mycobacteria   122, 159, 217
Mycoplasma   297
Mycotoxicosis   275
Mycotoxins   144, 269, 276
Myeloid:erythroid (M:E) ratio   200
Myeloperoxidase   89, 93, 109
Myelopoiesis   10, 141, 199

N-acetyl transferase   41
NADP reduction   205

Naloxone   45
Naproxen   274
National Center of Toxicology Research (NCTR)   294, 306
National Cancer Institute (NCI)   306
National Institute of Environmental Health Sciences (NIEHS)   306
National Institute of Occupational Safety and Health (NIOSH)   306
National Toxicology Program (NTP)   7, 231, 305
Natural killer cells   *See NK cells*
Neomycin   237
Nervous system, interaction with immune   54–57, 170, 231
Neuroendocine hormones   55–56
Neuromuscular disease   241–242, 246–247
Neuropeptides   107, 111, 170
Neurotransmitters   111, 115
Neuropharmacologic system   110
Neutralization   80
Neutralizing antibodies   299
Neutrophil chemotactic factor   96, 109
Neutrophils   87–90, 97, 181, 182, 194, 206
Neutrophils, defects   138, 139
Neutrophils, in IgE-mediated reactions   106, 109, 113
Neutrophils, in glomerulonephritis   116
Neutrophils, xenobiotic effects on   .150–152
Neutropenia   115, 138, 151
New Drug Application (NDA)   298
Nezelof's syndrome   138
Nickel   237, 265–266
Nicotinic acetylcholine receptor antibodies   115
Niemann-Pick disease   182
Nitrites   37, 41
Nitroblue tetrazolium test   194
Nitrofurantoin   131, 274
Nitrogen oxides   144, 256, 257, 267
Nitroglycerin   37
Nitrates   37
NK cells   10, 13, 79, 81, 91–93, 99, 100, 115, 167, 189, 192–193, 203, 204, 207, 304
NK cells, dysfunction   225, 227
NK cells, xenobiotic effects on   149–150
No effect level (NOEL)   46–47
Non-self, recognition   9
Nonsteroidal anti-inflammatory agents   61
Norepinephrine   38, 263–264, 279

Occupational asthma   269–272
Occupational Safety and Health (OSHA)   305
Ocular manifestations, immunotoxicity   239–240
Ocular phaco-anaphylaxis   129
Office of Pesticide Programs (OPP)   301
OKT3   177
Oncogenicity studies   293, 304
Ophthalmia, sympathetic   3
Opiates   253
Opportunistic pathogens   216, 298
Opsonization   80, 81, 85, 99, 195, 206
Opsonization, failure   138, 139
Oral contraceptives   183
Organ cellularity/weights   199–200, 298
Organic dust toxic syndrome   275
Organophosphates   128
Ovalbumin   202
Oxamiquine   42–43

Oxazolone 204
Oxidant injury 97
Oxisuran 198
Oxygen dependent/independent killing 89
Oxygen radicals (toxic) 89, 117, 145, 172
Oxyphenisatin 131
Oxytocin/Vasopressin 56
Ozone 267, 268

P-450, cytochrome enzyme system 142, 222, 249
PAF 45, 58, 61–62, 83, 88, 94, 95, 96, 97, 109
Pancytopenia 142
Panhypogammaglobulinemia 146
Papain 105, 240, 270
Parabenzoates 254
Parakeets 275
Paraphenylenediamine 237
Paraquat 35
Parasite immunity 95, 100, 105, 106, 203–204, 207
Parathorome 274
Passive cutaneous anaphylaxis 108, 229, 271
Patch testing 122, 124, 125
Pathology 2
Penicillamines 131, 151, 255
Penicillins 105, 115, 131, 195, 228, 253, 254, 270, 274, 294
Penicillins, semi-synthetic 151, 152
Penicillinase 274
Pentachlorophenol 247
Peptidoglycan 79, 160, 161, 162, 168
Perforin 92
Perfumes 237
Perinatal environmental risk factors 223–224
Pernicious anemia, pernicious 222
Peroxidase 95
Peroxide generation 88, 89, 139
Pesticides 40, 247–248
Peyer's patches 299
PGD$_2$ 31, 58, 60–61, 94, 101, 144, 170, 264
PGE$_1$ 96
PGF$_{2\alpha}$ 58, 60–61
PGG$_2$ 60
PGH$_2$ 60
PGI$_2$ (prostacyclin) 58, 60–61, 96
Phagocytic dysfunctions 138, 139
Phagocytosis 87–91, 182, 205–206
Phagocytosis, inhibition 117
Pharmacogenetics 33, 40, 221
Pharmacologic effect, as an endpoint 35
Phenacetin 151
Phenobarbital 37, 45, 145
Phenothiazines 115, 151
Phenotype variability 295
Phenylbutazone 151
Phenylthiourea 222
Phenytoin 115, 131, 145–147, 151, 222, 252, 255, 274, 294
Phorbol myristate acetate (PMA) 203
Phosphatidylinositol 51
Phosphodiesterase 112
Phospholipase 172
Phospholipase A 51, 59–60
Phospholipase C 51–52
Phthalic anhydrides 270
Physiologic responsiveness 221
Phytohemagglutinin (PHA) 143, 190, 203
Picric acid derivatives 237, 305
Pigeon droppings 119

Piperazine 270
Pitressin 274
PKC   See protein kinase C
Plant residue analyses 302
Plaque-forming cell (PFC) assay 201
Plasma cells 10
Plasmin 84, 86
Plasminogen activator 97, 122
Platelet activating factor   See PAF
Platelets 10, 86, 96, 114, 127, 129
Platelets, deficiency 138
Platinum salts 270
Plicatic acid 113, 270
Pneumococci 181
Pneumoconioses 127, 131, 215, 222, 279–281
Pneumocystis carinii 216, 239
Pneumonia 238–239, 265
Poison ivy 39, 105, 121, 122, 237
Pokeweed mitogen (PWM) 146, 187, 190
Pollen 224, 239
Polybrominated biphenyls 150, 243–245, 293
Polychlorinated biphenyls 245–246
Polycyclic aromatic hydrocarbons 249–250
Polymixin B 253
Polynucleotides 165
Polyoma virus 218, 297
Polysulfone 259
Popular perception 47
Population exposure estimate 298
Porphyria 221
Post-capillary venules 18
Post-splenectomy infection 282
Post-vaccinal encephalitis 130
Potency, definition 36
PPD 120
Practolol 131, 255
Precipitins, in hypersensitivity pneumonitis 117
Preclinical testing 295
Prednisolone 191
Premanufacturing Notice (PMN) 302
Primidone 131
Priming 44
Primrose, European 237
Procainamide 115, 131, 151, 294
Procoagulant 96
Progressive multifocal leukoencephalopathy 217
Prolactin 56
Propanolol 151
Properdin 83, 84
6–Propylthiopurine 40
Propylthiouracil 131, 151, 152
Prospective/Retrospective studies 296, 300
Prostaglandins 60–61, 94, 145
Protamine sulfate 273, 274
Protein A 128, 153, 202
Protein kinase C 29, 51–52, 54, 182, 203
Proteose-peptone 204
Public Health Service Act 294
Pulmonary disease anemia 272
Pulmonary infiltrative disease 254
Pulmonary lymphoid hyperplasia 217
Pulmonary manifestations, immunotoxicity 238–239
Purpura 254
PYB6 fibrosarcoma tumor 204, 207
Pyrazolone derivatives 115, 152
Pyrethrum 270
Pyrimethamine 151

Pyrogenic exotoxins   161
Pyrogenicity testing   297

Quinidine   115, 131, 151, 152
Quinine   114, 115, 151
Quinones   41

Rabies vaccine   130
Radiocontrast media   119, 258–260, 274
Radioimmunoassays (RIA)   184, 185
Radon   268
Ragweed   220
Raji cell assay   118, 194
RAST testing   108
Rat tumor models   207
Receptor site alteration   37
Receptor specificity   298
Receptors, acetylcholine   110, 054
Receptors, β-adrenergic   110, 111
Receptors, C5a   85, 90
Receptors, CD4   148
Receptors, CR1   84, 85, 86, 90, 96
Receptors, CR2   85, 87
Receptors, CR3   85, 86, 88, 90, 195
Receptors, CR4   85
Receptors, cholinergic   222
Receptors, cytokine   11
Receptors, Fc   14, 88, 90, 117, 193, 205
Receptors, Fc$_e$ 106
Receptors, Fc$_e$RI   94, 106
Receptors, Fc$_e$RII   106
Receptors, histamine   58–59, 152
Receptors, inhibition of   140
Receptors, IL-1   122
Receptors, IL-2   30, 176
Receptors, mannose   79, 90
Receptors, morphine   263
Receptors, muscarinic   110
Receptors, nitrate   37, 45
Receptors, T cell   26, 30
Receptors, T3–Ti   51
Receptors, TCDD   252
Recombinant DNA technology, safety evaluation   294
Recombinational activating genes   57
Recovery from effects   301
Red cedar, asthma   113
Redbook, FDA   294
Regulatory agencies   125
Regulatory concerns   294–297
    Antigenicity   295–296
    Autoimmunity   294–295
    Biochemical Pesticides   303
    Chemical Pesticides   304
    Inadvertent Reactions   296
    Immunomodulation   296–297
    Indirect Immunotoxicity   297
    Microbial Pesticides   303–304
    Sensitization   295
Regulatory functions, xenobiotic effects on   140
Relaxin   274
Relevance   113, 120, Chapter 10, 306
Respiratory syncitial virus   223
Reticular dysgenesis   138, 139
Retrovirus   297
Retrovirus structural protein p15(E)   182
Reversible or compensatory effect   305
Rh antigen   114, 256
Rheumatic fever   3, 114, 129, 130

Rheumatoid arthritis   129, 130, 218
Rheumatoid factor   118, 281
RhoGam   169
RIA   295
Risk assessment   45–47, 228, 297, 301, 308
Risk factors allergy,   214, 219–220
Risk factors, environmental   222–224
Risk factors, pharmacological   220–222
Risk, unreasonable   305
Rosettes, sheep erythrocyte   244, 263
Rosin   237, 270
Route of exposure   39–40, 298, 307
Rubella   2

Salicylate-induced asthma   119
Sarcomas   192
SCID-hu mice   298
Scleroderma   246
Scopoletin   195
Scratch testing   107, 111
Screening panel   303
Secretory piece   25
Secretory products, inhibition of   140
Sedormid   114, 115
Selenium   149, 150, 266
Sendai viruses   297
Sensitization   295
Sensitization index   204
Sensitization potential, chemicals   123
Sensitization ranking   124
Septic shock   99
Sequestered antigens   129
Serotonin   57–59, 96, 112, 121
Serum protein reduction   258
Serum sickness   116, 253
Severe combined immunodeficiency   138, 139
Seveso, Italy   250
Shingles   168
Shultz-Dale reaction   229
Shwartzman reaction   224
Sick building syndrome   268
sIgA   25
Signal transduction   52
Silica/silicosis   122, 144–145, 219, 279, 280, 281
Silver   237
Singlet oxygen   89
Skin   106, 109
Skin manifestations, immunotoxicity   236–238
Skin testing   194, 195
Slow reactive substance   94
Slow-releasing factor of anaphylaxis   58
Smokeless tobacco   262
Sodium dehydrocholate   274
Sodium zirconium lactate   238
Somatiform disorders   277
Somatostatin   56
Species differences   215
Sphingolipids   182
Spina bifida   275
Spleen   16–17, 299
Splenectomy   16–17, 164, 186, 282–284
Splenin   164
Sprague-Dawley rat, model of asthma   112
Sprue, celiac   127–128
SRS-A   58
Staphylococci   181
Staphylococcal enterotoxins   203
Stem cells   10, 298
Stem cells, defects   138

Stem cells, xenobiotic effects on 140, 141–143, 151
Stereochemistry 295
Stibophen 115
Stimulation index 191
Streptococci 182, 206
Streptokinase-streptodornase 194
Streptomycin 274
Stress related effects 198
Stromal cells, xenobiotic effects on 142, 143
Structure/activity relationships 33, 44, 298
Substance P 56, 107, 111, 141, 224, 272
Substances of abuse 262–265
Subtilisin 270, 305
Succinylcholine 41, 221, 222
Sulfa derivatives 115, 228, 253
Sulfamethoxazole 254
Sulfites 241, 254, 274, 305
Sulfobromphthalein 274
Sulfonamides 115, 131, 151, 152, 221
Sulfur dioxide 267, 268
Superantigens 99
Superoxide anion 89, 145, 194, 195, 204, 205
Superphysiological concentrations 296
SV-40 virus 218
Sympathetic ophthalmia 240
Synergism 44, 215, 224, 252
Systemic lupus erythematosus 188, 190, 196, 296
Szentivanyi theory 110, 111

T amplifier lymphocytes 12–13
T cell dependent antigen 198, 201
T cell dependent 300
T cell dysfunction 138, 217
T cell independent antigen 201, 202, 206
T cell receptor See TCR
T cell regulated antigens, type II 201
T cells, activated 203
T cells, cytotoxic/suppressor 189
T cells, enumeration 188–190
T cells, in late phase reactions 109
T lymphocytes, origin and development 12–13
T lymphocytes, xenobiotic effects on 147–149
T lymphocytes 164, 165, 167, 175, 199, 204, 207
Tachyphylaxis 37
T_c cells 13, 31, 91–93, 100, 166, 191, 192
T_c cells, in DTH 121
TCDD See Dioxins
TCR 26, 29, 169
T_{dth} cells 13, 121
Teichoic acid 160
Tetanus toxoid 185, 202
Tetracyclines 151, 270, 274
Δ^9-Tetrahydrocannibinol 262
Tetrahydroxyflavan 120, 128
T_h cell, defects 138, 139
T_h cells 12–13, 28, 29, 121, 160, 162, 168, 171, 175, 189, 196
T_h cells, depressions 148
Thalidomide 2
Theophylline 112, 150, 255
Therapeutic responses 37–38
Thiamine 274
Thimerosal 237, 240
Thiopental 254
Thiouracil 253
Thoracic duct 18
Threshold effect level 305

Thrombin 86, 118
Thrombocytopenic purpura 114, 115, 129, 130
Thromboplastin 122
Thrombospondin 96
Thromboxane 58, 94, 96
Thy-1, antibodies 203
Thymectomy 12, 16
Thymocytes 196
Thymopentine 164
Thymopoietin 12, 164
Thymosin 12, 56, 164
Thymulin 164
Thymus 15, 16, 138, 199, 299
Thyroid stimulating hormone receptor antibodies 115
Thyroiditis, Hashimoto's 129
Thyroxine 222
Tier testing 197–198, 303–304, 306–308
Times Beach 2, 235, 251
Tissue half-life 298
Tissue plasminogen activator 295
TNF, stimulation 142, 145, 148
TNF-α 88, 91, 93, 97, 129, 177, 259
TNF-β 69, 91
Tobutamide 151
Tolerance, immunologic 168–169, 171
Tolerance, toxicologic 37
Tolmetin 274
Toluene 37
Toluene diisocyanate (TDI) 113, 115, 128, 222, 270, 271–272
Total leukocyte count 199
Toxic effects, expression 34–45
Toxic oil syndrome 246–247
Toxic responses, immediate or delayed 38
Toxic responses, types 36–39
Toxic shock syndrome toxin 161
Toxic Substances Control Act (TSCA) 301–302
Toxicity, differentiating from hypersensitivity 5
Toxicity, factors affecting 39–45
  Age 42
  Characteristic of affected individual 40–43
  Dose 39–40
  Embryo/developmental effects 42
  Genetics 40
  Health/nutritional status 43
  Sex 42–43
  Species 41
Toxicity, predicting 3
Toxicologist, role of 33
Toxicology, developmental/reproductive 42
Toxicology, defined 33
Toxicology endpoints 199–200
Toxoplasmosis 2, 217
Transfer factor 168
Transforming growth factor-β 68, 101, 142, 170
Transfusion reactions 2, 273
Transgenic mice 299
Transplantation, rejection 296
Transplantation rejection, immunotherapy 171–177
Transplantation 2, 218
Tributyltin oxide 305
Trichophytin 194
Trimethoprim-sulfamethoxazole 151, 254
Trinitrophenol (TNP)-Ficoll 201

Trisomy 21   222
Trypan blue   199
Trypsin   270, 274
Tryptase   94, 106
Tryptophan   241
T_s cells   13, 31, 163, 169, 170, 175
T_s cells, increase   145, 146
T_s cells, in autoimmunity   129
TSCA   301–302
TSCA Regulated Chemicals   302, 304–305
Tuberculin reaction   120, 122
Tuberculosis   122, 168, 172, 182, 217, 239, 246, 280–281
Tubocurarine   274
Tuftsin   164
Tumor models   207
Tumor necrosis factor   65–66, 193–194, 197, 205
Tumor necrosis factor-β 121
Tumors   100–101, 115, 164, 171, 215
Tumors, therapy   167–168, 173

Ulcerative colitis   241
Unreasonable Risk   305
Uroshiol   237
Urticaria   236, 253, 258

Vaccines   294
Validation   306–307
Variation, normal   214
Vascular permeability   85, 96, 107, 121, 122, 139, 258
Vasculitis   117, 196, 246

Vasoactive intestinal peptide (VIP)   56, 117
Vasopressin   56
Venomous bites and stings   273
Vesicular stomatitis virus   205
Viability stains   199
Viability   299, 304
Vinyl chloride   40, 115, 131
Vinyl chloride   305
Viral infections   167
Virtual safe dose (VSD)   46
Vitamin B_{12}-intrinsic factor antibodies   115

Warfarin   41
Warning label   305
Wheal and flare skin reaction   105, 107
Whitlock-Witte bone marrow cultures   197
Wiskott-Aldrich syndrome   138, 168, 184, 191
Wolburn, litigation   293

Xenobiotics, adverse effects   10, 14, 27, 30
Xenobiotics, definition   5
Xenobiotics, interference by   86, 87, 97, 137, 140
Xenobiotics, toxic characteristics   43–45
Xenobiotics, types of responses   36–39
Xenobiotics, upregulating effects   150
Xylene   143

Yellow dye No. 5   305
Yu-cheng disease   245

Zinc   198, 266
Zirconium   237
Zomepirac   274